Promoting Safe and Effective Transitions to College for Youth with Mental Health Conditions

Adele Martel • Jennifer Derenne
Patricia K. Leebens
Editors

Promoting Safe and Effective Transitions to College for Youth with Mental Health Conditions

A Case-Based Guide to Best Practices

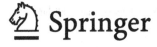

Editors
Adele Martel
Division of Child and Adolescent
Psychiatry
Department of Psychiatry and Behavioral
Sciences
Ann and Robert H. Lurie Children's
Hospital of Chicago
Northwestern University Feinberg School
of Medicine
Chicago, IL
USA

Jennifer Derenne
Division of Child and Adolescent
Psychiatry
Department of Psychiatry and Behavioral
Sciences
Stanford University School of Medicine
Lucile Packard Children's Hospital
Stanford, CA
USA

Patricia K. Leebens
Child Study Center
Yale School of Medicine
Yale University
New Haven, CT
USA

ISBN 978-3-319-68893-0   ISBN 978-3-319-68894-7   (eBook)
https://doi.org/10.1007/978-3-319-68894-7

Library of Congress Control Number: 2018932742

Printed on acid-free paper

This Springer imprint is published by the registered company Springer International Publishing AG part of Springer Nature
The registered company address is: Gewerbestrasse 11, 6330 Cham, Switzerland

Preface

The number of young people arriving on college campuses with preexisting mental health conditions and a history of prior treatment has been on the rise over the past two decades [1, 2]. These students have tremendous potential for success. However, their ability to adapt to the college environment may be compromised. Mental illness during childhood and adolescence can result in gaps or delays in psychosocial development making it difficult to manage transition stresses [3]. Ongoing characteristics of the illness itself and its interface with the college milieu may influence adjustment as well. Mental health providers, along with other key stakeholders, can help college-bound patients and their families identify the risks inherent in the transition and arm them with knowledge, skills, and attitudes to build resilience and hopefully make the transition to college safe, positive, and instructive.

How best to help college-bound psychiatric patients prepare for the transition to college, and how to incorporate that preparation into routine clinical care, has been the topic of various group discussions and continuing medical education (CME) programs at the American Academy of Child and Adolescent Psychiatry (AACAP) [4]. This book is modeled after a case-based program entitled "Promoting Safe Transitions to College Mental Health Services: Lessons Learned" which was presented at AACAP in 2011 and 2015. A similar program was presented to a multidisciplinary audience at the American College Health Association's annual meeting in 2013. In comparison to the CME program, the scope of this book has been broadened to include case examples with a range of clinical presentations and diagnostic entities which are commonly seen in the late adolescent and young adult period. We have also included cases of students representing some special populations on campus which may have unique experiences, vulnerabilities, and needs in the context of the transition to college. The selected cases provide sufficient examples of transition practices and campus supports and can inform an approach to those populations, clinical outcomes, and diagnoses not directly covered by separate cases.

The purpose of the book, which unfolds through varied, rich, and nuanced cases, is to (1) provide clinicians with knowledge, therapeutic strategies, and tools to better support the transition of their patients to college and into young adulthood, (2) help clinicians understand and interface more effectively with the campus system of care in the best interests of their patients, and (3) provide a framework to clinicians for evaluating and improving upon their own transition preparation and planning practices. It is expected that informed practitioners and prepared patients will both be at decreased risk for negative outcomes.

The book is primarily written by child and adolescent psychiatrists from across the country, in various stages of their professional development (trainees to near-retirees), who have worked with young people on both sides of the transition in private practice, college or university counseling centers, specialty clinics in academic settings, child welfare or juvenile justice facilities, and/or community mental health centers. We also welcome clinical case contributions from three of our general psychiatry colleagues who have spent much of their careers working with college students. Each author was asked to select a patient case in which he/she considered the transition to college to be suboptimal. Authors were encouraged to create composite cases to protect the identity of patients and to highlight teaching points. Authors were then challenged to retrospectively analyze the case, using a practice-based learning and improvement approach, to identify changes in their or their institution's practices regarding transition preparation and planning.

The clinical case chapters consist of five sections. The **Case History** section includes information on the patient's readiness for transition to college, the content and process of transition preparation and planning activities, the choice of college setting and type, and the transition care plans that were developed and a description of the patient's "transition outcome." In the **Analysis of Transition** section, the author reflects on factors in the patient's history predictive of a more positive transition outcome, those factors that suggest he/she was at risk for a negative transition outcome, and aspect(s) of transition preparation and planning which could have been approached differently to improve the outcome. The **Clinical Pearls** section provides take-home messages based on the author's review of the case, other clinical experiences, and areas of expertise. The **Brief Literature Review** section highlights issues and research trends related to the specific diagnosis or special population and the transition to college. The **Helpful Resources** section includes links to websites for clinicians, patients, and families, as well as office-based tools, related to transition to college. Though this case presentation format deviates from the standard psychiatric evaluation, it was created to focus on the patient's readiness for transition to college and transition preparation and planning.

Many young people with mental illness heading to college are well prepared and stable and initially make the transition to college and new mental health services with relative ease only to be derailed by some event or circumstance. For example, the sale of the childhood home, the tragic death of a high school friend, parental divorce, parental illness and death, a natural disaster (like a hurricane), a terrorist threat or attack, and a suicide on campus—all can exacerbate a student's symptoms and impact transition. Cases such as these are not presented here. However, we posit that transition preparation and planning, embraced as a wholistic endeavor, might help students through such difficult times.

This book is written for mental health professionals (physicians, psychologists, social workers, school counselors, advanced practice nurse practitioners, and others) who work with children, adolescents, and their families before, during, and/or after the transition to college. This book may also provide some guidance to high school staff as they work on educational transition planning and to university stake-holders as they develop programs and policies for young people transitioning to campus with a mental illness. By the end of this book, it should be clear that for the student heading to college with a psychiatric diagnosis, "the work of wellness promotion and prevention begins long before that student heads to campus" [4] and requires a collaborative, team-based approach.

References

1. Martel A, Sood B. Best practices and resources: national models for college student mental health. In: Sood B, Cohen R, editors. The Virginia Tech Massacre – strategies and challenges for improving mental health policy on campus and beyond. Oxford Oxford Press; 2015. p. 93–125.
2. Brunner JL, Wallace DL, Reymann LS, Sellers J, McCabe AG. College counseling today: contemporary students and how counseling centers meet their needs. J Coll Stud Psychother. 2014;28(4):257–324.
3. Skehan B, Davis M. Aligning mental health treatments with the developmental stage and needs of late adolescents and young adults. Child Adolesc Psychiatr Clin N Am. 2017;26(2):177–90.
4. Martel A, Derenne J, Chan V. Teaching a systematic approach for transitioning patients to college: an interactive continuing Medical Education Program. Acad Psychiatry. 2015;39(5):549–54.

Chicago, IL, USA   Adele Martel
Stanford, CA, USA   Jennifer Derenne
New Haven, CT, USA   Patricia K. Leebens

Acknowledgments

We are grateful to our contributing authors for the opportunity to work with them and to learn from them. Each author has not only presented a case but has retrospectively analyzed the outcome in the hopes that others, in addition to themselves, can learn from their experiences and enhance patient care.

We also appreciate the feedback and support of our colleagues and the patience of our significant others (RM, DH, CRS) during the creation of this book.

We would like to thank Caitlin Prim, Miranda Finch, Kaaviya Varadarajan, and Rajeswari Balachandran at Springer for their guidance and support in the preparation of this manuscript.

Disclaimer

The information provided in this book is intended as a guide and is not a substitute for professional medical advice or treatment for specific medical conditions. You should not use this information to diagnose or treat a health problem or disease without consulting with a qualified healthcare provider. Providers should use clinical judgment when caring for specific patients.

To protect privacy and maximize teaching points, the authors have de-identified case material and have combined the experiences of several patients into composite cases. In some cases, patients have also provided written permission to present their stories.

Contents

List of Contributors

Vivien Chan, M.D. Student Health Center, University of California Irvine, Irvine, CA, USA

Department of Psychiatry and Human Behavior, UCI Health, Orange, CA, USA

Ludmila De Faria, M.D. University Health Services, Florida State University College of Medicine, Tallahassee, FL, USA

Jennifer Derenne, M.D. Division of Child and Adolescent Psychiatry, Department of Psychiatry and Behavioral Sciences, Stanford University School of Medicine, Lucile Packard Children's Hospital, Stanford, CA, USA

Zhanna Elberg, M.D. Department of Psychiatry, Jacobs School of Medicine and Biomedical Sciences, University at Buffalo, Buffalo, NY, USA

D. Catherine Fuchs, M.D. Department of Psychiatry and Behavioral Sciences, Vanderbilt University Medical Center, Nashville, TN, USA

Dorothy E. Grice, M.D. Department of Psychiatry, Icahn School of Medicine at Mount Sinai, New York, NY, USA

Ashley Holland, D.O. Department of Child Psychiatry, University of Massachusetts Medical Center, Worcester, MA, USA

Doris Iarovici, M.D. Counseling and Mental Health Services, Harvard University Health Services, Cambridge, MA, USA

Daniel Kirsch, M.D. Department of Psychiatry, University of Massachusetts School of Medicine, Worcester, MA, USA

Elisabeth M. Kressley, M.D. Child Study Center, Yale School of Medicine, Yale University, New Haven, CT, USA

Patricia K. Leebens, M.A.T., M.A., M.D. Child Study Center, Yale School of Medicine, Yale University, New Haven, CT, USA

Basheer Lotfi-Fard, M.D. Department of Psychiatry and Behavioral Health, The Ohio State University, Columbus, OH, USA

Kirk Lum, M.D. Child and Family Psychological Services, Inc., Norwood, MA, USA

Adele Martel, M.D., Ph.D. Division of Child and Adolescent Psychiatry, Department of Psychiatry and Behavioral Sciences, Ann and Robert H. Lurie Children's Hospital of Chicago, Northwestern University Feinberg School of Medicine, Chicago, IL, USA

Ryan C. Mast, D.O., M.B.A. Department of Psychiatry, Wright State University, Boonshoft School of Medicine, Dayton, OH, USA

Jessica Moore, M.D. PGY5 Child and Adolescent Psychiatry, UT-Southwestern Medical Center, Dallas, TX, USA

Karen Pierce, M.D. Northwestern University, Feinberg School of Medicine, Chicago, IL, USA

Adelaide Robb, M.D. Psychiatry and Behavioral Sciences, Children's National Health System, Washington, DC, USA

A.L. Rostain, M.D., M.A. Perelman School of Medicine, University of Pennsylvania Health System, Philadelphia, PA, USA

Dara Sakolsky, M.D., Ph.D. Department of Psychiatry, University of Pittsburgh, School of Medicine, Pittsburgh, PA, USA

Western Psychiatric Institute and Clinic, University of Pittsburgh Medical Center, Pittsburgh, PA, USA

Brian Skehan, M.D., Ph.D. University of Massachusetts Medical School, Worcester, MA, USA

Timothy VanDeusen, M.D. Department of Psychiatry, Connecticut Mental Health Center, Yale School of Medicine, West Haven, CT, USA

Christina G. Weston, M.D. Department of Psychiatry, Wright State University, Boonshoft School of Medicine, Dayton, OH, USA

Part I

Background Chapters

The Practice Gap in Health Care Transition: Focus on Young People Heading to College with a Mental Health Condition

Adele Martel

What Is Health Care Transition?

Planned health care transition for young people with special health care needs [1], including those with emotional, behavioral, and developmental disorders, has been deemed a health priority both here in the U.S. [2] and abroad [3, 4]. In the health care literature, transition is described as a purposeful and planned process of change, moving adolescents with chronic health conditions from child-centered to adult-oriented models of health care. It is thought of as an active and dynamic process that addresses not only the medical needs of adolescents but their psychosocial, educational, and vocational needs as well [5, 6]. In reality, all adolescents, regardless of health status, will undergo transition to adult-oriented health services. For healthy youth and those requiring straightforward care, the transition is expected to be uncomplicated. The goal of transition in health care is to maximize lifelong functioning and potential by ensuring uninterrupted, developmentally appropriate, and comprehensive health care services as adolescents move into young adulthood [7].

Gaps in health care transition services continue to exist for youth with chronic conditions and, in particular, for those with emotional, behavioral, and developmental disorders, based on national survey data [8]. For those specifically headed to college with a pre-existing mental health condition (MHC), the inadequacy of transition preparation and planning is supported by clinical experiences of mental health professionals on both sides of the transition [9, 10, 11]. The results of a recent, web-based survey on the experience of students living with mental health

A. Martel, M.D., Ph.D.
Division of Child and Adolescent Psychiatry, Department of Psychiatry and Behavioral Sciences, Ann and Robert H. Lurie Children's Hospital of Chicago, Northwestern University Feinberg School of Medicine, Chicago, IL, USA
e-mail: adele.martel@gmail.com

© Springer International Publishing AG, part of Springer Nature 2018
A. Martel et al. (eds.), *Promoting Safe and Effective Transitions to College for Youth with Mental Health Conditions*, https://doi.org/10.1007/978-3-319-68894-7_1

conditions [12] also suggest gaps in transition services for college youth. Fifty-seven percent did not access academic accommodations through their school's office of disability services (ODS), with some citing reasons for not doing so as fear of stigma, not knowing that a MHC might qualify them for services, or that they had a right to receive accommodations. Forty percent did not receive clinical services on campus with some citing that there were no services on campus, they did not know how to access services on campus, and there were service caps or limits. Lastly, 64% of survey respondents who were no longer attending college because of a mental health-related issue noted that academic accommodations and connecting with mental health services might have helped them stay in school. In another, qualitative study, freshman with attention-deficit/hyperactivity disorder (ADHD) were found to lack medication self-management skills and to have inaccurate beliefs about ADHD and when medication was necessary [13]. Though this study was very small and based at only one school, its findings accurately reflect the experiences of many clinicians treating college-age youth.

Developmental Tasks of College-Bound Youth

When transitioning to college, young people are faced with challenges on multiple levels. They are expected to continue to work on normative developmental tasks such as consolidating identity (who you are and what you want to be), increasing self-reliance in day-to-day functioning, separating from parents and other key adults, and sustaining mature and intimate relationships. They are also expected to manage an increase in academic demands and structure their time by balancing academics with wellness, social, and online activities. Typically, they are exposed to and are expected to tolerate increased diversity in both their fellow students and in the ideas and viewpoints of others. Many also need to adjust to a new living environment with shared living spaces, easy availability of alcohol and drugs, and a sexualized atmosphere—all in the context of less structure, decreased adult oversight, and ongoing maturation of the brain. The transition to college is an opportunity for significant personal growth and is stressful for most young people.

Those students entering college with mental illness face additional challenges, when compared to their peers without mental illness, in regard to health care transition. They must have some understanding of how their illness might impact functioning in the college environment and what supports they need to aid academic and social success. They are expected to manage their illness more independently, advocate for themselves, develop relationships with new treatment providers, and navigate a new system of care. This is a tall order given that all young people, not just those with mental illness, are still developing and honing many cognitive, executive function, and social skills. This is also a life stage when denial of illness, limited insight, and striving for independence can be appreciated from a developmental perspective. Still, with careful preparation, planning, attention to continuity of care, and ongoing support, more of these young people can transition successfully to college.

College Student Demographics and Mental Health Issues

To gain some insight into the scope of the need for mental health care transition services for college-bound youth, it is helpful to review the prevalence of mental health disorders in the college-age population in conjunction with recent college enrollment statistics.

In 2015, the total undergraduate enrollment in 2-year and 4-year degree-granting postsecondary institutions in the U.S. was 17 million [14]. Based on a variety of student characteristics, the diversity on campus is impressive [15]. Each of these student groups brings different strengths, vulnerabilities, mental health needs, and approaches to help-seeking to campus.

- Female students outnumber male students 9.5 to 7.5 million, respectively [14]
- 10.6 million undergraduates were enrolled on a full-time basis and 6.4 million on a part-time basis [14]; those enrolled part-time were twice as likely to be involved in the workforce [16]
- Three million undergraduates were Hispanic, 2.3 million were Black, 1.1 million were Asian/Pacific Islander, and 132,000 were American Indian/Alaskan Native [14]
- Over 427,000 undergraduates were international students, representing nearly 41% of the total number of international students in the U.S. [17]
- Approximately 17.2% of incoming first-year students at baccalaureate or *4-year* institutions reported that they were first-generation college students [18]
- Veterans on campus reached about one million in 2013 [19]

Most of the 10.6 million full-time undergraduates in 2-year and 4-year degree-granting institutions in the U.S. are under the age of 25 [14]. Along with their peers attending part-time, they are at high risk of already having or developing a psychiatric disorder while in college, based on the findings of Kessler et al. [20] in the National Comorbidity Survey Replication, that between 50 and 75% of DSM-IV defined anxiety, mood, impulse control, and substance use disorders emerge between ages 14 and 24. College age students experience the full range of psychiatric disorders, with overall 12-month prevalence rates similar to their non-college attending peers; anxiety, depression, and substance use disorders being most common [21]. More specifically, about 40% of college students (ages 19–25) met DSM-IV criteria for at least one Axis I psychiatric disorder in the previous year [21]. Merikangas et al. [22] found that nearly 50% of a sample of youth ages 13–18, an age range which includes youth considering postsecondary education, had at least one class of psychiatric disorder and over 20% had a seriously debilitating mental disorder. Suicide is the second-leading cause of death among college students, with the overall rate about 7 per 100,000 students [23]. Lastly, 27% of college students [24] report having been treated or diagnosed with a mental health condition in the prior 12 months. These data highlight the challenges faced by institutions of higher education in meeting the volume and breadth of the mental health needs of students [25–27] and more specifically, the challenges faced by mental health practitioners working on transition care plans for a variety of patients.

In regard to the population of interest, those students entering college with an already diagnosed mental health condition and in some form of treatment prior to matriculation, there is a paucity of published prevalence and enrollment data. We can extrapolate from the data on college students in general. It is also valuable to view this group from a developmental psychopathology perspective. "College students who have their first onset of mental illness or initiate substance use during childhood or adolescence appear to have a more pernicious trajectory and course of illness" [26]. Early age of onset of mental health disorders can be associated with greater severity and chronicity of illness, an increased likelihood of developing comorbid disorders, and delayed or suboptimal young adult functional outcomes [26, 28, 29].

The Freshman Survey, conducted annually by the Higher Education Research Institute, offers some additional insight into the difficulties of entering freshman. In the 2016 survey [18], about 12% of first time, full-time incoming freshman (baccalaureate institution or higher) reported feeling frequently depressed in the prior 12 months. In comparison, over 50% of students who identified as having a psychological disorder (depression, etc.) endorsed feeling frequently depressed in the past year. Students who identified as having autism spectrum disorder (ASD), ADHD, or a learning disability also reported frequently feeling depressed at significantly higher levels than the national sample. A similar pattern was seen regarding the frequency of feeling anxious in the past year with 79.5% of those with a psychological disorder reporting frequent anxiety which was more than double that of the national sample (34.5%). Anxiety, depression, and stress are common in college and all college-bound youth need to be prepared to monitor levels of anxiety and depression and know when to seek mental health and related services although this is particularly critical for young people with already diagnosed mental health disorders.

Mental Health Help-Seeking Trends in Transitional Age Youth

The use of mental health treatment services, and health services in general, are low or declining in the transitional age youth (TAY) population [30]. Skehan and Davis [31] recently reviewed barriers and facilitators to mental health help-seeking in this age group. They suggest that improvements in comprehensive and developmentally appropriate transition services may facilitate help-seeking in TAY with mental illness [31], decreasing the disability, morbidity, and mortality associated with mental health disorders in this age group [32].

Developing Best Practices for Transitioning Patients to College

Research in the field of health care transition is in its early stages, and very few transition interventions or programs designed for youth with mental health conditions have been comprehensively evaluated in regard to outcome [33, 34, 35]. Likewise, the literature on best practices for specifically supporting the transition to college of youth with mental health conditions remains sparse. In the absence of a robust literature base, transition process and content should be grounded in knowledge of normal child, adolescent, young adult, and family development, concepts central to positive youth development [3], reports of expert committees [36], and clinical experience. In this volume, the principles of the systems of care model [37] guide the approach to mental health care transition planning for college-bound patients [38, 39, 40]. This model emphasizes youth voice; a strengths-based, ethically sound, culturally competent and individualized approach; developmentally attuned services and providers; multidimensional care provided in a coordinated and integrated fashion; natural and informal supports; and a public health approach [37]. The mental health provider is seen as an integral member of the team, as treater, consultant, advocate, team leader, program director, and/or policy maker [40]. We have also relied on core features of educational transition planning, such as self-determination, goal setting, the team approach, and good communication, to inform our work. Lastly, we have included a significant amount of anticipatory guidance in our approach to help prepare patients and their families for expected changes and stresses during this complex developmental transition [36, 38, 41].

The Role of Mental Health Practitioners in Health Care Transition

Mental health practitioners (CAP, psychologists, social workers, school counselors, advanced practice nurses, to name a few) working with adolescents and their families have important roles to play in facilitating positive transitions to college and remedying transition gaps. Whether youth are cared for over a period of years or only for a brief period of time, the goals of health care transition should be kept in mind. Practitioners must assess, monitor, and move patients forward in their readiness for transition in ways that help them feel empowered as partners in decision-making. They need to:

- Help patients understand, manage, and seek services for their conditions and highlight these tasks as opportunities for independence
- Involve families in the treatment of patients to promote mutual understanding, growth in autonomy, and safety
- Collaborate with patients in developing transition care plans, including relapse prevention, which support their mental health and postsecondary education goals

The remaining background chapters cover several essential topics, the understanding of which is necessary to conduct comprehensive transition planning and preparation with college-bound mental health patients: the late adolescent/young adult developmental stage, the functional demands of the postsecondary academic and social milieus, the range of available postsecondary options, privacy and disability laws as applied to college students, campus models of mental health service delivery, the campus system of care, and practice-based strategies for health care transition.

References

1. McPherson M, Arango P, Fox H, Lauver C, McManus M, Newachek P, Perrin JM, Shonkoff JP, Strickland B. A new definition of children with special health needs. Pediatrics. 1998;102(1):137–40.
2. https://www.healthypeople.gov/.
3. Canadian Pediatric Society. Transition to adult care for youth with special health care needs (Reaffirmed 2011). Pediatr Child Health. 2007;12(9):785–8.
4. McNamara N, McNicholas F, Ford T, Paul M, Gavin B, Coyne I, Cullen W, O'Connor K, Ramperti N, Dooley B, Barry S, Singh SP. Transition from a child and adolescent to adult mental health services in the Republic of Ireland: an investigation of process and operational practice. Early Interv Psychiatry. 2014;8:291–7.
5. Blum RW, Garel D, Hodgman CH, Jorissen TW, Okinow NA, Orr DP, Slap GB. Transition from child-centered to adult health-care systems for adolescents with chronic conditions. J Adolesc Health. 1993;14(7):570–6.
6. Paul M, Ford T, Kramer T, Islam S, Harley K, Singh SP. Transfers and transitions between child and adult mental health services. Br J Psychiatry. 2013;202:s36–40.
7. American Academy of Pediatrics, American Academy of Family Physicians, American College of Physicians. A consensus statement on health care transitions for young adults with special health care needs. Pediatrics. 2002;110(6):1304–6.
8. McManus MA, Pollack LR, Cooley WC, McAllister JW, Lotstein D, Strickland B, Mann MY. Current status of transition preparation among youth with special needs in the United States. Pediatrics. 2013;131(6):1090–7.
9. Martel A, Derenne J, Chan V. Teaching a systematic approach for transitioning patients to college: an interactive continuing medical education program. Acad Psychiatry. 2015;39(5):549–54.
10. Ascherman LI, Shaftel J. Facilitating transition from high school and special education to adult life: focus on youth with learning disorders, attention-deficit/hyperactivity disorder, and speech/language impairments. Child Adolesc Psychiatr Clin N Am. 2017;26(2):311–27.
11. Lee T, Morgan W. Transitioning to adulthood from foster care. Child Adolesc Psychiatr Clin N Am. 2017;26(2):283–96.
12. National Alliance on Mental Illness College students speak: a survey report on mental health. 2012. https://www.nami.org/getattachment/About-NAMI/Publications-Reports/Survey-Reports/College-Students-Speak_A-Survey-Report-on-Mental-Health-NAMI-2012.pdf.
13. Schaefer MR, Rawlinson AR, Wagoner ST, Shapiro SK, Kavookjian J, Gray WN. Adherence to attention-deficit/hyperactivity disorder medication during the transition to college. J Adolesc Health. 2017;60(6):706–13.
14. National Center for Educational Statistics—Undergraduate Enrollment. https://nces.ed.gov/programs/coe/indicator_cha.asp (undergraduate enrollment data).
15. Sood B, Martel A. Examining common failures in campus mental health systems. In: Sood B, Cohen R, editors. The virginia tech massacre—strategies and challenges for improving mental health policy on campus and beyond. Oxford: Oxford Press; 2015. p. 65–92.
16. Bureau of Labor Statistics. https://www.bls.gov/news.release/archives/hsgec_04282016.pdf.
17. https://www.insidehighered.com/news/2016/11/14/annual-open-doors-report-documents-continued-growth-international-students-us-and-us.
18. Eagan MK, Stolzenberg EB, Zimmerman HB, Aragon MC, Sayson HW, Rios-Aguilar C. The American freshman: national norms fall 2016. Los Angeles: Higher Education Research Institute, UCLA; 2017. https://www.heri.ucla.edu/monographs/TheAmericanFreshman2016.pdf. Accessed 1 June 2017.
19. https://www.mentalhealth.va.gov/studentveteran/studentvets.asp.
20. Kessler RC, Bergland P, Demler O, Jin R, Merikangas KR, Walters EE. Lifetime prevalence and age-of-onset distribution of DSM-IV disorders in the national comorbidity survey replication. Arch Gen Psychiatry. 2005;62:593–603.
21. Blanco C, Okuda M, Wright C, Hasin D, Grant B, Liu S-M, Olfson M. Mental health of college students and their non-college-attending peers. Arch Gen Psychiatry. 2008;65:1429–37.

22. Merikangas KR, He J-P, Burstein M, Swanson SA, Avenevoli S, Cui L, Benjet C, Georgiades K, Swendsen J. Lifetime prevalence of mental disorders in U.S. adolescents: results from the National Comorbidity Survey Replication-Adolescent Supplement (NCS-A). J Am Acad Child Adolesc Psychiatry. 2010;49(10):980–9.
23. Iarovici D. Perspectives on college student suicide. Psychiatric Times. 2015;32(7):27.
24. American College Health Association-National College Health Assessment II: Reference Group Executive Summary Fall 2016. Hanover: American College Health Association; 2017. http://www.acha-ncha.org/docs/NCHA-II_FALL_2016_REFERENCE_GROUP_EXECUTIVE_SUMMARY.pdf.
25. Riba M, Kirsch D, Martel A, Goldsmith M. Preparing and training the college mental health workforce. Acad Psychiatry. 2015;39(5):498–502.
26. Pedrelli P, Nyer M, Yeung A, Aulauf C, Wilens T. College students: mental health problems and treatment considerations. Acad Psychiatry. 2015;39(5):503–11.
27. Brunner JL, Wallace DL, Reymann LS, Sellers J, McCabe AG. College counseling today: contemporary students and how counseling centers meet their needs. J Coll Stud Psychother. 2014;28(4):257–324.
28. Leebens PK, Williamson ED. Developmental psychopathology: risk and resilience in the transition to young adulthood: risk and resilience in the transition to young adulthood. Child Adolesc Psychiatr Clin N Am. 2015;26(2):143–56.
29. Copeland WE, Adair CE, Smetanin P, Stiff D, Briante C, Colman I, Fergusson D, Horwood J, Poulton R, Costello EJ, Angold A. Diagnostic transitions from childhood to adolescence to early adulthood. J Child Psychol Psychiatry. 2013;54(7):791–9.
30. IOM (Institute of Medicine) and NRC (National Research Council). Investing in the health and well-being of young adults. Washington, DC: The National Academies Press; 2015.
31. Skehan B, Davis M. Aligning mental health treatments with the developmental stage and needs of late adolescents and young adults. Child Adolesc Psychiatr Clin N Am. 2017;26(2):177–90.
32. Gore FM, Bloem PJ, Patton GC, Ferguson J, Joseph V, Coffey C, Sawyer SM, Mathers CD. Global burden of disease in young people aged 10–24 years: a systematic analysis. Lancet. 2011;377(9783):2093–102.
33. Prior M, McManus M, White P, Davidson L. Measuring the "triple aim" in transition care: a systematic review. Pediatrics. 2014;134(6):e1648–61.
34. Singh SP, Tuomainen H. Transition from child to adult mental health services: needs, barriers, experiences and new models of care. World Psychiatry. 2015;14(3):358–61.
35. McManus M, White P. Transition to adult health care services for young adults with chronic medical illness and psychiatric comorbidity. Child Adolesc Psychiatr Clin N Am. 2017;26(2):367–80.
36. American Academy of Pediatrics, American Academy of Family Physicians, American College of Physicians—Transitions Clinical Report Authoring Group. Supporting the health care transition from adolescence to adulthood in the medical home (Reaffirmed 2015). Pediatrics. 2011;128(1):182–200.
37. Stroul B, Blau G, Friedman R. Updating the system of care concept and philosophy. Washington, DC: Georgetown University Center for Child and Human Development, National Technical Assistance Center for Children's Mental Health; 2010. https://www.psy0-18.be/images/SOC_Brief2010.pdf.
38. Martel A, Sood B. Best practices and resources: national models for college student mental health. In: Sood B, Cohen R, editors. The virginia tech massacre—strategies and challenges for improving mental health policy on campus and beyond. Oxford: Oxford Press; 2015. p. 93–125.
39. Chan V, Rasminsky S, Viesselman J. A primer for working in campus mental health: a system of care. Acad Psychiatry. 2015;39(5):533–40.
40. Winters N, Pumariega A. AACAP Practice Parameter on child and adolescent mental health care in community systems of care. J Am Acad Child Adolesc Psychiatry. 2007;46(2):284–99.
41. Young CC, Calloway J. Transition planning for the college bound adolescent with a mental health disorder. J Pediatr Nurs. 2015;30:e173–82.

Essential Domains in Transition Planning and the Roles of Various Constituents

Patricia K. Leebens

Starting the Transition Process: The CAP as Choreographer

As noted previously the CAP has a unique role in helping choreograph the transition to college of youths with special needs. As experts in the biopsychosocial needs of developing children and adolescents, CAPs can use their additional knowledge of complex psychiatric conditions and developmental psychopathology to help shape college transitions which meet the needs of an individual youth and his/her family. This process of preparing for the college transition will involve the youth, parents, as well as multiple stakeholders (i.e., teachers and other educational personnel, therapeutic, and medical professionals), and, possibly, other significant persons in the life of the student. While exploring possible colleges, the adolescent and parent will also become familiar with college services, which will be important in a youth's successful transition to college. Ideally, youths will be moving, with confidence and manageable anxiety, from a familiar world that they have successfully negotiated to a new setting, using skills and knowledge that they have mastered or have begun to master during adolescence and the transition process.

As each transition is based upon the needs, resources, and interests of the student and his/her family, a good place to start this process is following the initial psychiatric assessment, when the CAP presents a review of the youth's and family's strengths and vulnerabilities, the youth's diagnostic formulation, including DSM-5 diagnoses, and recommended treatment interventions. If the initial psychiatric evaluation occurred many months or years prior, a review of the youth's diagnoses, strengths and vulnerabilities, current treatment and educational supports, and post-high school hopes and plans would help.

P.K. Leebens, M.A.T., M.A., M.D.
Child Study Center, Yale School of Medicine, Yale University, New Haven, CT, USA
e-mail: patricia.leebens@gmail.com

© Springer International Publishing AG, part of Springer Nature 2018
A. Martel et al. (eds.), *Promoting Safe and Effective Transitions to College for Youth with Mental Health Conditions*, https://doi.org/10.1007/978-3-319-68894-7_2

Depending upon the age, capabilities, and wishes of the teen and of the parents, the meeting could occur with the patient and the parents separately and then reviewed again in a joint meeting of patient and parents. If appropriate, other stakeholders (i.e., child welfare worker, mental health, or school personnel) might be involved in this feedback process as well, depending upon the location of the evaluation (private practice setting, IOP, inpatient setting, school, etc.). The information presented at the feedback meeting would be an interactive process and would adjust to the needs, and ability to tolerate feedback, of the youth and parents. When the young person and family understand his/her mental health condition and ongoing treatment needs, the value of looking at the available mental health services on-campus visits hopefully becomes more obvious. Also, a more realistic and frank discussion of various post-secondary education options can take place. Table 2.1 is a provider checklist for this meeting(s).

Providing a one- or two-page feedback sheet which summarizes the information from the feedback meeting will help as a general roadmap for future therapeutic interventions and skill development. This roadmap would be reinforced

Table 2.1 How readiness assessment interfaces with post-secondary education planning

Conduct a global review (or re-review) of youth's current functioning
• Review youth's post-secondary career interests, educational goals, and dreams • Review youth's strengths and limitations • Clarify diagnosis and prognosis • Review current level of support from family, school, friends, tutors, coaches, agencies, providers • Discuss short- and long-term treatment goals and needs • Discuss/emphasize timing of medication discontinuation trials (suggest complete by April 1 of senior year in high school) • Develop plans to remedy gaps in readiness for college
Encourage youth and family to consider full range of post-secondary options based on global review, emphasizing everyone's path is different
• Type of school (2-year, 4-year, vocational/technical) • Geographic location (live at home, close to home, out of state) • Full-time or part-time college • Work-school combination • Gap year program or plan • Delayed matriculation option • Size, student diversity, available majors, social life, costs
Encourage youth and family to explore availability of mental health and disability resources on/near campus based on youth's identified needs
• Types of counseling services including how to access, session limits, fees, and wait times • Psychiatric services including criteria to access, fees, and wait times • Location of services on/near campus and transportation availability • Access to emergency services on/off campus • Availability of intensive or specialized mental health services (inpatient, IOP, substance abuse treatment, etc.) • Student health insurance available and/or acceptance of family's current insurance plan • Disability services • Documentation required for accommodations (update testing if necessary) • Student-driven mental health support/advocacy groups • Wellness groups • Students of concern committee

and/or amended over the course of treatment, and as issues arise in the youth's development and evolution of health conditions and educational issues. From this general roadmap evolves specific transition readiness tasks which further outline necessary information and skills (See the Transition Readiness Assessment and Action Plan in Chap. 5 Appendix) that will help the youth meet the new demands of college life and greatly assist the youth in making a successful transition to college.

What We Know About the Demands and Challenges of College Life for Youth with Mental Health Conditions: The Six Domains

In order to assess a young person's readiness for college—and the transition process—one has to appreciate the demands and challenges that await students in a college environment. We have devised six important domains of function which will help focus the skill development and body of information needed for a successful transition to college for this special population [1]. The six domains are:

- Health Condition Knowledge and Skills
- Self-Advocacy Knowledge and Skills
- Independent Life Skills
- Psychosocial Development
- Academic Skills and Executive Function
- Anticipatory Guidance

In each section below is a brief discussion of each domain with examples of how function within a domain interfaces with the college environment and having a mental health condition. A composite chart of the six domains with examples can be found in the chapter appendix.

Health Condition Knowledge and Skills

The first domain focuses on a crucial area of responsibility for youth with mental health conditions with/without educational needs. Understanding their mental health condition(s), the symptoms seen with the condition(s), how to seek help when the symptoms are worsening, and what lifestyle choices need to be made to improve their overall health and stability are crucial areas of knowledge for the college-bound youth. Setting up and keeping medical and mental health appointments, taking medications regularly and as directed, signing medical releases so that all treaters past and present can communicate, understanding the effects of poor sleep, poor diet, and drug and alcohol use—are necessary to maintain stability and effectiveness as a college student. Hopefully, these good health practices would also help avoid relapse, academic and social difficulties, academic probation, and an unexpected medical leave from college. The CAP can play an instrumental role in helping college-bound youths (and their parents) understand their diagnoses, know the names and doses of their medications and why they are taking them, and ways to minimize their risk of relapse.

Self-Advocacy Knowledge and Skills

As important as health maintenance and relapse prevention is the college student's ability to advocate for him/herself in the new university environment. The student needs to know federal laws that oversee the institutional supports for students with mental health and/or educational needs. Obtaining and maintaining accommodations through the Office of Disability Services (ODS) and then distributing accommodation letters to professors each semester is the responsibility of the new student. Seeking help from professors, tutors, treaters at home or on campus, or the ODS is at the initiation of the student. Learning to advocate for oneself may take some time for some youths and should best begin during the high school years if not before.

Independent Life Skills

Many new college freshmen find the "freedom" of college exhilarating—stay up all night playing video games, leave the dorm at will, drink beer as much as you want, sleep late—until they find out their hard-earned grades are being lowered because of absences from class. Managing the day to day demands of independent living is challenging for many young adults, but for college youth with mental health or executive function difficulties, getting to class or other appointments on time is often very difficult, particularly without the assistance of a parent or caretaker. Managing a schedule which might change each day and which might be full of a variety of commitments—class, seeing a therapist, stopping by the disability office, dropping off the laundry, meeting a professor to give them an accommodations letter, picking up meds at the pharmacy, meeting a friend for lunch—can be overwhelming. Tasks such as taking medications on time, managing money, choosing healthy food options, and keeping the dorm room or apartment clean can be difficult to get done consistently, even if one has the ability to complete the tasks.

Not learning/practicing some fundamental daily life skills before heading to college, such as setting and responding to a wake-up alarm and doing laundry, can contribute to stress and can also lead to a relapse of a mental health disorder. Visiting a relative who is in college and living in a dorm, talking to friends and siblings who attend college, reading materials about college life—may all be helpful for the high school student selecting colleges, so they can see the variety of college campuses and think about their own hopes and needs for a healthy college experience. Parents [2], school counselors, and the therapeutic team can all be instrumental in helping young people develop life skills prior to leaving home, so that this aspect of college life is not so overwhelming.

Psychosocial Development

Higher education offers stimulating intellectual pursuits as well as opportunities to challenge one's own values, beliefs, religion, identity, and way of life. Being away from home and being exposed to new cultures and ways of behaving may disrupt old roles and relationships, creating conflicts with family and friends from home. For many youths, this exposure to ideas and chances to experiment with new behaviors or roles is exhilarating. For others, particularly those with psychiatric illnesses, being prodded out of one's "comfort zone" may be overwhelming and destabilizing.

Exposure to a variety of holistic or complementary health interventions may challenge the youth's compliance with therapies and medications that have been effective for the student prior to college. Youths who have been protected by caretakers from independent activities in their community may be more immature and insecure than agemates and may have difficulty navigating the complex relationships with peers and adult professionals on a college campus.

Parents, teachers, treaters, and other stakeholders can encourage psychosocial development by offering opportunities to take on responsibilities at home, school, and in the greater community. Doing chores at home, volunteering or taking on age-appropriate jobs, interacting effectively with others to seek information or lodge a complaint, planning social dates with peers, and discussing emotional topics with caring adults—all are experiences and skills that can be practiced before college and contribute to a youth's maturity and confidence. Learning to drive a car, caring for younger siblings, preparing meals for family members, managing the use of a credit card, participating in traditional school rituals such as "prom" and graduation are activities that are benchmarks of maturity and help the youth learn to negotiate the greater world and gain experience, even if such activities are not always "successful."

Academic Skills and Executive Function

As college is fundamentally a center of rigorous intellectual pursuits, advanced academic and executive function skills are necessary for academic success. For acceptance to college, students demonstrate academic achievement in their high school setting; however, many students with mental health or educational needs may have received multiple supports—in the form of tutors, a structured home setting, medications to help with attentional disorders, accommodations in school, etc.—in order to perform at high levels required to complete college admission requirements.

Some describe college as "high school with the training wheels off." College requires increased cognitive demands: writing longer and more complex papers; synthesizing large amounts of information; using primary source materials which may require interpretation and synthesis; participating in rigorous classroom discussions; giving complex presentations—all while juggling multiple simultaneous demands. Though accommodations and resources may be available to help the college student with special needs, the relentless and sometimes overwhelming pace of college academic demands can be daunting. Developing skills and good work habits such as writing down assignments, keeping up with course demands, managing deadlines, writing complex papers, asking for help when needed, and studying for exams can be developed over the course of a student's academic life *prior* to college.

Anticipatory Guidance (Safety Issues and Thinking Ahead to College)

The vast array of opportunities for new experiences in college is also an important part of college life—often shaping new interests and relationships that can last a lifetime. However, these same opportunities for making choices can sometimes lead to daily hassles, traumatic events, legal problems, unwanted pregnancies, and chronic addictions, which can derail any young adult from completing a college education. Parents, as well as school personnel, CAPs, and other treaters play an instrumental role in helping a young person with mental health needs anticipate possible problems or temptations in college life, including those that may contribute

Table 2.2 Anticipatory guidance

Some possible barriers to treatment compliance on campus
A normal developmental desire to shed old identity and start fresh on campus
Avoiding contact with providers, family, and old friends in your new-found independence
Worries about confidentiality
Worries about stigma
Reluctance to start over and see new providers
A false sense of stability during the easier times of the academic year and stopping treatment
Trouble distinguishing college adjustment issues from symptom exacerbation
Thinking it is okay to skip medications so that you can drink
Choosing to self-medicate with substances as an alternative to prescribed medications
Staying up late to fit in with peers and not getting enough sleep

to treatment non-compliance (Table 2.2). Coping with roommate hassles, dealing with emotional and sexual intimacy, encountering classmates of other races or cultures, who may have different values or behaviors, can lead to positive growing experiences or psychiatric relapses.

Colleges, too, play a significant role in helping students adapt to college demands and communal living, by providing a proficient, available, and adequate system of care on campus and by creating a "healthy living" atmosphere in the overall college community. Understanding a college's values and "ethos" during the college selection process can also help students and parents select a college campus that can provide services for routine and emergent psychiatric issues, as well as an overall atmosphere that encourages and expects tolerant and responsible citizenship, while providing a quality education.

Who Does What When?

Just as each TAY has his/her own unique abilities, skills, interests, and vulnerabilities, parents, treaters at home and in college communities, school personnel, and college campuses themselves have unique characteristics that need to be considered in crafting a transition plan for a college-bound youth. Though the transition *process* will be similarly structured for each youth, the transition plan will differ for each person, depending upon type and severity of diagnoses, ability to self-advocate, educational strengths and deficiencies, developmental maturity, and supports available at home and in college. For youths with psychiatric disorders with/without educational needs, a CAP and other stakeholders, along with the youth, can identify the interests, needs, and wants of the college-bound youth and work to identify important skills that need to be practiced to be best prepared for college in general and for a specific campus. The plan can also identify which stakeholder(s) will take the lead in guiding the youth in gaining new knowledge about college life and the system of care on campus.

For example, a first-generation immigrant teen who has played a significant role in maintaining the family household may possess adequate life skills (cooking, cleaning, laundry, budgeting), but may be unfamiliar with the system of care available on college campuses or be unskilled in asking for academic and/or emotional support. Likewise, a college-bound youth with autism spectrum disorder may need a unique campus that can provide adequate intellectual stimulation within a structured framework, while providing mentors or "buddies" for negotiating complex social settings on campus. Financial need, distance from home, health of parents at home, the medical needs of the student, desires for specialized studies (i.e., oceanography, mechanical robots, acting, working with hearing impaired), etc. may all be factors which inform the college selection process, but also the content and focus of transition planning.

Given what can be the complex nature of transition preparation and planning, we have provided in the chapter appendix a template which "assigns" suggested transition tasks to the college-bound student, the parents/guardians, and the CAP (or other therapeutic team members, depending upon the student's current treatment venue) before, during, and after the college selection process. A two-page article, entitled "Launching our Patients to College" is also in the chapter appendix and may be useful to offer patients and families.

These appendices are based upon child development, knowledge of youth with special needs, and years of clinical experience from seasoned psychiatric practitioners on college campuses and in the greater psychiatric community and are a source of possible best practices.

Summary

Just as we clinicians need to understand the strengths, desires, needs, and vulnerabilities of our students/patients, we, along with their parents and other stakeholders must assist them with the development of knowledge and skills to survive in the new college environment. Like a unique biome, each college or university campus has its own characteristics which can be nurturing or harsh for an individual student. Ideally, the transitioning youth with mental health needs will be matched with a "nurturing biome," and will obtain the necessary skills and knowledge to survive the college climate and the "flora and fauna" of the new environment. An opportunity to visit or experience his/her new "biome"—by participation in pre-matriculation summer programs, a comprehensive new students' week, or even an on-campus program at another campus—will provide a new student a chance to put into practice new knowledge and skills (i.e., sharing a dorm room, doing laundry, deciding what to do with free time, asking for help from strangers) *prior* to starting freshman year. As the semester unfolds, the new college freshman, with helpful supports from the home team and college resources, has a chance to become an effective resident of the new environment. Repeated practice improves proficiency and, ideally, increases confidence to try greater challenges. For most college students, and particularly for students with mental health conditions, a successful transition to college serves as a bridge to further growth and development, in order to leave childhood and negotiate effectively the increasing challenges and opportunities of adulthood.

Chapter Appendix

- Readiness Domains and Sample Tasks for Youth with Mental Health Needs Transitioning to College (1 page)
- Sample Transition Preparation and Planning Tasks Assigned to Key Stakeholders when Youth Heading to College with a Mental Health Condition
  - Patient Tasks (1 page)
  - Parent/Guardian Tasks (1 page)
  - Child and Adolescent Psychiatrist and/or Other Mental Health Professional Tasks (1 page)
- Launching Our Patients to College ("Reprinted with Permission from the American Academy of Child and Adolescent Psychiatry, © All Rights Reserved, 2017") (4 pages)

Readiness Domains and Sample Tasks for Youth with Mental Health Needs Transitioning to College

Health Condition Knowledge and Skills	Self-Advocacy	Independent Life Skills	Psychosocial Development	Academic Skills and Executive Function	Anticipatory Guidance
– Identifying and monitoring main symptoms and reaching out for help when needed – Managing stress – Healthy lifestyle – Taking medications as directed and obtaining refills in timely fashion – Keeping medical and mental health appointments – Understanding impact of poor sleep, poor diet, lack of exercise, use of drugs and alcohol, poor medication compliance on risk of relapse – Signing medical releases and permissions for medication and medical interventions – Deciding about emergency contacts and possible parental access to treaters	– Participate in IEP meetings in high school – Understanding laws: IDEA, ADA, FERPA, HIPAA – Contacting Office of Disability to obtain accommodations – Informing profs of accommodations – Setting up support system on campus – Communicating with former or ongoing treaters from home – Recognizing need for and accepting help in a timely fashion, ideally BEFORE crises arise – Advocating for self with professors, peers, roommates	– Managing schedule of classes, assignments, jobs, and social activities – Handling life tasks (sleep, getting up, eating, meds, hygiene, clean-up, finances, laundry) – Making and keeping appointments with tutors, counselors, profs, physicians, disability office – Balancing relationships with home (when to go home? How often? Stay how long?) – Managing bills/credit cards – Arranging transportation from home to school	– Learning to drive – Holding down a job or regular volunteer job – Coping with others with different lifestyles and values – Taking courses out of comfort zone – Trying out new roles with friends and family, as well as new college acquaintances – Coping with the exposure to politics, religions, philosophies, and ways of living that may challenge the status quo – Handling exposure to treatment interventions which may challenge current mental health treatment	– Handling multiple simultaneous demands – Breaking down big assignments into manageable tasks – Increase use of primary source materials requiring interpretation and synthesis – Managing greater cognitive demands – Writing longer complex papers – Synthesizing large body of information – Evaluating ideas – Speaking up in class	– Coping with roommate hassles and expectations – Dating and intimacy challenges – Living with people of varied cultures, religions, races, genders – Managing challenges to academics: sex, alcohol, drugs, porn, social networks, video games, lack of sleep, intense relationships, over-commitment – Handling legal access to alcohol – Dealing with adult legal system – Signing contracts and leases – Practicing stress management (i.e., yoga, meditation, exercise, contact with nature, art, music)

Sample Transition Preparation and Planning Tasks Assigned to Key Stakeholders when Youth Heading to College with a Mental Health Condition

	Before College Selection Process	During College Selection Process	After College Has Been Selected	Post-Matriculation
Patient Tasks	– Identify types of colleges desired – Identify preferred locations – Identify how often come home – Identify biggest hopes/worries about going to college – Identify biggest hopes/worries about being away from home – Identify HS requirements needed for most colleges – Give best effort on SAT/ACT and HS classes, and test prep courses – Comply with and participate in mental health treatment as outlined below – Attend IEP or 504 meetings – Complete cognitive/educational testing if recommended to obtain accommodations for national tests and college classes – Work on healthy choices and independent life skills prior to college (i.e., drive a car, do laundry, manage credit or debit card, get a job, do basic cooking, seek help from others, good medication compliance, limit drug and alcohol use, get exercise)	– Check out whether college has a disability center and can offer accommodations – Check out available mental health services on campus as well as off campus – Check out insurance coverage at college; whether home insurance can be used or new insurance needed – Check out availability of writing lab/tutors/support services/mentors for ASD, ADHD, LD students, etc. and if part of tuition – Check out transportation needed to get to mental health treatment – Check out if special interest groups/support groups are available (i.e., LGBT, AA/NA campus meetings, sex abuse survivors, multicultural groups, religious groups, political activism, mental health advocacy groups)	– Obtain accommodations with disability center – Identify mental health treaters at college, in community, or at home – Clarify insurance coverage – Sign releases for old and new treaters to communicate with parents – Sign releases for home CAP and therapist to communicate with treaters and other important personnel on campus – Attend special programs for new students and/or special interests – Clarify how to get meds (on-campus MD via health center, community psychiatrist call in to local pharmacy, at home provider calls pharmacy, parents mail meds) – View college website with parents and CAP to become familiar with locating services on campus	– Sign releases if not done – Meet with disability counselor and advisor(s) – Distribute accommodation letters to professors and learn attendance policy for each class – Introduce self to resident advisors and/or student advisors in dorm – Set up schedule for meals, exercise, mental health appointments, tutors, etc. – Secure location for meds in living setting, and set up system for daily med reminders – Set up appt(s) with new treater(s) and check in with old treater(s) if needed – Identify who to call for any after-hours emergency and provide number to parent, trusted friend, and roommate, if appropriate – Review budget with parents, if appropriate

	Before College Selection Process	During College Selection Process	After College Has Been Selected	Post-Matriculation
Parent or Guardian Tasks	– Help child apply for accommodations for SAT/ACT through school – Identify hopes and worries about child going to college – Identify possible financial contributions of parents – Clarify mental health coverage for child if out of state – Identify how often would child like to come home – Clarify any non-college family responsibilities that parent expects of child – Support and participate in child's mental health treatment – Encourage age-appropriate independence and healthy living practices in child (i.e., manage money, setting and waking up to alarm, medication compliance, getting driver's license, manage stress in healthy ways, get job or do volunteer work, good personal hygiene, doing own laundry) – Arrange for child to have cognitive testing done or repeated if not done within 2–3 years of college matriculation	– Assist child with above tasks – Check out insurance coverage at college and whether home insurance can be used or new insurance needed; parent may find that taking out the student insurance, in addition to parent's insurance, may help child with better mental health coverage for local hospitals and providers – Check out possible transportation costs to and from school, considering how many trips to and from school are anticipated – Check proximity and quality of nearby general hospitals and whether there are available emergency psychiatric services in the hospital – Attempt to develop a reasonable budget for child based on family funds and possible costs for college expenses and transportation to school, prior to meeting with child and provider	– Assist child with above tasks – Help child apply for accommodations with disability center if one available – Clarify insurance coverage and consider paying for college student insurance if provides access to local treaters – Review with child basic consumer information and legal issues (i.e., signing up for credit cards, signing leases or loan agreements, hosting parties where minors are drinking alcohol or using drugs, driving under the influence, date rape, transporting drugs of abuse, etc.) – Discuss with child what they (parents) expect of their child in order to have them (parents) pay for education: treatment compliance; weekly check-ins; pass all classes; seek help when needed; respect budget limits; practice healthy living	– Assist child with above tasks – Visit counseling center and disability center with child if child agrees – Inquire about possible emergency services that may be available via counseling center and presence of a student of concern committee – Obtain names and contact information for child's on-campus mental health team, treating psychiatrist, resident advisor, student advisor, roommates or floormates – Attend first appointment with new mental health provider with child's permission, if appropriate – Notify treaters and/or college personnel (student of concern committee) of any concerns about their child's mental status changes or level of functioning

	Before College Selection Process	During College Selection Process	After College Has Been Selected	Post-Matriculation
CAP and/or Other Mental Health Professional Tasks	– Assist parent and patient with their tasks noted above – Discuss patient's diagnoses with parent and patient, and treatments needed to improve symptoms and outcome – Discuss factors which increase risks of relapse/worsen symptoms and factors which may be protective or decrease risks – Discuss meds (i.e. names, purpose, side effects, how best taken, security needed with meds when away from home, how to obtain refills, when to call CAP with issues) – Discuss drug and alcohol use, impact on mental health, interactions with meds, risks (and possible experienced benefits) involved in drug/alcohol use – Discuss sexual/reproductive health and possible impact of diagnoses and medications on sexual experience and fetal health if taking medications or using alcohol and/or illicit substances – Discuss with patient and parent recommended therapeutic supports needed in college	– Assist parent and patient with their tasks noted above, including review of budget and parent/patient financial expectations – View websites of one or two possible college choices with patient and parents to help them locate counseling services, medical services, disability center, academic supports, and after-hours emergency services or emergency process – If patient plans college out of state, check in with your malpractice provider about coverage and HIPAA issues if using telepsychiatry to continue treating patient – Clarify with patient your preference (yes or no or joint with college treater) about continuing to treat patient when in college; discuss rationale (distance to college, disease severity, h/o lethal behaviors, availability of appropriate treatment on/near campus, self-care abilities)	– View college's website with patient and parent to help them locate counseling center info and/or disability center info, and what to do if after-hours emergencies – Assist parent and patient in deciding following: – Student's allowance and what can money be spent on – Grades expected to remain at college – Grades expected for parent to pay for college – How often come home – How often parents visit – How often communicate – Discuss transition to college and possible issues (roommate hassles, social pressures, drug/alcohol use, dating/sex, how to seek help, pressure to share meds, etc.) – Contact new mental health treater if identified and coordinate care; clarify with patient and parent who is in charge during holidays and summers – Contact heads of counseling and disability services	– Check in with patient to see if they believe they can work with on-campus mental health team; make changes early on if poor fit; indicate to patient that you are going to check in with parents and current treatment team after a month – After first month of college contact members of new mental health team, including psychiatrist, to make sure that patient is attending appointments – After first month of college check in with parents and with current treaters to see if they have any questions or concerns about current services or emergency plans that have been put in place – If psychiatric management is shared with home psychiatrist and college practitioner, check in with patient during visits home and during vacations; coordinate care with college practitioner

Launching Our Patients to College[1]

Vivien Chan, MD, Jennifer Derenne, MD, Adele Martel, MD, PhD, and
Patricia K. Leebens, MD

At any given time in our practice, we have adolescent patients visiting colleges, applying to universities, entering post-secondary education, and leaving home. Preparing for college success is a process that starts, ideally, much earlier. The child and adolescent psychiatrist can play an active role in helping patients plan and prepare for these transitions.

Post-secondary Education Options

Many post-secondary options exist. Students with special needs sometimes consider going to technical, vocational, or two-year community colleges. Community college can be a stepping-stone toward attaining a bachelor's degree. Four-year colleges vary in size and diversity of student body, fields of study, geographic location, part-time study options, and a mix of graduate degrees offered. Paths to success without launching directly to college include volunteering, entering the work force, taking a "gap" year, and going abroad. Incorporating regular clinical assessments with personalized discussions of *pro et contra* are important tasks for the child and adolescent psychiatrist. For example, attending college locally while living at home can gradually increase independence in life skills and allows local support and medical relationships to continue. Community college education may allow for a more flexible curricular approach and the ability to work part-time. Transferring to a new campus after attending community college can offer more incremental change but may be problematic, especially for patients with limited social abilities, as making new friends where peers have already resided for 2 years can be difficult. Campus-specific "bridge" programs are designed to facilitate transition from high school to college. Some programs are for any transitioning student while others are by invitation-only, designed for special populations (e.g., first-generation college, disadvantaged backgrounds, at-risk, academically underprepared, autism spectrum) (U.S. Department of Education website). Each college-bound patient and family should consider all viable options given the young person's mental health needs.

Disability Laws After Grade Twelve

Parents and patients need to be prepared to identify and document special needs and to expect changes from previous levels of support. After graduation from high school, the Individuals with Disabilities Education Act (IDEA), which specifically

---

[1] Originally published in *AACAP News* 2014;45(5):193–94. Reprinted with permission from the American Academy of Child and Adolescent Psychiatry, ©All Rights Reserved, 2017.

directs funding to local school districts for students with disabilities, no longer applies; individualized education programs (IEPs) do not continue through college. Instead, emotional, academic, and physical needs are treated as disabilities that require workplace accommodations under Section 504 of the Rehabilitation Act (when federal funds are received by the institution) and the Americans with Disabilities Act (ADA) which extends the mandate of Section 504 beyond recipients of federal funds. At the federal level, these disability laws are enforced by the Department of Justice and the Office for Civil Rights, respectively.

Students are discouraged from making individual negotiations with professors about academic needs for chronic conditions. Patients who desire any type of accommodation, like extended time, isolated testing, or special housing, must self-identify at their college disability office. Whether called "Office of Student Support" or "Disability Services Center," this office ensures campus compliance to ADA and Section 504. Practitioners can help patients by working on self-advocacy skills, investigating how and when patients need to register, discussing the need for updated neuropsychological assessments or psychological testing, and providing the appropriate documentation for requested accommodations.

Mental Health Services on Campus

Most campuses, large and small, offer counseling services. Learning about resources available for psychotherapy and psychiatric needs, fees and limits to services, ease in accessing care and managing prescriptions, and availability of specialty providers (for more complicated diagnoses) is essential before transition. Some staff personnel designated as "counselors" may not be mental health professionals (e.g., academic, housing, financial, or disability counselor). Also, registering at one unit or building at college may mean just that—registering for one supportive service. While some campuses highly coordinate services for individual students, this sophisticated level of management should not be expected. Patients and families need to be guided early in their college search to include availability of appropriate psychiatric services as a "deal breaker" for college choice.

Safety on Campus

As national attention has increased about safety and danger at college, many campuses have developed a multidisciplinary team comprising deans and professors, legal staff, campus security, and health and counseling staff who meet to review at-risk students. While the name of this team may vary ("behavioral intervention," "crisis," or "consultation" team), risk management meetings occur regularly to discuss and assist these students. At some campuses, students may be unaware that they are reviewed, and at others, affected students are directly involved. For serious concerns about a patient, it may take a few phone calls or Internet links by a community provider to identify this resource. Parents should be made aware of this resource as well.

Federal Privacy Laws

An investigation following the Virginia Tech incident in 2007 (**www.oig.virginia.gov/documents/VATechRpt-140. pdf**) found overly rigid and individual interpretations of privacy laws. Medical professionals are familiar with the Health Insurance Portability and Accountability Act (HIPAA). The Family Educational Rights and Privacy Act (FERPA) governs the privacy of educational records at institutions which receive federal funds. Essentially, these laws protect privacy while permitting disclosure when necessary and in the case of emergencies. For example, under FERPA observations by campus personnel of aberrant behaviors can be shared with appropriate others. The overlap and interpretation of HIPAA, FERPA, and state laws on campus is complicated. Further guidance from the U.S. Department of Education has been published (U.S. Department of Education website).

Transition Planning

When anticipating a transition, it is helpful for the adolescent psychiatrist to have a clear sense of treatment goals and safe practice limits. Useful discussions include knowing and talking about the diagnosis, assessing mental stability during the college application process, and determining ongoing treatment needs. Establishing a transition plan is crucial. If remaining with the current psychiatrist, review the frequency of future appointments. If attending college at a distance, clarify the physician's opinions of phone appointments, texts, and emails, and practice of telemedicine across state lines (pending medical license and malpractice carrier regulations). Transfer of care to a new physician also takes planning, and determining who is "in charge" of treatment for shared cases, especially for unstable patients or during holiday breaks is critical. Ensuring that appropriate authorizations for communication exist in advance decreases barriers when urgency arises. Creating a portable healthcare summary, preferably a joint effort by the patient, physician, and family, is a very valuable way for health communication to be conveyed.

Sample Transition Checklist
Middle School

- Review the need for a 504 Plan or an IEP and continuing one through high school
- Review socialization, interests, and hobbies (foundations now prime for later success)
- Discuss responsibility for basic ADLs (like grooming, sleep hygiene, nutrition, personal electronic use)

Early High School (Grades 9–10)
- Based on ability, begin exploring career goals and academic interests
- Discuss the diagnosis and impact of the condition on functioning; explore patient's knowledge of diagnosis
- Discuss the differences between high school versus higher education (class sizes, time spent in class, independent study, amount of unstructured time)
- Review the differences in types of higher education (differences in degree, duration and types, public vs. private institutions, in-state vs. out-of-state, or international)
- Update testing (typically 3-years current) required to support accommodations for entrance examinations and disability services on campus
- For students with special circumstances, look for college "bridge" programs

Late High School and After Graduation
- Review post-secondary education choices with attention to available mental health resources on campus; specifically, navigate websites with patients and parents
- If a high degree of support is currently used for academic function, explore ways to duplicate support on campus
- Practice *instrumental* ADLs (like managing medication, shopping, cooking, tracking finances, scheduling and keeping appointments, driving, using public transportation
- Work on a portable healthcare/psychiatric summary and/or transition "portfolio"
- Discuss changes (or not making changes) to treatment in anticipation of transition

Managing the Transition
In addition to typical developmental issues, such as wishing for a "fresh start" by abandoning prior diagnoses, sharing space with a roommate, developing intimate relationships, homesickness, and using drugs and alcohol, attention specifically to mental health care during the college transition can smooth the way for success. For those interested in further resources, AACAP *Facts for Families* specific to college-bound patients are newly available (#111, 114, and 115) and educational programs are offered at the AACAP Annual Meeting each October.

References
Commonwealth of Virginia. **www.oig.virginia.gov/documents/VATechRpt-140.pdf**
U.S. Department of Education. **www2.ed.gov/about/offices/list/ovae/pi/cclo/brief-1-bridge-programs.pdf**
U.S. Department of Education. **www2.ed.gov/policy/gen/guid/fpco/doc/ferpa-hipaa-guidance.pdf**
U.S. Department of Education. **www2.ed.gov/policy/gen/guid/fpco/brochures/post-sec.pdf**

References

1. Martel A, Derenne J, Chan V. Teaching a systematic approach for transitioning patients to college: an interactive continuing medical education program. Acad Psychiatry. 2015;39(5): 549–54.
2. Fuchs DC. Managing Health/Mental Health Independently and Communication Parameters for Families; 2017. https://www.settogo.org/managing-healthmental-health-independently-and-communication-parameters-for-families/

The Range of Postsecondary Options and Thinking About the Differences Between High School and College

3

Jennifer Derenne

In the not too distant past, college was reserved for those who were exceptionally academically gifted or wealthy. Times have changed, and some post-high school training is now generally necessary to enter the workforce. In many communities, attending college immediately following high school is the norm and is considered the expected developmental path for many young people. Parents, teachers, coaches, and even physicians often assume that young people want to go to college, and that they should do so right away. Students and families may resist deviating from this path, as many tend to want to stay in step with their peers. They may also feel pressure to attend a parent's alma mater, or to follow a similar path as older siblings or extended family members. However, not every student is cut out for college, and others benefit from careful planning to facilitate a successful transition. It is important for family and medical providers to understand this and to be receptive to considering alternate pathways.

Because adolescents and young adults differ in their readiness for college, it is important for clinicians to be aware of different options, and to bring these up early and often in the discussion of future plans. It is not unreasonable to start planting seeds about academic planning as early as the middle school years. Some parents and teens may be sensitive to any insinuation that the young person is not intelligent or mature enough to pursue the more traditional 4-year college track. However, when framed as the clinician's attempt to identify future challenges and pitfalls to promote successful transition, patients and families tend to be more receptive to the discussion.

J. Derenne, M.D.
Division of Child and Adolescent Psychiatry, Department of Psychiatry and Behavioral Sciences, Stanford University School of Medicine, Lucile Packard Children's Hospital, Stanford, CA, USA
e-mail: jderenne@stanford.edu

© Springer International Publishing AG, part of Springer Nature 2018
A. Martel et al. (eds.), *Promoting Safe and Effective Transitions to College for Youth with Mental Health Conditions*, https://doi.org/10.1007/978-3-319-68894-7_3

Undergraduate Postsecondary Education Options

Postsecondary institutions of higher education (IHE) in the U.S. can be categorized using various characteristics (Table 3.1) such as size (number of enrolled students), level of degree granted, proportion of residential students vs. commuters, part-time or full-time student status, percent of entering students transferring from other IHE, level of research activity, and public, private for-profit or private nonprofit [1]. Geographically, they are located along the spectrum of urban to rural. Some colleges focus on students with special interests (arts, for example) and others focus on special student populations (historically black colleges and universities and Hispanic-serving institutions, for example) And, typically, they are divided into 4-year and 2-year institutions. All of these features reflect aspects of the campus environment, the student population, how institutions meet the needs of their students (including their mental health needs), impact tuition costs, and should be taken into consideration by all college applicants. College navigator is a free online tool to help youth and parents review the characteristics of nearly 7000 schools in the U.S. [2].

Four-year schools, typically colleges or universities, offer baccalaureate degrees (earned in the course of 4–5 years or longer if there are breaks or periods of part-time study). Some schools have limited courses of study, focusing on business or liberal arts or engineering, while others, typically the universities, have a broader range of majors and degree options available. Some majors offer (or even require) internships or cooperative (co-op) experiences so that graduates have practical work experience under their belts to make them more attractive to potential employers and to develop workplace competencies (Table 3.2). Co-ops involve students leaving the classroom and working full-time in an organization or company to gain practical skills and experience. They are generally paid for their work and typically do not pay tuition while they are working, which may be attractive to students who are concerned about the financial stresses of higher education. For our patient population, attention should be given to options to continue with student health insurance while involved in a co-op experience. Internships tend to be more flexible; placements may be limited to a summer or a few months, and some students complete multiple experiences in the course of schooling. Internships may also be paid or unpaid, full or part time. For some of our patients, who find classroom academics particularly stressful, the insertion of practical experiences into degree requirements can be appealing.

Table 3.1 Undergraduate postsecondary education options

	Description	Residential or commuter	Degree
Four-year college or university	Usually completed in 4–5 years, major in liberal arts, science, business, engineering, etc.	Either	Baccalaureate Some give associate
Community or junior college	Usually completed in 2 years, less expensive per credit hour, general studies credits may transfer to 4-year institution	Commuter	Associate or certificate
Vocational/trade or technical or career school	Focus on mastery of a skill or trade (automotives, medical technology, welding)	Commuter	Associate or certificate

Table 3.2 Co-op vs. internship vs. apprenticeship vs. work study

	Description	Paid position	Tuition
Internship	Work experience relevant to field of study. Variable in length (months to years) and commitment (full or part time). Student may complete more than one over the course of education	Yes/no	Yes/no
Apprenticeship	Working full-time and learning a skilled trade under the supervision of a licensed tradesman (plumbing, masonry, etc.)	Yes	Usually no
Co-op	Working full-time in an organization to gain practical skills and knowledge while still enrolled in a course of study	Yes	Usually no

Community or junior colleges are generally 2-year programs in which students earn an associate's degree. They tend to be more affordable per credit hour than 4-year IHE, and offer a wide array of courses, including general studies requirements. Some have agreements with local universities that will allow a student to transfer to a 4-year program as long as they have completed general studies successfully and are in good academic standing. Others offer associate degrees or certification in career-related subjects. Some community colleges work with high school students who are finishing their high school degrees in an alternative setting while also taking some college level courses ("middle college" programs). Students at community colleges tend to live off campus and many take classes while also holding down full- or part-time jobs to support themselves. Attending a community college and living at home may be a good alternative for a young person with mental illness who may need to maintain home supports while getting their feet wet in the higher education setting or who had a mental health setback close to high school graduation and needs more time for stabilization.

Vocational/Trade or Technical or Career Schools offer associate degrees or certificate programs that allow students to master the skills necessary for competence in trades like automotive repair, ultrasound technology, dental hygiene, medical coding, or welding. These programs may be 2 years in duration or less. Apprenticeship programs may be associated with technical schools and generally involve learning a skilled trade like plumbing, carpentry, or masonry under the supervision of a licensed tradesman. Apprentices are working and earning money while learning on the job (Table 3.2). For some youth, including those with mental illness, these type programs would be the best personal fit and should be considered.

Alternative Postsecondary Pathways (Table 3.3)

Work

Some young people feel pressure to start earning money, and may decide against more formalized education or training and elect to enter the workforce straightaway. Others may need to earn money to support themselves and to afford school, so they may combine work with enrolling in a class or two at a time. Still others may need to spread college academics out over time to avoid burnout.

Table 3.3 Post-secondary educational and alternative options

Post-high school education options
College or university
Community college
Vocational/trade or technical or career schools
Alternative postsecondary options
Gap year
Workforce
Military

Gap Year

It is becoming more common for teens to take a gap year between high school and college to travel domestically or abroad, volunteer, work, or complete an exploratory internship in a field of potential interest. Some choose to defer admission to their college of choice and participate in formal gap year transition programs that are affiliated with their IHE. Others postpone applying to college and join organized programs such as the Peace Corps [3] or AmeriCorps [4]. More colleges are encouraging accepted students to take a gap year. Some students benefit from stepping off the academic treadmill to recharge while for others a gap year helps them focus on their interests and possible fields of study. For college-bound mental health patients, a carefully planned and structured gap year might promote psychosocial maturation, increase self-confidence, and/or extend a period of stabilization before entering the college milieu.

Military

For those who crave external structure and support, camaraderie, and the opportunity to build a career and travel internationally, the military can be an attractive option. The GI bill provides incentive for soldiers to seek higher education with tuition reimbursement at a later point.

Programs for Special Populations

As increasing numbers of students with pre-existing mental health needs are pursuing higher education, universities are recognizing the need for transition programs to help support at-risk students who may require extra support with transition to college or who may not have had adequate preparation. These so-called "bridge" programs provide special structure and support to help successfully transition students with diagnoses like ADHD, ASD, and LD. These programs could be held in the summer or they could be built into the academic year. Colleges may also reach out to first-generation students and those from disadvantaged backgrounds to offer summer programs aimed at helping students get a head start on the college experience. They are able to gradually get settled on campus, meet peers, learn about the available resources, and meet with mentors and advisors during the slower summer months. University websites are a great place to research whether such programs are available, as are patient advocacy groups such as CHADD, Autism Speaks, and the Learning Disabilities Association of America. Information for first-generation college students is available at http://www.imfirst.org/, and for foster youth at https://www.casey.org/media/SupportingSuccess.pdf and http://www.nccwe.org/downloads/info-packs/CohnandKelly.pdf. Please see the clinical case chapters for further information.

Differences Between High School and College

Academic Expectations and Managing the Daily Schedule

Students and families often fail to appreciate the magnitude of the differences between high school and college (Table 3.4) and this can lead to suboptimal transitions. It is important to acknowledge that high school education is mandatory, while college is voluntary. In high school, school days are generally structured by parents, teachers, and coaches. Parents often make sure that the teen is out of bed on time, has breakfast, and makes it to school with the appropriate materials in hand. They may remind their child to complete hygiene and may take care of laundry, cooking, and other household tasks for them.

Once at school, teachers monitor attendance in class, grade class participation, and remind students to hand in assignments. There are typically somewhere between 15 and 30 students in each class, the teacher gets to know them well, and parents are usually notified if there are concerns about academics. Students may have study hall or free periods that offer protected time to complete homework or study for exams in a structured setting. Guidance counselors help students pick their courses and

Table 3.4 Differences between high school and college

	High school	College
Enrollment	Mandatory	Voluntary
Class size	Usually 15–30	Intro classes may be >100
Teachers	Available before and after school for questions	Professors may have limited office hours
Structure	Parents and teachers structure day, make sure that student gets to classes, social activities, extracurricular activities	Student must design schedule, make sure that they have adequate time to get to and from class
Class attendance	Monitored closely by parents and teachers	Likely not monitored in large lecture halls. May be monitored in small group sessions (labs or discussion groups) or not at all
Grading	Typically a mix of homework, exams, and class participation. Parents may have access via online monitoring programs	May be based solely on exams and large projects.

make sure that the student is on track to graduate with the appropriate credits in place. Teachers are usually available before and after the school day for questions and concerns. Online programs allow parents to monitor assignments, grades, and the class syllabus without having to involve the student at all. There is a dedicated lunch break, and after-school activities generally finish before dinner. After school, parents may resume organization tasks, reminding teens to study, making sure that appropriate forms are signed and returned, and shuttling their children to and from appointments, social events, after-school activities, and sports.

In college, the responsibility for organization and structure shifts to the student. Many college-bound youth seamlessly internalize these skills throughout the high school years and are independent with morning alarms, laundry, appointments, maintaining wellness, and juggling activities. Others still rely quite significantly on parents, nannies, coaches, and teachers to keep them accountable, and it may require a concerted effort on the part of adults to help the student master these skills. College students need to set up a reasonable schedule of classes, make sure that they are able to wake up on time, get enough sleep, and manage their time effectively. They have access to academic advisors who will help them plan their schedules, but there is more onus on the student to keep track of degree requirements. Higher-level classes may be limited to 10–20 students, but introductory courses are often held in lecture halls holding hundreds of people so professors are not able to get to know each student personally, they may not take attendance, and grades may be based entirely on exams. Class may meet every other day, or once a week for night class, and professors may hold office hours only 2 hours per week. Often, the first exams do not take place until almost halfway through the semester, so students do not have any tangible feedback on how well they are keeping up with reading and retaining information. In addition, the amount of reading and out of class work required is exponentially larger than most students are accustomed to. Students can find themselves in the unfamiliar position of needing to be strategic with reading to be sure to cover "high yield" materials in detail [5].

Student Rights and Responsibilities

Section 504 of the Rehabilitation Act of 1973 mandates that individuals with physical or mental impairment that limits major life activities are to be included without discrimination. Subsequent legislation, most recently the Individuals with Disabilities Education Act (IDEA) of 1997, provided federal funding for individualized special education programs for students ages 6–21 as well as early childhood intervention programs. IDEA entitles all elementary, middle, and secondary school students to a free and appropriate public education in the least restrictive environment. Children with a disability (physical, emotion, intellectual) that substantially interferes with their educational progress are eligible for special education services. The onus is on the state to identify students at risk and in need of accommodations, and these are most often identified by parents, teachers, global school screenings, and health professionals. By the time they get to high school, students with disabilities should have had some experience working with school staff and parents to develop and modify their individualized education programs (IEPs). By the time the student turns age 16 (states may mandate a younger age) and is approaching graduation, the IEP must include a mandatory transition plan. Students with health conditions (physical or mental) that do not meet criteria for an IEP may still be eligible for reasonable program and classroom modifications and accommodations through 504 Plans that enable the student to get more benefit from the educational program.

Often, students and parents do not realize that IEP and 504 Plan accommodations do not automatically transfer to the college setting (Table 3.5). In fact, IEPs are not recognized at IHE, and the school is no longer responsible for identifying individuals at risk. Students must advocate for themselves, which means that they need to be organized and self-aware enough to arrange an appointment with the Office of Disability Services (ODS) (sometimes called the Office for Accessible Education or by other titles). Understandably, this can be challenging, especially for students who would prefer to have a "fresh start" and are hopeful that they will be able to forgo the accommodations that were needed in high school. Given the disabilities of some of our patients, students may need coaching and support in these endeavors. In college, accommodations are covered under Section 504 and the Americans with Disabilities Act (ADA). Colleges must make reasonable accommodations (Table 3.6) supported by testing and medical necessity that do not substantially change the academic program. Writing and tutoring services are also generally available. The student and family are required to obtain and submit the

Table 3.5 Disability laws and self-advocacy

	High School	College
Disability Laws	Individuals with Disabilities Education Act (IDEA) Section 504 of the rehabilitation act of 1973	Americans with Disabilities Act (ADA) Section 504 of the rehabilitation act of 1973
Identification of need for accommodations	Parents, teachers, health professionals, health screenings	Student self-advocates
Oversight	Special education	Office of Disability Services
Management of accommodations	Reviewed annually, re-evaluated every 3 years, mandatory transition plan as student approaches graduation	College can offer accommodations based on documentation. Must connect with professors each semester

Table 3.6 Examples of common college accommodations

Note taking services
Extra time on tests (time and a half or double time)
Flexible deadlines for papers and projects
Taking exams in separate classroom to reduce distraction
Tape recording lectures
Oral exams
Use of calculator, scratch paper, spell check
Reader or scribe
Use of audio and visual instructions

appropriate testing and supporting medical documents. Patients and families need to be counseled to look into the services available when researching and applying to schools, and should be in close communication with the ODS early in the process to make sure that a solid and supportive plan is in place from the start. If the student does not initially choose to use accommodations, the groundwork is in place for future use.

References

1. The Carnegie Classification of Institutions of Higher Education. About Carnegie classification. (n.d.). http://carnegieclassifications.iu.edu/index.php. Retrieved 18 Aug 2017.
2. National Center for Educational Statistics. College Navigator. (n.d.). https://nces.ed.gov/collegenavigator/. Accessed 18 Aug 2017.
3. Peace Corps. (n.d.) https://www.peacecorps.gov/. Accessed 18 Aug 2017.
4. Corporation for National Community Service. Ameri Corps. (n.d.). https://www.nationalservice.gov/programs/americorps. Accessed 18 Aug 2017.
5. Southern Methodist University. Transitioning to life at SMU: how is college different from high school? 2017. http://www.smu.edu/Provost/ALEC/NeatStuffforNewStudents. Accessed 18 Aug 2017.

Understanding Campus Mental Health Services and the Campus System of Care

4

Vivien Chan

For mental health practitioners already working with college-bound patients and families, part of necessary transition work includes helping patients and parents early in the college selection process become familiar with mental health and supportive services at each college being considered. Even within the same geographic region and within similar college types, there is incredible variability in services offered. The proactive provider will actively support patients and families in identifying the college with services that best match the needs of the young person transitioning to college.

Campus Responsibilities for Emotional Health

Some believe that the role of higher education is firmly rooted in academic learning, solely to foster critical thinking and to prepare students for occupational careers. Others realize the importance of fostering mental health and that the entire campus (students, faculty, and staff) benefits from robust mental health services but need to juggle the financial business of education. It is important to recall however, that unlike elementary and high school, higher education is *voluntary*. Its approach for students needing more help places responsibility firmly on the adult-student, even if the learner is still an underage minor, which means that students must disclose their need for services and access those services through the appropriate on-campus office.

Families and professionals need to understand the value in asking explicit questions about the available mental health services on campus beyond what may be

4

V. Chan, M.D.
Student Health Center, University of California Irvine, Irvine, CA, USA

Department of Psychiatry and Human Behavior, UCI Health, Orange, CA, USA
e-mail: Vchan1@uci.edu

© Springer International Publishing AG, part of Springer Nature 2018
A. Martel et al. (eds.), *Promoting Safe and Effective Transitions to College for Youth with Mental Health Conditions*, https://doi.org/10.1007/978-3-319-68894-7_4

published on higher education websites. Colleges can promote mental health through *outreach*: generally, health promotional campaigns and awareness-raising events; *screening*: brief surveys, either mass or targeted, designed to identify and highlight areas of concern, like depression, eating disorders, and substance use disorders; *interventions*: professionally delivered triage, individualized case management and referral (including crisis evaluation and referral), brief counseling and psychotherapy, topical peer group offerings, classroom or dormitory based prevention-type mental health and self-care learning (mindfulness, meditation, yoga, nutrition, exercise); and *treatment*: licensed professional identification of medical and mental health illness/diagnosis with developed treatment plan to resolution or stability of condition. However, campus websites sometimes blur the lines between *outreach, screening, interventions*, and *treatment,* and may consider all to be mental health services on campus. Even within the category of *treatment*, campus ethos (and funding) may limit what can be capably and appropriately handled.

Health Insurance

The positive impact of the federal Paul Wellstone and Pete Domenici Mental Health Parity and Addiction Equity Act of 2008 (MHPAEA) on requiring equal coverage for mental health and substance use conditions cannot be overemphasized [1]. Combined with the federal Patient Protection and Affordable Care Act (ACA) of 2010 [2, 3] which requires health care coverage and allows for youth up to age 26 years to remain covered on their parents' insurance, there are limited scenarios where a young adult may arrive to college uninsured or underinsured. These include non-citizen immigrant students, students who are financially independent and purchase a high deductible plan, or families who have selected a plan from an employer with under 50–100 employees as the MHPAEA only applies to large group health plans.

Some colleges and universities mandate proof of adequate health insurance as a condition of matriculation. Some offer student health insurance plans while others do not. Some health insurance entities are limited to certain geographic service areas, providers, facilities, and usage rules. Medicaid may also have state-specific restrictions and benefits that vary by county of enrollment. It is important to be aware of these limitations and plan for this early in the college transition process.

Finding Mental Health Treatment on or Near Campus

Often, the introduction to health and mental health services on campus is done at an orientation presentation, but the knowledgeable provider and family will have completed their homework much earlier. Required physical and immunization health information forms may prompt incoming college students to think about health needs. Some campuses directly solicit mental health information from incoming students and reach out to self-identified, at-risk students in order to smooth transitions. Students and families should explore routine care, as well as resources available for higher levels of care and emergency situations.

Not surprisingly, one of the largest barriers to comprehensive mental health treatment is transportation. A student who has the ability to easily drive or ride a 5–20 mile distance has many more options than the student who must walk or bicycle 1–3 miles for ongoing care. Parents and students should investigate whether medical and mental health services, like student health centers, exist on campus, as well as their staffing and hours of availability. Students attending small institutions may not have access to any campus-based health services and may need to rely on their health insurance and off-campus medical offices for care.

At some student health services, mental health care is delivered exclusively by primary care doctors or mid-level practitioners. At others, a mental health specialty service is also available. Some facilities are quite basic, while others contain urgent care, laboratory, pharmacy, and radiology services. It is critical for families to understand how these programs are funded (via student fee or by insurance), whether there are copayments for services, and which insurance is accepted. Additionally, families should investigate how emergency and after-hours care are handled, as well as access to specialty care and the nearest receiving hospitals.

Mental health services may also be delivered in a dedicated mental-health counseling (and usually, psychological and psychiatric) service. Counseling centers, often exclusively staffed by mental health professionals, are *different* than academic counselors and may deliver a range of brief-to-comprehensive services. It is imperative that a prospective student determine the following: who delivers the service, what level of complexity of treatment does the service offer, and whether there are any time or session limits on treatment. How well a service is staffed often reflects its scope [4]. They should also inquire about the practicalities of filling prescriptions, obtaining laboratory and neuropsychological assessments, and coordinating with medical services.

The majority of student medical and mental health services nationwide are organized by hierarchy through the Division of Student Affairs, but a few are organized with medical schools, university medical centers and Health Affairs. Counseling centers may be located and function separately from the student health center, while other institutions have co-located but independent counseling and student health services. Still others are fully integrated, with mental health and medical services provided in one location using shared record keeping. Models of service provision and staffing ratios have been described in detail elsewhere [4].

Regionally, there can be variations in how psychiatric emergencies are handled. The location and quality of the nearest psychiatric inpatient facility is something that prospective students often neglect. Patients and families are often shocked by the cost of ambulance services. While forward-thinking students and families may explore routine care, learning about available escalated care, such as intensive outpatient, sober living and supports, specialty-track disorders, partial hospitalization, inpatient psychiatric hospitalization, and emergencies are also part of transition planning.

Once they have learned about campus services, providers and families will need to make decisions about who is in charge of the student's mental health care and for how long. Some local practitioners have enduring relationships with their patients and may find it reasonable to continue to provide medical care, even if at a distance. Others set clear boundaries about when someone is considered an active patient and may require regular face-to-face appointments in order to render safe and ongoing care; they may otherwise insist on terminating care and should prepare summaries of past care for the next care team. Individual practitioners need to keep in mind that most professional licenses do not extend to inter-state treatment and that the Centers of Medicare and Medicaid Services, often used as a benchmark for standards, has outlined specific guidance on telehealth services [5]. This can become even more complex when working with international students and with domestic students who wish to travel afar and abroad.

In managing risk, it is helpful to keep in mind that any medical decision-making or evaluation one would feel comfortable doing in the usual scope of practice without the benefit of an in-person examination may be reasonable to make at a distance. However, if the professional advice given would require an in-person examination and assessment to render appropriate and safe care as a minimum standard (e.g., diagnosis; the results of a medication initiation or titration), then care should not be delivered unless face to face. The health care team(s) may also need to explicitly communicate and collaborate, planning ahead for extended holiday breaks and summer hiatus treatment. A note about underage minors and mental health treatment: even though an enrolled student is treated as an adult for educational purposes, some states require parent or legal guardian consent for the administration of psychotropic medication.

Mental Health Treatment and Privacy Laws on Campus

Practitioners may be surprised to learn that the records generated by student health and counseling services at schools receiving federal funds administered by the U.S. Department of Education and which exclusively serve students are not governed by HIPAA (Health Insurance Portability and Accountability Act of 1996) but are held to FERPA (Family Educational Rights and Privacy Act) according to a joint guidance [6]. State privacy laws may be more lax or more stringent than federal ones. Some campus-based providers may be hybrid entities, following HIPAA for non-enrolled students, faculty, and staff, and FERPA for enrolled students. In practicality, most health organizations hold themselves to the more stringent HIPAA standard, and it compels licensed providers who work for campus entities to be well versed in their local regulations. In some past misreading of the law, unreasonable and excessive interpretations of privacy led to withholding of necessary information for continuity of care and for emergency treatment. All privacy laws permit exemptions that allow for sharing of information in emergency and crisis situations to facilitate treatment and in medical consultation. Not sharing information when authorized consent exists may be grounds for reporting to professional licensure boards. Given the many campus offices involved in students' lives, an authorization for consent for *each* campus office may be required to coordinate routine, comprehensive care. Chan and colleagues [6] prepared a summary table comparing and contrasting HIPAA and FERPA in campus health care.

The Campus Community "System of Care"

Often conceptualized as a self-contained village, there are many campus offices and services that can assist students in meeting their mental health needs. In order to advocate effectively for their college-bound patients, mental health providers should understand the campus system of care in order to serve as guides "to the network of services that help students to function optimally at college or university" [7]. While the campus system of care organization has been written about in detail elsewhere [7], some campus units that often support at-risk students are briefly described in Table 4.1.

Table 4.1 Some campus offices and services that can assist students in meeting their mental health and other needs

Campus unit	General features
Academic Staff: Professors, Academic Counselors, Teaching Assistants	Assist students in enrolling for coursework; set grades and curricula. Notify students about passing or failing grades, or being in academic jeopardy
Residence Life, Dorms and Housing	Staff, often including a Dean of Residence Life, overseeing the campus living environment; may be customized by special interests
Disabilities Services	This office registers students and coordinates/delivers necessary accommodations based on diagnosed disability
Conduct or Judicial Affairs	Provides a base code of conduct for the community and enforces violations, including academic dishonesty and social transgressions
Financial Aid	Assists students with aids, grants, loans, and annual financial disclosure filings
Campus Social Services	When available, often staffed by social workers who can aptly navigate the campus structure and community resources
Dean of Students	Includes student activities and groups, organized around cultural, social, charitable, athletic, gender, political topics; student government and leadership roles; student-run mental health support/advocacy groups
Career services	Links students to work opportunities, including work-study; helps prepare students for post-graduate careers
Students of Concern/ Behavioral Intervention Teams	An interdisciplinary group of campus professionals convening to identify, monitor, and discuss the management of at-risk students
Wellness, Recreation and Dining Services	Prevention in the form of regular exercise and appropriate healthy nutrition; health education about wellness, sexual, physical, and emotional health
Title IX Office	Every campus receiving federal funds must respond to and remedy hostile educational environments, including those of sexual, gender, and identity discrimination. Often encompasses counseling and resources for intimate partner and sexual violence

Mental Health Care on Campus

Families and individuals already working with mental health providers have an inherent advantage by being in treatment. Ideally, the treatment includes planned, thoughtful, individualized transition planning well in advance of matriculation to college. Looking ahead at a transition includes making early decisions about health insurance, transportation, and actively learning about a prospective campus's offerings. By heavily researching available online resources and by asking to schedule a brief telephone call with a health administrator or practitioner to learn about the breadth and limits of services, patients and providers can find out more about what actually exists before narrowing down school choices.

References

1. Centers for Medicare and Medicaid Services. The Mental Health Parity and Addiction Equity Act. (n.d.). https://www.cms.gov/cciio/programs-and-initiatives/other-insurance-protections/mhpaea_factsheet.html. Accessed 2 April 2017.
2. HealthCare.gov. Patient Protection and Affordable Care Act. (n.d.). https://www.healthcare.gov/glossary/patient-protection-and-affordable-care-act/. Accessed 2 April 2017.
3. U.S. Department of Health and Human Services. About the Affordable Care Act. (n.d.). https://www.hhs.gov/healthcare/index.html. Accessed 2 April 2017.
4. Chan V, Feliciano E, Mitchell T. A decade of observations from within the U.S. college mental health psychiatry listservs. J Psychiatry Mental Health. 2016;1(1). 10.16966/2474-7769.101.
5. https://www.cms.gov/Outreach-and.../Medicare-Learning.../TelehealthSrvcsfctsht.pdf. Accessed 2 April 2017.
6. U.S. Department of Health and Human Services and U.S. Department of Education. Joint Guidance on the Application of the Family Educational Rights and Privacy Act (FERPA) and the Health Insurance Portability and Accountability Act of 1996 (HIPAA) To Student Health Records. 2008. https://www2.ed.gov/policy/gen/guid/fpco/doc/ferpa-hipaa-guidance.pdf. Accessed 2 April 2017.
7. Chan V, Rasminsky S, Viesselman J. A primer for working in campus mental health: a system of care. Acad Psychiatry. 2015;39(5):533–40.

Adaptation of Pediatric Health Care Transition Guidelines for Use with Youth Heading to College with Mental Illness: Building a Toolkit

5

Adele Martel

Transition discussions and related activities need to be integrated into clinical practice in a way that addresses the needs of youth with psychiatric illness headed to college, supports their families during the transition, and is practical and sustainable for clinicians. Using a structured transition process on a routine basis should allow for more comprehensive *transition planning* and potential transition success.

In 2011, the American Academy of Pediatrics, the American Academy of Family Physicians, and the American College of Physicians published a clinical consensus report [1], providing recommendations for health care transition (HCT) planning for all youth beginning in early adolescence. This report offers practical guidance and activities to support practice-based *transition planning*, and encourages medical subspecialists to adapt the process to their settings, populations, and situations. A hallmark figure in this report is a health care *transition planning* algorithm which outlines a protocol for managing the transition process. Salient take home points from this algorithm include:

1. Transition is a process that is accomplished over time, it is not an event
2. Transition is a collaborative process with youth participation fundamental to that process
3. When possible, start *transition planning* early, preferably by age 12
4. Action steps, which include tasks for the youth, family, and providers, are connected to different age ranges and should proceed in a linear fashion
5. Concentrated efforts may be necessary to move transition forward, when for example, a patient is first seen in late adolescence

A. Martel, M.D., Ph.D.
Division of Child and Adolescent Psychiatry, Department of Psychiatry and Behavioral Sciences, Ann and Robert H. Lurie Children's Hospital of Chicago, Northwestern University Feinberg School of Medicine, Chicago, IL, USA
e-mail: adele.martel@gmail.com

© Springer International Publishing AG, part of Springer Nature 2018
A. Martel et al. (eds.), *Promoting Safe and Effective Transitions to College for Youth with Mental Health Conditions*, https://doi.org/10.1007/978-3-319-68894-7_5

Table 5.1 The six core elements of
health care transition (Got Transition™)

• Transition Policy
• Transition Tracking and Monitoring
• Transition Readiness
• Transition Planning
• Transfer of Care
• Transfer Completion

Embedded within the algorithm, and published by Got Transition™ [2] are the *Six Core Elements of Health Care Transition*. These six basic components of transition and the associated clinical tools essentially translate the consensus report into a series of steps for implementation in clinical practice (Table 5.1).

Recognizing that gaps still exist in the health care transition process for youth with mental health conditions, we have adapted and elaborated upon the *Six Core Elements of Health Care Transition* [2] and created a set of transition tools, for use in routine practice by CAP, specifically with college-bound psychiatric patients in mind. Often, customization of the Six Core Elements focuses on a selected chronic illness [3]. We have approached this task more broadly, taking into consideration the wide range of diagnostic entities and frequent psychiatric comorbidity seen in the college-age group and in the general practice of CAP. Given the academic demands of college, it is important to assess learning issues in the transition process, and recognize that they may be related to the primary diagnosis, a symptom of another diagnosis, or related to medication side effects. Likewise, with the complex social demands of the college environment and possible delays in psychosocial development for many patients, it is important to examine psychosocial maturation and its implications for transition interventions and post-secondary choices. It would also make sense if health care *transition planning* for college-bound patients was temporally aligned with mandated educational *transition planning* efforts for special education students and with the college application process. For patients treated by both a CAP and a therapist, in a split treatment model, transition efforts need to be coordinated. Lastly, whether there is a comorbid medical condition or not, there should be communication with the PCP about the psychiatric transition plan.

In the following section, the features and intent of each of the Six Core Elements are described [2] and are labeled HCT, followed by comments on adaptations for college-bound students with mental health conditions, labeled COLLEGE. Sample office-based tools are described (TOOLS) and are included in the chapter appendix. These tools were first presented by the author as part of a continuing education program at the 2013 annual meeting of the American Academy of Child and Adolescent Psychiatry.

Core Element #1 Transition Policy

HCT A key first step is to develop a *transition policy* or statement for the practice. This policy introduces the concept of transition, explicitly describes the practice's approach to health care transition including if and when a patient ages out of the practice, and provides information on privacy and consent. The *transition policy*, for example, can state the practice's commitment to a smooth transition from

Table 5.2 Some things to think about when deciding to provide care for patients away at college

Take into consideration
• Patient's treatment goals and preferences
• Stability of patient
• Geographic location
• Readiness to manage mental health needs
• Readiness in other domains of functioning
• Licensing and malpractice coverage if patient is out-of-state
Under what circumstances/condition
• Trials off medications completed and assessed by April 1 of senior year
• Follow-up appointments on all school vacations or minimum of every 3 months
• Means of communication established for between appointments
• Only with shared treatment and communication with campus/local providers
• Releases signed prior to departure for providers, disabilities services, and possibly parents

adolescence to young adulthood and what that might look like in the course of treatment. The goal is to eliminate misunderstandings, foster teamwork, and hopefully get the youth involved. All staff are made aware of the policy and should understand the practice's approach to transition. The policy is introduced to the youth, as early as age 12 and preferably by age 14, and to the family.

Many CAP naturally talk about these developmental issues with patients and families but do not frame it as "transition." However, the goal is for practitioners to be more cognizant of and deliberate about health care transition with patients and families.

COLLEGE For college-bound patients, the transition care plan requires collaboration and deliberation among the provider, patient, family, and others and is a highly individualized process based on provider practice approach and attitudes, the patient's status, and the services available at the IHE. So, the *transition policy* also needs to address if patients can be followed after they leave for college and under what conditions or circumstances (Table 5.2).

TOOL A sample two-page *transition policy* for a child and adolescent psychiatric practice is in the chapter appendix. The second page of the *transition policy* specifies the practice's policies regarding ongoing care of college-bound patients. It provides a more complete list of things for providers to think about when agreeing to continue care from afar and serves as a guide for patients and parents as to what to expect moving forward. Unlike the general office *transition policy*, the addendum can be discussed with college-bound patients and their families during junior and senior years of high school versus at age 12.

Core Element #2 Transition Tracking and Monitoring

HCT The purpose of this transition component is to track a patient's progress through the steps of health care *transition planning*. A patient first has to be identified as belonging to the target group of patients, again preferably starting at age 12, and entered into a "registry."

COLLEGE For our purposes, it is suggested that the practitioner focus on the intent of *transition tracking and monitoring* and keep it simple. So, if the youth is planning on post-secondary education, then a tracking sheet is prominently placed in the patient's chart. Or, tracking could be accomplished through meaningful use of the electronic medical record. Importantly, the *transition tracking and monitoring* sheet serves as a reminder for the provider to complete all steps no matter when the patient is first seen even if the time frame needs to be collapsed.

TOOL A sample *transition tracking and monitoring* sheet for transitioning psychiatric patients to college is in the chapter appendix. This tracking sheet is organized by the Six Core Elements. Of note, suggested ages and grades for completing tasks have been listed to align this tracking sheet with steps in the college application process. The provider may repeat steps as needed for a particular patient. The shaded areas of the sheet show additional considerations related to readiness for college and decision-making about college and are discussed next.

Core Element #3 Transition Readiness

HCT Starting at age 14, the provider begins more formally to identify the goals and needs of the youth in regard to independent management of their health care. *Transition readiness* assessments, completed on a regular basis with the youth and parent or caregiver, not only track the youth's health knowledge and skills, but provide a basis for jointly establishing actions to move the youth forward in readiness for transition to adult-oriented health care. Several general HCT readiness assessment tools are available and can be used with college-bound psychiatric patients (Table 5.3). Many pediatric hospitals have created their own HCT readiness assessments so providers should check their institutional resources. These tools include statements such as "I know where my pharmacy is and how to refill my medicines" [2]. Some tools have parent/caregiver versions as well [2, 3].

COLLEGE For college-bound youth with MHC, readiness for transition to college needs to be assessed in multiple domains of function relevant to college success with independent management of health care and self-advocacy serving as the foundation.

TOOL With this in mind, we have created a specialized *Transition Readiness Assessment and Action Plan for Youth Heading to College with a Mental Health Condition* (See the chapter appendix). A version of this tool and a brief description of how it was developed were first published in 2015 [4]. This checklist is intended for use by the CAP in routine practice and includes items related to mental illness in general and some items that are illness specific. The tool is organized by important domains of function (described in Chap. 2) which are essential for preparing patients for life beyond high school. It also includes a list of topics for anticipatory

Table 5.3 Readiness assessment tools

Some General Health Care Transition Readiness Assessments
Center for Health Care Transition Improvement www.gottranstion.org Transition readiness assessment for parents/caregivers (25 questions) http://www.gottransition.org/resourceGet.cfm?id=240 Transition readiness assessment for youth/young adults (25 questions) http://www.gottransition.org/resourceGet.cfm?id=239
Transition Readiness Assessment Questionnaire TRAQ 5.0 (20 questions) © Wood, Sawicki, Reiss &, Livingood, 2012 http://www.hscj.ufl.edu/jaxhats/docs/traq_5.0.pdf
UNC TRxANSITION (32 questions) http://pediatrics.med.unc.edu/transition/files/trxansition-scale-version-3
Some College Readiness Assessments
Landmark College http://www.med.upenn.edu/pan/documents/CollegeReadinessGuide.pdf Looks at five areas that are critical for college success: Academic skills, self-understanding, self-advocacy, executive function, and motivation/confidence
Virginia's College Guide for Students with Disabilities http://www.doe.virginia.gov/special_ed/transition_svcs/outcomes_project/college_guide.pdf Are you ready for the responsibility? Pp. 20–21
Specialized Transition Readiness Assessment and Action Plan for Youth Heading to College with a Mental Health Condition
• Published as supplemental material in 2015 Academic Psychiatry 39(5): 549–554 • Published in appendix with permission

guidance. Within each domain, items are somewhat arranged in a developmental fashion. The goal is for the patient to have increasing responsibilities and information as they move into and through adolescence.

The checklist is comprehensive and lengthy, and consideration should be given to assessing one or two domains at a time. Providers are also encouraged to individualize the use of the tool, focusing on sections of most relevance to a patient's situation and needs. This tool is designed to serve multiple purposes, as a readiness assessment tool, a task assignment or action planning tool, and a transition "cheat sheet" for the provider.

College readiness assessment tools (Table 5.3) are available which focus predominantly on academic and executive functioning skills, and ask questions such as "What academic accommodations are helpful to you?" These may be used in a parallel process of transition preparation and planning by the high school. There are some transition toolkits available for ADHD, learning disabilities, and autism spectrum disorders. These are typically developed by patient advocacy groups or state departments of education, for use by parents, educators, and youth but they can be helpful to the CAP as well. Please see the helpful resources sections in the clinical case chapters.

Given the nature of psychiatric practice and important nuances in the college application and selection process for youth with MHC, it is recommended that a face-to-face global review of the youth's current functioning and needs (see Chap. 2) be done in addition to using paper or online readiness assessment tools. We suggest that this meeting(s) takes place during the junior year of high school if possible and be repeated as necessary. A description of transition planning and preparation—its rationale, process, and content—written specifically with patients and families in mind, is available and may be helpful information to offer prior to or at the time of the face-to-face meeting [5].

This face-to-face meeting(s) is essential for youth with MHC heading to college and can set the tone for the entire college application and selection process. The *transition tracking and monitoring sheet* (chapter appendix) provides a checklist for this meeting(s).

Core Element #4 Transition Planning

HCT *Transition planning* should flow naturally from *transition readiness* assessment and takes place roughly between the ages of 14 and 17. Prioritized actions and plans to address the transition needs of the patient are developed collaboratively by the patient, family, and providers, and completed over time. Assigned tasks, which often come directly from the readiness assessment form, are adjusted as readiness assessments are updated. *Transition planning* also involves revisiting how the model of health care changes when the patient turns age 18, discussing *transfer of care* plan options including the timing of transfer and whether the young person needs/wants to change providers, and discussion of health insurance. It may be useful to review the practice's *transition policy* again, including the special considerations for college-bound patients (chapter appendix). The patient, with the provider's help and structure, should begin to prepare a Medical Summary. This task may help the patient recognize the course of his/her condition and help the patient identify strategies for relapse prevention.

COLLEGE *Transition planning* requires a few enhancements for college-bound psychiatric patients. It may be necessary to involve the high school team in action plans to address the transition needs of some patients, particularly those who utilize academic accommodations and other supports. The Mental Health and Medical Summary should go beyond a list of medications and include the items listed in Table 5.4. A sample, two page, Mental Health and Medical Summary is in the chapter appendix. Patients should also begin to build a Transition Portfolio containing documents that may be necessary for obtaining disabilities services on campus

Table 5.4 Suggested information to include in a mental health and medical summary

Identifying information and contact information
Diagnosis (mental health conditions and other medical conditions)
Allergies to medications
Current mental health treatment services
Past mental health treatment history (diagnostic studies, medication trials, hospitalizations, etc.)
Past and current educational supports
Emergency contacts designated by patient
Comments section

Table 5.5 Suggested contents of a transition portfolio for disabilities services

Copies of educational, psychological, neuropsychological evaluations
Current or most recent IEP or 504 plan
List of accommodations and services student may need in college
Letters in support of student's request for accommodations
Mental health and psychiatric treatment summary
ACT or SAT scores
Copy of official letter from standardized testing service granting accommodations

(Table 5.5). The provider/patient/family may find it helpful to review some of the Transition Portfolio documents as to provide psychoeducation and promote insight into needed support services once at college. The youth, family, and providers should begin to take a realistic look, not only at options of continuing psychiatric care once at college, but at the range of post-secondary options that are available.

TOOL The specialized *Transition Readiness Assessment and Action Plan for Youth Headed to College with a Mental Health Condition* (chapter appendix), as previously noted, serves as an office-based tool for assigning readiness tasks to key constituents and tracking progress. ("What can I do to practice or prepare? Who can help?")

Core Element #5 Transfer of Care

HCT At age 18, all youth transition to an adult model of care; the young adult is in charge of his/her care and ongoing involvement of the parent and/or others requires consent (exceptions exist with court-appointed guardianship). As part of this Core Element, "Address any concerns that young adult has about transferring to adult approach to care. Clarify adult approach to care, including shared decision-making, privacy and consent, access to information, adherence to care, and preferred methods of communication, including attending to health literacy needs." [2].

Depending on the structure and policies of the practice, an actual *transfer of care* to another provider may or may not take place. In either case, ongoing *readiness assessment*, care planning, and updating the Mental Health and Medical Summary continue to occur. In the event of a *transfer of care*, a new provider is identified, authorized communication takes place between providers to exchange information and to clarify date of transfer and roles of each provider, and a Transfer Package is prepared. The sending provider should confirm with the receiving provider that the Transfer Package was received.

COLLEGE *Transfer of care* planning for college-bound psychiatric patients can be a challenge. Planning is interwoven with the college application process and once a young person receives acceptance letters and selects a college, there may not be much time left for planning (early decision candidates and wait list candidates have different timing scenarios). The stress of the college application process and its developmental meaning can destabilize the young person as well. The "downtime" between applications being sent in and acceptance letters being received can be used to further *transition readiness*. The patient and provider can continue to collaboratively work on the Mental Health and Medical Summary and Transition Portfolio which should enhance self-advocacy and may prove of evolving interest to the late adolescent/young adult. Parent–child activities to increase independence in important domains of function can be practiced during this time as well. This is also an important time for offering anticipatory guidance about college life and potential obstacles to treatment compliance on campus as noted on the *Transition Readiness Assessment and Action Plan for Youth Heading to College with a Mental Health Condition* (chapter appendix).

Once acceptance letters are received, it is important to review, once again, the mental health goals and treatment needs of the patient and justify them with the office *transition policy* and the available services on various campuses. Then, only after a hopefully "best fit" college is selected, can the CAP work with the youth and family to identify new providers, on and/or off campus.

For our purposes, a *transfer of care* plan or transition care plan refers to the plan that is established for ongoing mental health treatment and educational supports for the young person once he/she has started college. Will the student see all new mental health providers? Will home-based providers continue to be involved? Will the Office of Disability Services be involved? Is the new therapist on campus or off campus? When both home and school providers are involved, who manages an emergency and who is in charge? Some young people have the choice to continue to see their home provider(s) when they attend college and many prefer this arrangement, while others are obliged to find care on/near campus.

TOOL Sample transition care plans and accompanying cover letters are shown in the chapter appendix. One care plan is for the case when a complete *transfer of care* to new providers takes place. The other is for the situation when home-based and school-based providers share treatment, which is often the case given the need for care during school breaks, including summers. Transition care plans should be reviewed with and signed by the patient with the patient receiving a copy. The cover letter and the transition care plan should be incorporated into the Transfer Package along with other key items (Table 5.6). A sample Emergency Plan and a sample

Table 5.6 Suggested contents of a transfer package

Cover letter
Current mental health and medical summary
Transition portfolio (if applicable)
Final transfer of care or transition care plan
Emergency care plan
Legal documents such as signed releases of information and advanced directives [6, 7]
Contact information of all providers
Transition readiness: Pending actions and ongoing concerns
Additional health records (appropriate lab reports, imaging studies, etc.)

Pending Actions and Ongoing Transition Needs form can be found in the chapter appendix. Ideally, the Transfer Package is sent to the new provider(s) prior to *transfer of care*. Patients transitioning to college may not know who their new providers are until a few weeks after they arrive on campus and should be prepared to deliver the Transfer Package. The Transfer Package is a helpful tool but is not a substitute for direct telephone communications between old and new providers.

Core Element #6 Transfer Completion

HCT The final step in the general health care transition guidelines, *transfer completion*, focuses on communication. The sending or pediatric provider contacts the young adult and family (with prior permission) to verify that care has transferred to the new adult provider. The pediatric provider also contacts the adult provider to ensure success of transfer and continuity of care and offers to remain a resource to the adult provider. Feedback about the transition process is solicited from all involved and the *transfer of care* is deemed complete by both the sending and receiving providers. The suggested time for follow-up is 3 months after the last pediatric visit. Patients and families may find this period of overlapped care very helpful as they try to traverse care systems.

COLLEGE For college-bound youth with MHC who are transferring all mental health care to on or near campus, no more than 1 month should pass without follow-up to determine if the young person has met with the new provider(s), including meeting with the ODS. One month is approximately 25% of a semester and concerns or lack of continuity of care should be identified early. The sending provider may choose to remain a resource for 3 months, check in one more time to ensure continuity of care, and then *transfer of care* should be deemed complete. If the transition care plan involves shared treatment among home and campus providers, *transfer completion* would refer to the establishment of functional and regular communication between providers.

TOOL There is no new transition tool for this step. The home-based provider should document *transfer completion* on the *transition tracking and monitoring* sheet (chapter appendix).

Summary

CAP, and other mental health professionals, are encouraged to adapt all or parts of this toolkit to their particular practice needs and develop a standardized approach to transitioning patients to college. Transition preparation and planning takes time but it makes developmental sense, is preventive in its intent, and can be incorporated into regular mental health visits. Given that health care transition is a national priority, reimbursement for transition services is being reviewed in [8].

The case studies that follow confirm the value of proactive, developmentally based, and structured *transition planning* approaches.

Chapter Appendix

- Transition Policy for a Child and Adolescent Psychiatric Practice with Special Considerations for College-Bound Patients (2 pages)
- Health Care Transition Tracking and Monitoring Checklist: Transitioning Psychiatric Patients to College (1 page)
- Transition Readiness Assessment and Action Plan for Youth Heading to College with a Mental Health Condition (4 pages)
- Mental Health and Medical Summary (2 pages)
- Transition Care Plan: Transfer of Treatment to Campus Providers and/or Near-Campus Providers

  – Cover Letter (1 page)
  – Transfer of Care Plan PROVIDER Copy (1 page)
  – Transfer of Care Plan PATIENT Copy (1 page)

- Transition Care Plan: Shared Treatment by Home Providers and Campus Providers

  – Cover Letter (1 page)
  – Transfer of Care Plan PROVIDER Copy (1 page)
  – Transfer of Care Plan PATIENT Copy (1 page)

- Sample Emergency Care Plan (1 page)
- Pending Actions and Ongoing Transition Needs Form (1 page)

TRANSITION POLICY FOR A CHILD AND ADOLESCENT PSYCHIATRIC PRACTICE

(Please check one box or customize depending on your practice structure)

Dear Patients and Families,

Welcome to our practice.

We are committed to providing you with quality psychiatric care and to helping you make a smooth transition from adolescence into young adulthood. This process requires that we all work together – you, your families, your medical team, and other supportive individuals that you want on your transition team.

We will encourage you to take on increasing responsibility for your own health care and other aspects of your life. We will encourage your parents/guardians to provide you with opportunities and experiences to support your efforts to be more independent. For example, we will meet with you alone for at least part of each office visit. By age 18 years, you will participate in your own care as an adult and we will need your consent to discuss any personal health information with your family or anyone else (except in certain emergency situations).

Transition preparation and planning is a "roadmap to independence". The goal is to empower you to be able to care for your health needs, advocate for yourself at school or at work, and be better-prepared for the many exciting challenges of young adulthood.

☐ *Given that our practice sees youth through high school graduation or up to but not including age 19, part of this transition process will be to help you smoothly transfer your care to new providers and the adult healthcare system. For those of you heading to college, we will work with you to develop a transfer of care plan that includes providers on/near campus.*

☐ *Given that our practice sees youth up to but not including age 26, part of this transition process will be to help you smoothly transfer your care to new providers and the adult healthcare system. For those of you planning to go to college, we will be happy to discuss participating in your ongoing care.*

☐ *Other...*

Please let us know if you have any questions. We look forward to working with you.

Sincerely,

_____

(insert name of practice)

TRANSITION POLICY: SPECIAL CONSIDERATIONS FOR OUR COLLEGE-BOUND PATIENTS

We are happy to continue to help you plan for your ongoing mental health care while you attend college. We want to know your preferences in moving forward. We will discuss alternatives and provide you with information to inform your choices. Please feel free to ask us questions.

Based on feedback from our patients and on our experiences with other young people heading to college, we have established some guidelines to facilitate the development of safe and productive transition care plans. Our practice policy includes the following:

(1) We will take into consideration how stable you are, how prepared you are to manage your mental health needs independently, and how far away you will be as we discuss alternatives and work together to develop your care plan.

(2) At the time of your college acceptance, we will encourage you to carefully consider your academic, emotional, and financial needs in conjunction with the campus resources/supports that are available at various institutions in making your final decision as to which school is the "best fit" for you.

(3) In most cases, it is our recommendation that all major medication changes, especially **trials off** medication, be completed and assessed by April 1st of your senior year.

If we are to remain involved in your care then:

(4) *At a minimum*, we will ask you to attend appointments at least every three months and/or during your school vacations/breaks.

(5) We will establish with you a confidential means of communication between appointments.

(6) We will help you devise an emergency plan for when you are away from your family's home; this may involve having an introductory consultation with an on/near campus provider.

(7) We may request that your care be shared with providers on/near campus which will necessitate that you sign releases of information for these members of your college support system.

(8) We may recommend that you disclose your disability and obtain accommodations through the campus disabilities office (with our assistance).

(9) We may ask that you sign a release of information for us to contact your parents. We will discuss those emergency situations for which a release is not required.

HCT TRACKING and MONITORING CHECKLIST
Transitioning Psychiatric Patients to College

Use this sheet to track transition planning steps for your patients. The asterisk *
indicates a suggested time by which to complete the task. Repeat tasks as necessary
given strengths, vulnerabilities, and stability of each patient.

Patient Name	D.O.B.			
Age/Grade	12-13 Middle School	14-15 Grades 9-10	16-17 Grade 11	17-18 Gr 12 & Beyond
TRANSITION POLICY Introduced				
General Office Transition Policy	*			
Considerations for College-Bound Patients			*	
TRANSITION TRACKING and MONITORING Checklist incorporated into chart				
Youth age 12 or older and interested in pursuing postsecondary education	*			
Do HCT Readiness Assessment & Action Plan *(Multiple assessments with updated Action Plans should be completed)*	*	*	*	*
Do College Readiness Assessment & Action Plan if necessary *(School system may do this)*		*		
Meet with youth and family to: O Conduct global review of youth's current functioning including goals, strengths, limitations, diagnosis, prognosis o Review current level of formal and informal support (from family, providers, school, friends, agencies, private tutors, coaches, etc.) ☐ Discuss short- and long-term treatment goals and service needs			*	
Based on youth's identified needs: O Discuss range of post-secondary options (gap year, community college, work+school, four-year school, delayed matriculation, etc) O Make a list of criteria for selecting a college including availability of mental health and disability resources on/near campus based			*	
TRANSFER of CARE				
Complete and send Transfer Package				*
TRANSFER COMPLETION				
Confirm young adult met with new provider				*
Evaluate success of plan and continuity of care with young adult, other providers (& family)				*
Deem transition/transfer of care complete				*

TRANSITION READINESS ASSESSMENT and ACTION PLAN
For Youth Heading to College with a Mental Health Condition [1]

As you plan for your transition to young adulthood and post-secondary education, you will need to know about your psychiatric condition, how to manage your condition independently and how to advocate for yourself. You, your family, your provider, and others (teachers, tutors, etc.) can develop plans to address gaps in your knowledge and skills as identified by this checklist. Your doctor may complete this checklist with you in order to focus on those items most related to your condition and age and needs. Your parents may be given this or a similar checklist to complete.

NAME DATE OF BIRTH DATE OF ASSESSMENT	I know this or I do this	I need practice	What can I do to practice or prepare? Who can help?
TRANSITION CONCEPT and POLICY			
I understand how healthcare transition relates to my transition to college/work/independent living			
HEALTH CONDITION- KNOWLEDGE			
I know the name of my condition/disability			
I know how my condition impacts my social and community functioning			
I know what to do in case of an emergency			
I know the warning signs/symptoms of a relapse			
I know the circumstances and conditions which have led to trouble for me (destabilization and/or relapse) in the past			
I know how alcohol/drugs might affect my health condition			
I know how sleep (or lack it) affects my condition and know how to make sure I get enough sleep			
I know how pregnancy might affect my health condition			
I know what strategies and tools have helped me stabilize in the past			
I understand how my family's cultural beliefs might affect health care decisions			
I know pertinent family medical and psychiatric history			
MEDICATION - KNOWLEDGE			
I know if I am allergic to any medications, foods or things in the environment			
I know the names and purposes of my medication(s)			
I know my baseline eating, sleeping, elimination patterns			
I know the general side effects of my medication(s)			
I know the sexual side effects of my medication(s)			
I know the follow-up and blood work needed for my condition and medication(s)			
I know what would happen if I abruptly stopped taking my medication(s)			
I know to ask about possible medication interactions			
I know how substance use may affect my medication(s)			
I know how my medication(s) would be harmful to an unborn baby			
I know about the abuse, misuse, and diversion of medications			

HEALTH INSURANCE			
I know why it is important to have health insurance			
I carry my insurance card and know about copays			
I made/have a plan for health insurance after age 18			
HEALTH CONDITION - SKILLS			
I meet privately with my doctor for part of each office visit			
I can present acute concerns to my provider(s)			
I can name my providers(s) and reach them			
I make and keep track of my own appointments			
I can read a prescription bottle			
I take my medications independently			
I keep track of and fill my prescriptions			
I store my medications in a safe location			
I can explain my condition in a few sentences			
I can present my treatment history or have access to it (electronic mental health and medical summary)			
I complete/sign medical forms (health history, permission for treatment, release of records, HIPAA Policy, etc.)			
I discuss short- and long-term treatment goals with my provider			
I have checked out available mental health resources on various campuses (online, on college tours, phone inquiry)			
Once I turn 18, I will meet alone with my doctor unless I have signed consent forms (except guardianship or conservatorship)			
I have decided about emergency contacts and possible parental access to providers after I turn 18 years old			
SELF-ADVOCACY KNOWLEDGE			
I know the purpose of accommodations			
I know how my condition/disability impacts learning/working			
I know the accommodations which work best for me to participate at school and in the community as others my age			
I know how my condition/disability relates to future plans and setting goals			
I know the rights and responsibilities of an individual with disabilities (e.g., disability and privacy laws that apply in higher education settings: ADA, 504, FERPA, HIPAA)			
I know the pros and cons of disclosure to school, employer, roommates, friends			
I know the documentation that is required to receive accommodations at most post-secondary institutions			
I know the date of my most recent educational, psychological or neuropsychological testing			
SELF-ADVOCACY SKILLS			
I ask for help when needed			
I can explain to others in a few sentences how my condition/disability impacts me in various settings/situations			
I can describe to others the strategies and accommodations which work for me			
I participate in 504/IEP meetings and read related documents			
I maintain a portfolio of documents relative to my disability			

I have read my testing results (educational, psychological, neuropsychological, vocational, etc.)			
I have applied for accommodations for standardized college entrance examinations			
I have arranged to update my testing (if necessary)			
I have reviewed helpful websites on how and when to disclose my disorder/disability			
ACADEMIC SKILLS and EXECUTION FUNCTION			
I know my academic strengths and weaknesses			
I have a system for keeping track of projects, books and papers			
I have a system for preparing for tests and exams			
I have a system for taking notes			
I set aside time for school work			
I complete steps of a project in a timely fashion			
I use a computer for typing and word processing			
I know what classes I need to take to graduate from high school			
I know what classes are required to apply to most colleges			
I can describe how college academics differ from high school			
INDEPENDENT LIFE SKILLS			
I direct my own personal hygiene			
I eat a balanced diet			
I balance my time between work/social/leisure activities			
I set and respond to a wake up alarm			
I manage my own time with TV/social media/video games			
I do my own laundry			
I do simple cleaning tasks at home (sweep, wash dishes, etc)			
I have a driver's license and/ or use public transportation			
I manage basic finances (bank account, debit card, credit card)			
I shop for groceries and cook simple meals			
I comfortably communicate by phone and computer			
I use the internet efficiently for finding information			
PSYCHOSOCIAL DEVELOPMENT - EXPLORING IDENTITY and SOCIAL RELATIONSHIPS			
Family Interactions			
I have regular chores			
My parents give me opportunities to make decisions			
I can communicate my needs and wants to my family			
I can express feelings in my family			
I participate in cultural traditions			
Peer Interactions			
I hang out with friends			
I have friends who are supportive			
I have resolved conflicts with peers			
I can take the perspective of others			
I have strategies to deal with peer pressure			
I have strategies to deal with bullying			
I have had some dating experiences			

School and Community Involvement			
I participate in extracurricular activities (clubs/sports/religion)			
I have volunteer experiences in helping others			
I have held a part-time job			
Planning for the Future			
I have some personal interests and dreams			
I can discuss my strengths and limitations			
I set goals and accomplish them			
I can identify some of my personal values			
I have hobbies/leisure activities			
I have explored various career options			
I have explored various post-secondary education options (gap year, 2-year school, 4-year school, tech school, work, military)			
I have a list of criteria for selecting a college including availability of mental health and disability resources			
SAFETY ISSUES & THINKING AHEAD to COLLEGE ANTICIPATORY GUIDANCE	**Yes**	**No**	**Still Need To Do**
My healthcare provider has discussed the following with me:			
Strategies to promote health and mental wellness (nutrition, exercise, sleep hygiene, help-seeking, stress reduction)			
Internet/social media safety issues			
Tobacco, energy drinks, alcohol and drugs, including legal access to alcohol and cannabis			
Safe driving habits (drinking and texting while driving)			
Dealing with the adult legal system			
Ways people protect themselves from unwanted pregnancies and STDs when they are sexually active			
Date rape			
Possible obstacles to treatment compliance for young adults (stigma, invincibility of life stage, fresh start, confidentiality concerns, ebb and flow of the academic year and possible false sense of stability)			
Common factors impacting academic performance (sleep, stress, work, anxiety, medical illness, depression, etc)			
Typical college adjustment issues (homesickness, roommate difficulties, time management, eating choices, staying connected with old friends, managing new temptations)			
Challenges to the familiar and sense of self (exposure to new lifestyles, values, ideas, treatments)			
Staying connected with family/friends (phone, internet, visits)			
How my relationship with my family will change			
OTHER ISSUES and NOTES			
I would like to talk with my provider about…			
I would like to talk with my provider about…			

[1]Published as supplemental material in Academic Psychiatry 2015 39(5). Revised July 2017.

MENTAL HEALTH AND MEDICAL SUMMARY

Name _____ Birthdate _____

Phone _____ E-Mail _____

Emergency Contacts

#1_____Phone _____Relationship _____

#2_____Phone_____ Relationship _____

PCP at home _____ Phone _____

Health Center at school _____ Phone_____

Pharmacy at home _____ Phone_____

Pharmacy at/near school _____Phone_____

Health Insurance

ID# _____Phone_____ Insured _____

ID# _____Phone_____ Insured _____

DIAGNOSIS (Include Psychiatric and Medical Conditions)

OUTPATIENT TREATMENT SERVICES (last 6 months)

	Provider/Program	Phone
Individual Therapy		
Outpatient Med. Management		
Educational Supports (IEP/504/tutor)		

EXPECTED/PLANNED CAMPUS (on/near) OUTPATIENT TREATMENT SERVICES

	Provider/Program	Phone
Individual Therapy		
Outpatient Med. Management		
Disability Services		

PAST OUTPATIENT TREATMENT SERVICES (prior to last 6 months)

Type of Service	Provider/Program	Date(s)

INPATIENT/PHP/IOP TREATMENT SERVICES HISTORY

Service Type and Date	Reason for Admission	Hospital/Program

ALLERGIES: _____

CURRENT MEDICATIONS

Medication	Dose	Frequency	Medication	Dose	Frequency

PAST MEDICATION TRIALS

Medication (Include Highest Dose)	Date	Response	Medication (Include Highest Dose)	Date	Response

DIAGNOSTIC STUDIES

Test	Date of Most Recent	Comments
Lab work		
EKG		
EEG		
Brain CT/MRI/Other		
Psychological/Neuropsychological Testing		
Other		

Family Psychiatric History

_____

_____

_____

Psychiatric Advanced Directive: yes _____ no _____

Special Circumstances/Comments Youth/Family Wants to Include
(Examples: common presenting problems, circumstances & conditions which
have led to destabilization and/or relapse, helpful strategies & tools to help
stabilize, safety concerns, activities to be avoided, dietary restrictions, etc.)

_____

_____

_____

Patient Signature_____ Date_____

Provider Signature_____ Date_____

Date updated _____ Date updated _____ Date updated _____

COVER LETTER

Transfer of Treatment to Campus Providers and/or
Near-Campus Providers

Dear Receiving Provider,

John M. is an 18-year-old who will be matriculating at *R and M College* and transferring to your care. *I have provided individual therapy and medication management to John since he was in 10th grade* and I appreciate your willingness to take over *his* care.

The purpose of this cover letter and Transfer Package, which *John and his parents (and/or other trusted individual(s), such as case worker)* have helped prepare, is to introduce *him* to you, summarize the transfer of care plan we have discussed, provide important documents to you, and note some transition issues that may require more immediate attention or follow-up. Enclosed, please find:

- Current Mental Health and Medical Summary, with an electronic version available from *John* for easy updating
- Transfer of Care Plan, mutually agreed upon and signed by *John*
- Pending Actions and Ongoing Transition Needs form
- Emergency Care Plan, with contact information for *John's* selected emergency contacts and all of *his* providers
- Legal Document(s): a signed release of information authorizing our communication and an Advanced Directive *(if available)*
- Additional Health Records: *lab reports, imaging studies, etc.*

I have recommended to *John* that, if possible, *he* not make any changes in *his* medication regimen for the first (quarter/trimester/semester) and to do so only under the care of a physician. *John's* last appointment with me was on *August 15, 2017. He* was given prescriptions for all of *his* psychiatric medications with **one** additional refill.

John and *his* home treatment team have collaborated to make this challenging transition go as smooth as possible. This student has many areas of strength as well as some ongoing transition needs. Please note the list of pending actions that may require your more immediate attention.

I will contact you, and/or *John*, and/or *his* family in about one month to check in on how the transition to college is going and to ensure continuity of care has taken place.

Please let me know when you receive this Transfer Package. And, please do not hesitate to contact me with any questions/concerns. Thank you for your support.

Sincerely,

Home Provider (Sending Provider)

TRANSFER OF CARE PLAN (PROVIDER COPY)

Transfer of Treatment to Campus Providers and/or Near-Campus Providers

Patient's Name _____ Date of Birth _____

1. You will be taking over this young adult's ongoing mental health care in its entirety or you are taking over this young adult's psychiatric medication management with _____ as therapist.

2. As the referring provider, I will remain a resource for you during the initial phases of the transition.

- I will contact you, the young adult (and perhaps the family) in about one month to assess continuity of care.
- I will close this case in three months.

3. *I am* **OR** *I am not* able to see this young adult in consultation if you deem it necessary *(Some practices end care after high school graduation or when the patient turns 18.)*

4. A copy of the signed Release(s) of Information to allow our communication is enclosed.

5. I will notify you of any changes in treatment that take place just prior to this young adult's departure or any items that require follow-up, such as lab work, disability services assistance, etc.).

6. *Unless I notify you otherwise*, I will provide _____ with prescriptions for all of his psychiatric medications with one additional refill for each medication.

TRANSFER OF CARE PLAN (PATIENT COPY)

Transfer of Treatment to Campus Providers and/or Near-Campus Providers

Place signed copy of care plan in the chart. Give patient a copy of the plan.

Patient's Name _____ Date of Birth _____

1. Dr. _____ will be taking over your ongoing mental health care in its entirety **or** Dr. _____ will be taking over your psychiatric medication management with _____ as therapist.

2. As the referring provider, I will remain a resource for you during the initial phases of your transition.

   - I will contact you, your new provider and your family in about one month to check in and assess continuity of care
   - Your case will be closed in three months.

3. *I am* **OR** *I am not* able to see you in consultation if it is deemed necessary. *(Some practices end care after high school graduation or when the patient turns 18.)*

4. You have signed Release(s) of Information to allow me to communicate with your new provider and your family.

5. I will notify your new provider of any changes in treatment that take place just prior to your departure or any items that require follow-up, e.g., lab work, disability services assistance, etc.).

6. *Unless otherwise noted,* I have provided you with prescriptions for all of your psychiatric medications with one additional refill for each medication.

_____
Patient Name PRINT

_____   _____
Patient SIGNATURE   Date

COVER LETTER

Shared Treatment by Home Providers and Campus Providers

Dear Receiving Provider,

John M. is an 18 year old who will be matriculating at *R and M College. I have provided individual therapy and medication management to John since he was in 10th grade* and I appreciate your willingness to share in *his* ongoing care.

The purpose of this cover letter and Transfer Package, which *John and his parents (and/or other trusted individual(s), such as case worker)* have helped prepare, is to introduce *him* to you, summarize the transfer of care plan we have discussed, provide important documents to you, and note some transition issues that may require more immediate attention or follow-up. Enclosed, please find:

- Current Mental Health and Medical Summary, with an electronic version available from *John* for easy updating
- Transfer of Care Plan, mutually agreed upon and signed by *John*
- Pending Actions and Ongoing Transition Needs form
- Emergency Care Plan, with contact information for *John's* selected emergency contacts and all of *his* providers
- Legal Document(s): a signed release of information authorizing our communication and an Advanced Directive *(if established)*
- Additional Health Records: *(lab reports, imaging studies, etc.)*

I have recommended to *John* that, if possible, *he* not make any changes in *his* medication regimen for the first *(quarter/trimester/semester)* and to do so only under the care of a physician. *John's* last appointment with me was on *August 15, 2017. He* was given prescriptions for all of *his* psychiatric medications with **one** additional refill. *His* next appointment with me is *during Thanksgiving Break.*

John and *his* home treatment team have collaborated to make this challenging transition go as smooth as possible. This student has many areas of strength as well as some ongoing transition needs. Please note the list of pending actions that may require your more immediate attention.

I will contact you, *John,* and/or *his* family in about one month to check in on how the transition to college is going and to ensure continuity of care has taken place.

Please let me know when you receive this Transfer Package and please contact me with any questions/concerns. I look forward to hearing about your first meeting with *John.*

Sincerely,
Home Provider (Sending Provider)

TRANSFER OF CARE PLAN (PROVIDER COPY)

Shared Treatment by Home Providers and Campus Providers

Patient's Name _____ Date of Birth _____

1. We will be sharing this young adult's ongoing mental health care in its entirety or we will be sharing this young adult's psychiatric medication management with _____ as therapist.

2. We will communicate on a regular basis **(phone or fax or e-mail)**, including but not limited to, when medication changes are made, when there are items to follow-up with (such as lab work, disability services assistance, etc.), or there are concerns.

3. A copy of the signed Release(s) of Information to allow our communication is enclosed.

4. *At a minimum*, we each expect to see this young adult every three months.

5. We will advise the young adult (and family) to consider his/her actual physical location (at home or at school) to determine which one of us is in charge at any moment in time or in the event of an emergency (understanding that in a crisis either of us will respond and then collaborate). The care of students who choose to study abroad will require additional planning.

6. *Unless otherwise notified*, we will provide our shared patient with prescriptions for psychiatric medications which include only one additional refill for each medication. We acknowledge that co-prescription of controlled substances will require additional monitoring/communication.

TRANSFER OF CARE PLAN (PATIENT COPY)

Shared Treatment by Home Providers and Campus Providers

Place signed copy of care plan in the chart. Give patient a copy of the plan.

Patient's Name _____ Date of Birth _____

1. I will be sharing your ongoing mental health care in its entirety with Dr. _____ **or Dr.** _____ and I will be sharing your psychiatric medication management with _____ as therapist.

2. We will communicate on a regular basis **(phone or fax or e-mail)**, including but not limited to, when medication changes are made, when there are items to follow-up with (such as lab work, disability services assistance, etc.), or there are concerns.

3. You have signed Release(s) of Information to allow me to communicate with your new provider and your family.

4. *At a minimum*, we each expect to see you every three months.

5. At any moment in time or in the event of an emergency you and your family are to consider your actual physical location (at home or at school) to determine which one of us is in charge, understanding that in an emergency either of us will respond and we will collaborate in your care plan. If you choose to study abroad we will need to do additional planning.

6. *Unless otherwise notified*, we will provide you with prescriptions for psychiatric medications which include only one additional refill for each medication. You understand that co-prescription of controlled substances will require additional monitoring/communication.

_____
Patient Name PRINT

_____   _____
Patient SIGNATURE   Date

EMERGENCY CARE PLAN

Patient Name _____ Date of Birth _____

In the case of an emergency, if you are in crisis, and/or if you are having suicidal thoughts please call any of the trusted individuals you have listed below. Please enter numbers into your cell phone for easy access.

You can also call 9-1-1, text the crisis line 741741, go to your nearest emergency room, and/or call the Suicide Hotline at 1-800-273-TALK

Please share this information with your emergency contacts.

CONTACT INFORMATION of MENTAL HEALTH PROVIDERS

	Name	Office Phone	Other Phone
Home Therapist			
Campus Therapist			
Home Prescriber			
Campus Prescriber			
Other			

CAMPUS EMERGENCY NUMBERS

Security		
Resident Assistant		
Counseling Center		
Health Center		
Other		
Other		

EMERGENCY CONTACTS

Name	Relationship	Phone #1	Phone #2
	Parent		
	Parent		
	Significant Other		
	Friend		
	Sibling		
	Other		
Suicide Hotline		1-800-273-TALK (8255)	
Emergency Services		9-1-1	
Crisis Text Line		741741	

TRANSITION READINESS: PENDING ACTIONS and ONGOING TRANSITION NEEDS

(Attach this form to the cover letter)

Patient Name _____ Date of Birth _____

Pending Actions

Yes   No   N/A   Young adult has scheduled an appointment with you

Yes   No   N/A   Young adult has made disclosure to Office of Disability Services

Yes   No   N/A   Young adult has Portfolio of documents for Office of Disability Services

Yes   No   N/A   Young adult is aware of how to fill prescriptions on/near campus

Yes   No   N/A   Young adult has health insurance and carries insurance card

Yes   No   N/A   Young adult requires follow-up lab work

Yes   No   N/A   Young adult has established a regular communication plan with guardians/family

Yes   No   N/A   Young adult has discussed likely challenges in and out of the classroom including: academic expectations, possible obstacles to treatment compliance once on campus, stress management, sleep hygiene, alcohol and other substance use

Ongoing Transition Needs *(personalize for your patient, examples in italics)*

Health Care Knowledge and Skills: *Area of strength; may need support with distinguishing symptom relapse from typical transition stress*

Self Advocacy Knowledge and Skills: *Will need encouragement to contact the Office of Disability Services and follow through with professors*

Independent Living Skills: *Area of strength though struggles to manage online gaming time*

Psychosocial Development: *Has struggled with peer relationships so may be susceptible to peer pressure to use substances to fit in on campus*

Academic Skills-Executive Function: *Area of strength; however, abilities dramatically falter when symptom exacerbations occur*

References

1. American Academy of Pediatrics, American Academy of Family Physicians, American College of Physicians. A consensus statement on health care transitions for young adults with special health care needs. Pediatrics. 2002;110(6):1304–6.
2. www.GotTransition.org
3. American College of Physicians. Condition-Specific Tools; 2017. https://www.acponline.org/clinical-information/high-value-care/resources-for-clinicians/pediatric-to-adult-care-transitions-initiative/condition-specific-tools. Accessed 18 Aug 2017.
4. Martel A, Derenne J, Chan V. Teaching a systematic approach for transitioning patients to college: an interactive continuing medical education program. Academic Psychiatry. 2015;39(5):549–54.
5. Martel A. Planning Ahead for Your Mental Health Care as You Transition to College, 2017. https://www.settogo.org/cardstack/planning-ahead-for-your-mental-health-care-as-you-transition-to-college/#card=1. Accessed 18 Aug 2017.
6. Mental Health America. Psychiatric Advanced Directives: Taking Charge of Your Care. 2017. http://www.mentalhealthamerica.net/psychiatric-advance-directives-taking-charge-your-care. Accessed 18 August 2017.
7. National Resource Center on Psychiatric Advanced Directives. 2015. http://www.nrc-pad.org/. Accessed 18 Aug 2017
8. American Academy of Pediatrics. Coding and Reimbursement Tip Sheet for Transition from Pediatric to Adult Health Care, 2017. https://www.aap.org/en-us/Documents/coding_factsheet_transition_coding.pdf Accessed 18 Aug 2017.

Part II

Clinical Cases Focusing on Diagnosis

Perplexed in Translation: Bringing a Language Disorder to College

Karen Pierce

Case History

Ann is a 17-year-old high school senior female in a small urban school who was in special education throughout her school years for issues with language and reading. She presents with worsening anxiety in the fall of her senior year as she was in the process of applying to college. She began to panic as the first quarter exams approached and developed insomnia. Her presenting diagnoses are Adjustment Disorder with Anxiety DSM-5 309.24 (F43.22), Reading Disorder (F81.0), and Language Disorder DSM-5 315.39 (F80.9). She had adequate internal language to know to request help making her transition to college successful.

Ann is the oldest of a family of three, residing with her younger brother and sister, who had no known learning challenges, and two working parents. She had the same fulltime caretaker since birth. Her birth was unremarkable and her milestones were on target, except for delayed speech. Ann initially presented at age 3, after a referral from her preschool teacher, with a paucity of vocabulary and mild articulation issues. She received early speech and language instruction that quickly improved her articulation, but her language issues persisted with speaking slowly, word retrieval problems and with single word answers. She had difficulty learning to read and in first grade reading, spelling, and math were below grade level. Her 3 year IEP reviews continued to qualify her for services for Reading Disability and Speech and Language Impairment. She continued to see the learning specialist in school and her parents helped her with homework.

Despite her language difficulties, she had friends of both genders. She admitted to some difficulty in listening in group conversations. She excelled in team-based

K. Pierce, M.D.
Northwestern University, Feinberg School of Medicine, Chicago, IL, USA
e-mail: karenpierc@gmail.com

© Springer International Publishing AG, part of Springer Nature 2018
A. Martel et al. (eds.), *Promoting Safe and Effective Transitions to College for Youth with Mental Health Conditions*, https://doi.org/10.1007/978-3-319-68894-7_6

sports, playing both school and competitive club teams. She enjoyed volunteering in a local kindergarten and an afterschool tutoring program, time permitting.

In high school, Ann received content-based tutoring once weekly for science, history, and English plus some help with writing. She had two to three optional resource periods per week at school. Her teachers gave the entire class keywords or vocabulary lists for each of the units and the day's notes in most subjects. She used extended time for exams when she thought she needed more time, and had a reader for science and sometimes in history, if she chose to use it. She rarely asked her Learning Disabilities (LD) teacher and other staff for help or accommodations as they knew her well and would offer help proactively. She took a foreign language immersion and culture class for 3 years but had no formal foreign language instruction. She was doing fair in a lower level math class and science lab. If science was not presented with a lot of visual information, she easily got confused and had to ask for some help. She was organized, did her homework daily, and could keep track of her schedule. She regularly used her school's excellent website to check current homework assignments, her grades, or missing work.

Her most recent neuropsychological testing showed high average verbal comprehension and perceptual reasoning skills with average working memory and processing speed. She was superior in similarities and visual puzzles and average in coding and digit span. Reading scores showed average oral reading fluency, oral reading rate, and essay composition. Oral reading accuracy was borderline. On a timed reading test, she scored at the 13th %ile (grade 6.3) but when given double time, she improved to the 87th %ile (grade 16.1). She scored high for anxiety on a self-rating scale. Her parents or teachers did not rate her for symptoms of ADHD or poor executive functioning. She had no prior history of mental health treatment. She had no medical problems and used topical medicine for acne. She did not use vitamins or supplements. There was no history of trauma in her life or her family.

On exam, Ann was a pretty female with fair eye contact. When she was thinking, she looked away and had trouble holding the examiner's attention. She was slow to respond to questions and her answers were with circumlocutions or with one or two words. There were many pauses, "umms" and "I don't knows" when questioned. She did not ask the speaker to slow down nor re-explain a question. She did ask about vocabulary words when it appeared that she did not get the exact meaning. She looked anxious when discussing college but could not identify reasons. She denied symptoms of depression, panic attacks, suicidal or homicidal ideation, guilt, or thought disorder. She would occasionally drink 1–2 beers on weekends, once or twice a month with her friends without blackouts or inappropriate behavior. She denied using marijuana, cigarettes, or other drugs. She was currently not dating but had a preference for men. Her period was regular without changes in her mood or anxiety. She admitted being worried most of the time with difficulty falling asleep 2–3 nights a week. She had some nightmares that woke her up but she could not recall the content.

The CAP diagnosed Ann with Adjustment Disorder with Anxious Mood and noted her trouble with language skills and reading comprehension. Ann and her parents accepted that she was anxious but were perplexed that she may still have trouble with communication and reading. Weekly therapy was recommended to help Ann manage her anxiety, understand her abilities and challenges, and how they might translate to the college environment. She agreed to therapy with her CAP and consented to involvement of her parents, school, and tutor.

Ann, her parents, and her school had little insight into how her language difficulties impacted her and the automatic and invisible accommodations that she was receiving at school and with her parents. Transition preparation and planning focused on Ann, her parents, and her school support team.

INDIVIDUAL work was initiated to develop a narrative about her strengths and weaknesses including taking a look at her cognitive style and what she did to accommodate it. Ann began to notice speech hesitancies, her trouble telling her story when there was no one supporting the details in what she was discussing, and when she gave up looking for answers. She became more articulate and aware of the language she was missing. She discovered that her use of online school and texting with her friends was a great way to compensate for the oral exchange of language.

Ann engaged in CBT for her anxiety with deep breathing, cognitive reframing, and how to recognize anxiety when it started. These skills were easily learned and implemented with relief in her anxiety. She discovered that her anxiety was in fact triggered by many language experiences and learned to ask more questions to understand content.

As Ann began to learn more about her learning style and emotional regulation, she was surprised when discussing what services she might need in college. Though she knew about her language and reading disorders she thought they did not interfere with her schooling. Ann agreed to work with her school staff and CAP to develop a list of her learning strengths, weaknesses, and what accommodations she might need. Ann learned about the Americans with Disabilities Act as a contrast to her Individualized Education Plan (IEP) that was predominantly developed by the adults in her life. Her rights to services with accommodations were discussed and self-advocacy skills were enhanced.

FAMILY The family sessions began with the permission of the patient to discuss "senior strategies" and to decrease their behaviors which undermined their daughter's independence. "Senior strategies" are a series of observations and behaviors that are used with all families with a transitioning youth to help promote a successful transition to college.

"If you see it, don't say it." When a youth is at college, parents will not generally be able to see their child's environment (although the use of face time/video conferencing can be used after the transitioning). The parents must begin to notice when and how they facilitate functioning, i.e., if a lunch or homework is left behind with a parent's awareness, no reminders are given. If the shampoo/shaving cream is low, do not replace it without asking. For Ann, Mom realized that each morning she would remind her to take her backpack that was at the door. When Mom realized this, she did not remind Ann one day with Ann calling Mom mid-day because of forgotten work. Mom did not drive the backpack to school and Ann had to face the consequences. In therapy, she began to work on the language to advocate for herself. Since she had rarely forgotten anything, the teacher gave her an extension.

"Teaching Sleep Hygiene, No wake up calls, reminders, or holding carpool for a late sleeper." College youth are often sleep deprived as the nonstop socializing and the poor time management make for late nights. Learning to use an alarm for both morning awakenings and after naps is a necessary skill. As Ann worked very hard in school, she often stayed up late and had trouble getting up. Both parents facilitated this with gentle awakenings or last minute rides. Eventually, Ann learned to wake up with an alarm and get to bed at an earlier hour. She served some detentions for tardiness which was an incentive for her to learn to use an alarm.

"Adult Skills" Ann's parents did not teach Ann about using money or budgeting. Ann's parents often handed her cash or allowed use of their credit card. Ann was instructed on how to use an ATM instead of asking parents for cash. She learned to use her own credit/debit card. Ann had to develop a budget, as the freedom of the credit card resulted in over-buying. Activities of Daily Living like shopping for toiletries, doing laundry, and preparing food were discussed. None of these skills are difficult but all of these skills need time management to succeed. Ann had never done any of these skills and felt overwhelmed at more to do besides school work, social life, and sports. Parents and she discussed how to accomplish these tasks by using reminders, multi-tasking (putting in a load of laundry while she was studying), and breaking it down into chunks. At first, she would enter stores, not find what she needed, and leave. Ann needed to develop language to ask store clerk for help to find things.

Her parents explored Ann's language disorder and how unwittingly they had compensated for her, to "speak" for her, reacting to what was needed without words. Letting her initiate her needs was difficult as they felt that this was the last chance to teach her before she went away. Mom recognized that she too often struggled with words but she was great at "seeing" what needed to be done and not recognizing how she was enabling Ann. Eventually, they allowed her to struggle with finding her words and asking for help. The parents had great faith in their daughter but they too expressed some anxiety about her ability to navigate all these new adult skills.

SCHOOL The CAP attended a school staffing for engagement of the school in the transition. The school unintentionally had enabled some of Ann's expressive language difficulties despite her IEP describing advocacy goals. Ann was surprised to learn of all the automatic accommodations that had been put in place. She recognized her pattern of using extended time accommodations for language-rich subjects like history and English but not for some science units and never for math. Ann learned strategies to improve her reading comprehension. She was encouraged to meet with teachers, pre-read notes, and ask for visual explanations with examples around key concepts. She was taught to highlight vocabulary and review it before reading. The LD clinician began to wait for Ann to ask for help rather than diving in. The CAP helped Ann develop a written learning plan based on the school meeting to present to colleges.

Ann was accepted to several schools including her first choice, the one she considered the "best." She admitted that the "best" might not meet her learning needs. She discovered that the learning services at her "choice" school were not as comprehensive as those she had been receiving in high school. Services with a resource person were offered only once weekly and peer tutoring was available for class content. Ultimately, she decided that this was sufficient and accepted admittance. With encouragement, Ann took charge of informing the college about her disability, gathered all necessary reports from her school, tutors, and CAP for the school's review process (despite having access to these reports, Ann, had not looked at them carefully). She met with the disabilities office at the college. After her needs were approved, she was instructed that she was responsible for asking each professor for accommodations. Her anxiety abated and she was using CBT skills to manage her anxiety. No recommendation was made for therapy to continue at school and Ann could always call the CAP as needed.

Ann started her freshman year but began to struggle at midterms. She was overwhelmed by the task of simultaneously writing two papers and studying for two exams. She realized that she did not have enough support at school. Her poor sleep returned. Her anxiety came at times when complex language was presented, when she had to negotiate her services or explain her learning challenges. The reading was overwhelming and she did not understand most of what she read. She had not asked her professors for the accommodations that she had identified which had been helpful to her in the past. She recognized that she struggled with the language on exams and would answer poorly or incompletely. In consult with CAP and the learning center at college, she was encouraged to meet weekly with her professors and ask for help to explain concepts. She also had neglected the college foreign language requirement that her cultural high school class did not fulfill. She was constructively able to initiate help from her high school language teacher, her high school IEP, and her neuropsychologist to write letters waiving her college language requirement. Ann recognized that she did not fully understand the need for a good learning resource center at college. She finished the semester but transferred to a community college near her home that provided daily resource help, was less difficult, and registered for only three classes.

Analysis of Transition

Ann was a high functioning youth in the context of a comprehensive support network while in high school and living at home. To all she seemed well adjusted with a minimal impact of her language learning disability. With the transition to college, the language skills needed and the separation from home and school brought her disability and her anxiety into focus.

Positive predictors of success were many: Ann was fortunate that her learning issues were identified early, getting educational support throughout her education. She and her family sought CAP support immediately when they realized that this transition may be stressful. The parents and the school were involved and worked to help Ann be successful. Ann had solid executive functioning skills, a high self-esteem, and many friends and could engage successfully in team-based sports. She responded readily to CBT and showed that she could use these strategies under stress. Her confidence and skills improved with intervention before she transitioned.

Despite her progress and preparation, Ann's insight and understanding of her disability was rudimentary and left her unprepared for a college setting. She had significantly less support than she received in high school. She was unable to transfer to the college setting how little language she used, and without others speaking for her, she failed. Although Ann developed a narrative of her disability and asked her CAP for what she needed, ultimately she was unable to apply this skill with her college professors. Despite best intentions, the high school unwittingly played into this by not teaching Ann about her challenges early on and doing some of the translation works for her. The accommodations and the level system of instruction in high school compensated for Ann's weakness ultimately undermining her true abilities for college. Her school had adapted the reading curricula with many supports embedded so Ann had no idea how limited her reading comprehension would be without this scaffolding. In choosing her college, she minimized her need for services. Once weekly resource sessions were not enough for her to understand the college curricula.

There are special considerations for transitioning patients with language disorders to college as spoken and written language are critical for communication. Most of learning at college is language based so good skills in this area are critical. Helping the student navigate *with language*, a narrative of their learning strengths and weaknesses can be helpful yet a challenge as the words to describe this process are often lacking in a language-challenged youth. Whatever benefits a patient derives from understanding their learning issues, they must feel empowered to be assertive in advocating for their accommodations and finding mentors to help them through the college process. They must learn that asking for help is effective and the struggle to be understood is important. Many language-challenged youth rely on their visual skills to help with through but the individuality of each college student fails to give them a visual context to navigate through classes and classwork. There is a tendency for helpers to want to compensate for the disability but care must be engaged so that the student is not dependent on this help.

Clinical Pearls

- One cannot assume that if a student is diagnosed with an LD and receiving services that this prepares them for the transition to college. The impact of their deficits varies with setting. A student needs to have a clear understanding of how their learning issues will translate to the college environment.
- The practicing clinician has an important role to play in facilitating collaboration among the student with learning challenges, the family, and the special education staff at the high school to ensure a realistic and solid understanding of the student's learning challenges and strengths.
- Begin as early as 8th grade to educate a student about their learning strengths and weakness and to require the student to practice self-advocacy skills in order for them to get the services they need.

- Parents must recognize the ways in which they may enable their child's dependence. In accepting their child's learning challenges, families often become unwitting collaborators in the deception that there is little impact of this in their child's life.
- Families must support their child's independence and give them the confidence to navigate the college world ahead. College transitions can recreate the fear of sending their learning challenged youth away unprepared and they must be supported to let go and believe that the services that were provided will become tools of the future.
- Often the accommodations and the level system of instruction in high school compensate for a student's weakness ultimately disabling them at the transition to college. High schools need to be aware that their accommodations and adjustments to curricula may not be available at most colleges.
- Transition preparation and planning involves more than arranging for services at the post-secondary institution. It involves helping the student develop skills and strategies to manage learning issues, practicing self-advocacy skills, and working with the student to create a portable learning plan that can be taken to college.
- Life skills like using money, getting up by one's self and taking care of daily tasks should be taught and encouraged early.
- CAPs should screen all patients for a language disorder, including those who first present to treatment early in their college years with "new" academic difficulties in the college setting.
- CAPs should review and understand IEPs, testing, and transition plans in order to translate this to the patient and their families. CAPs should seek consultation with speech and language therapists to help them understand any testing a child brings to the evaluation.

Brief Literature Review

Speech and language disorders significantly impact a youth's quality of life and education status. Mild to moderate language impairments can be subtle and difficult to detect. When young people with disabilities transition to adulthood, there is very likely impact on post-secondary education, social communication, and ultimate employment.

Recently, a report declared that "approximately two children in every class of 30 pupils will experience language disorder severe enough to hinder academic progress" [1]. Language is the main tool for communication and when this is lacking or insufficient, communication suffers. Despite early intervention, there are no clear evidence-based treatments for language disorders and the etiology varies widely. When compared with typically developing peers, fewer individuals with language impairment complete high school or receive an undergraduate degree [2]. Self-report data from the 2016 Fall National College Health Assessment [3] reveals that

4.2% of students reported being diagnosed or treated for a learning disability in the last 12 months and 0.9% reported speech/language disabilities [3]. The majority of young adults with specific language impairment who pursue education after high school seek vocational rather than academic qualifications [4]. In addition, individuals with speech and language impairment tend to be employed in lower-skilled jobs and lower levels of post-secondary educational attainment than their typically developing peers [2, 4]. The data on educational and vocational outcomes for individuals with speech and language disorders highlight the need for continued support to facilitate a successful transition to young adulthood.

Most youth with a language disorder have another specific learning disorder. Ann suffered from a reading disorder that interfered with her ability to read, understand, and keep up with college reading. One needs oral language skills, decoding, and fluency to master the synthesis of reading.

Since 1990, IDEA [5] has mandated transition services for students receiving special education to improve post-secondary outcomes. Students with all disabilities, including those with language disorders, experience a higher dropout rate, poor post-secondary educational attainment, and continued dependence on parents [6]. Only 28% of youth identified with a disability in high school disclosed that disability to their post-secondary institution [7]. The student should be at the center of this process that ideally starts with the transition to high school. CAPs should be aware of this process for all the youth that they work to ensure that it is done early and realistically.

Helpful Resources

Resources for Clinicians

- Ascherman LI, Shaftel J. Facilitating transition from high school and special education to adult life, child and adolescent psychiatric clinics. 26(2):311–27.
- Beitchman J, Brownlie EB. Language disorders in children and adolescents. Cambridge, MA: Hogrefe & Huber; 2014.
- Law J, Dennis JA, Charlton JJV. Speech and language therapy interventions for children with primary speech and/or language disorders (Protocol). Cochrane Database Syst Rev. 2017;(1):Art. No.: CD012490. doi: 10.1002/14651858.
- Newman, Lynn, et al. "omparisons across time of the outcomes of youth with disabilities up to 4 years after high school. A report of findings from the National Longitudinal Transition Study (NLTS) and the National Longitudinal Transition Study-2 (NLTS2). NCSER 2010–3008. *National Center for Special Education Research*. 2010.
- Schuele CM. The impact of developmental speech and language impairments on the acquisition of literacy skills. Ment Retard Dev Disabil Res Rev. 2004;10(3): 176–83.

Resources for Families

- The Center for Parent Information and Resource. http://www.parentcenterhub. org/repository/speechlanguage/
- The Learning Disabilities Association of America. https://ldaamerica.org/types-of-learning-disabilities/language-processing-disorder/
- National Parent Center on Transition and Employment. http://www.pacer.org/ transition/learning-center/planning/college-planning.asp
- Patricia W. Newhall. Language-based learning disability: what to know. http:// www.ldonline.org/article/56113/

References

1. Norbury CF, Gooch D, Wray C, Baird G, Charman T, Simonoff E, et al. The impact of non-verbal ability on prevalence and clinical presentation of language disorder: evidence from a population study. J Child Psychol Psychiatry. 2016;57(11):1247–57.
2. Johnson CJ, Beitchman JH, Brownlie EB. Twenty-year follow-up of children with and without speech-language impairments: family, educational, occupational, and quality of life outcomes. Am J Speech Lang Pathol. 2010; 19(1):51–65. doi: https://doi.org/10.1044/1058-0360(2009/08-0083). Epub 2009 Jul 30.
3. American College Health Association. American College Health Association-National College Health Assessment II: Reference Group Executive Summary Fall 2016. Hanover: American College Health Association; 2017. http://www.acha-ncha.org/docs/NCHA-II_FALL_2016_ REFERENCE_GROUP_EXECUTIVE_SUMMARY.pdf.
4. Conti-Ramsden G, et al. Adolescents with a history of specific language impairment (SLI): strengths and difficulties in social, emotional and behavioral functioning. Res Dev Disabil. 2013;34(11):4161–9.
5. Individuals with Disabilities Education Act, 20 U.S.C. § 1400. 1990.
6. Newman L, et al. Comparisons across time of the outcomes of youth with disabilities up to 4 years after high school. A report of findings from the National Longitudinal Transition Study (NLTS) and the National Longitudinal Transition Study-2 (NLTS2). NCSER 2010-3008. National Center for Special Education Research; 2010.
7. Newman L, Wagner M, Knokey A.-M, Marder C, Nagle K, Shaver D, Wei X, Cameto R, Contreras E, Ferguson K, Greene S, Schwarting M. the post-high school outcomes of young adults with disabilities up to 8 years after high school. A report from the National Longitudinal Transition Study-2 (NLTS2) (NCSER 2011-3005). Menlo Park: SRI International; 2011.

"There Is My Way … and Then There Is My Way": College Transition Challenges for a Student on the Autism Spectrum

7

Kirk Lum

Case History

Peter is a 19-year-old Caucasian male with Autism Spectrum Disorder (ASD), the only child of a middle-class family, who lives with his biological mother in the suburbs of a large Northeastern city. He graduated from a public high school where he received special education services. Peter's home life was complicated by the loss of his father to colon cancer when he was age 11. His mother had limited financial resources requiring her to work full-time outside of the home. Otherwise, she devoted herself to Peter, and they developed a very close relationship. Peter's mom was a willing and generally cooperative participant in his care. While she did not appear to be on the autism spectrum, she could sometimes be quite literal and rigid in her interpretation of directions and in following recommendations from care providers.

Peter had difficulties with attention and behavioral regulation in kindergarten and was diagnosed in the 1st grade with ADHD. He was prescribed stimulant medications by his primary care doctor. His mom reported a clear improvement in response to stimulants and elementary school report cards reflected the same. Early school reports indicated that Peter was good natured and liked by teachers. He had some unusual behaviors and did not consistently engage with his peers in play. He received accommodations through a 504 plan including attempts to minimize classroom distractions and additional time to complete schoolwork and tests. In 5th grade, school personnel recommended additional evaluation in the context of declining academic performance and persistent atypical behaviors: inappropriate touching of others, inflexibility around routines, rocking in his seat, and licking

K. Lum, M.D.
Child and Family Psychological Services, Inc., Norwood, MA, USA
e-mail: klum@cfpsych.org

© Springer International Publishing AG, part of Springer Nature 2018
A. Martel et al. (eds.), *Promoting Safe and Effective Transitions to College for Youth with Mental Health Conditions*, https://doi.org/10.1007/978-3-319-68894-7_7

classroom walls. He had few friends and was the target of bullying at school. Neuropsychological testing revealed average cognitive ability but executive function weaknesses. Overall results, in conjunction with Peter's clinical presentation, supported a diagnosis of Asperger's Disorder (now Autism Spectrum Disorder). He also received a diagnosis of Generalized Anxiety Disorder based on clinical evaluation and testing. As a result, Peter was deemed eligible for special education services. His IEP afforded him services for social and emotional support including a social skills lunch group and weekly individual sessions focused on coping skills with the guidance counselor.

Through middle and high school, Peter's mental health care was provided by community practitioners in a split treatment model. He worked with one consistent therapist, a psychologist who provided a combination of supportive therapy and CBT, as well as parent guidance to his mother. Medication management, which shifted to a child and adolescent psychiatrist (CAP), included trials of stimulants, atomoxetine, guanfacine, and sertraline. A trial of an atypical antipsychotic was considered in middle school due to some behavioral dysregulation and aggression. But his most challenging behaviors were in reaction to teasing from peers, and he eventually responded well to support and behavior modification focused on development of his social skills. Sertraline was helpful in reducing Peter's underlying anxiety and some of his avoidant tendencies. It also had some benefit for his perseverative thinking though he remained cognitively rigid. Peter was cooperative with his treatment but had some medication compliance issues starting in junior year of high school when his mom agreed to give him more responsibility for taking his medications independently.

With significant support from his IEP and a devoted high school counselor, Peter graduated from high school "on time" with commendable grades. Throughout high school, homework demands were minimal as his IEP included time in the resource center where he received daily help in completing his work while at school. At home, Peter's mom provided a great deal of support: getting him up for school in the morning, dispensing his medication, cooking for him, and cleaning up after him. She made sure he attended to his hygiene. Though it was challenging to get Peter to change his routine and try new things, she drove him to any activities he was willing to try. Peter inflexibly refused to learn to drive during high school. His mom did not encourage him to try to find a part-time job believing it was more important that he focus on academics and a few extracurricular activities. He participated in Anime and Dungeons & Dragons clubs at school and took archery lessons for a time. Social involvement with peers was limited during high school though he made some casual friends. He struggled with reciprocity in interactions and peers often viewed his unwillingness to compromise as being "stubborn."

Peter was set on going to a 4-year college and living on campus. During the college application and selection process, Peter showed little interest in learning about and preparing for the transition to college. He resisted psychoeducation about the needs of college students with ASD, what academic and social challenges he might face in the college milieu, and the variability in supports and programs offered at different colleges. He developed some insight into the rigidity of his thinking as an aspect of his ASD, often joking that "There is my way—and then there is my way," but he still did not identify as having a disability. He was adamant that he was ready for college and did not want to be treated differently from his non-ASD classmates. At the insistence of his mother, Peter attended a college transition workshop offered by a local ASD support organization but this did not appear to have much impact due to his resistance.

Concerned that Peter was not yet ready to live independently, particularly in the less structured setting of college, his high school counselor and treatment team presented additional options. These included taking a structured gap year or starting his postsecondary education at a community college and commuting to school from home. Summer bridge programs that offer social and academic support for students with ASD were discussed but were rebuffed by Peter and his mom as being either unnecessary or too expensive. Despite the treatment team's concerns, Peter's mom shared his optimism that he would be fine "going off on his own" based on his high school success.

Peter and his mom visited a few small colleges within driving distance of his home that had reputations of being "Asperger's friendly." He was accepted to two of these colleges and made "accepted student" visits accompanied by his mom, during which they learned about student health, counseling, and disability services. He selected a school a 3 h drive from home. During the summer freshman orientation program, Peter and his mom met his academic advisor who had experience working with ASD students and she helped them connect with the student disability center and would facilitate Peter connecting with his professors at the start of the semester to discuss his learning needs. They also met his peer mentor who would help orient him to campus life and activities and offer coaching on the "unwritten rules" for college students. They submitted paperwork and a supporting letter from his CAP for a single room given his sensory sensitivities and anticipated difficulties sharing a living space. Concerns he could become socially isolated were mitigated by the expectation for him to eat in the dining halls as required by his meal plan.

Peter, his mom, home mental health providers, and the college's counseling center director decided together that his home CAP would continue medication management. This made sense given Peter's alliance with his CAP, stability on his medications, and plan to come home frequently with the college nearby in his home state. Therapy would be with a new therapist at the campus counseling center. Peter signed releases authorizing communication among his home providers, the counseling center, and his mom.

In the meantime, still struggling to accept that he had a disability, Peter worked halfheartedly with his therapist on preparing for the college social milieu. They discussed dating and sexuality and risky social situations he might encounter in college, particularly as related to alcohol and drugs. They talked about his inflexible thinking and rigid adherence to rules and how this might create problems living cooperatively with peers in a dormitory. Peter and his CAP talked about strategies for managing the anxiety expected with the move from home to college, with a focus on being safe and compliant with his medication.

Over the summer, Peter threw a major curve into the planning. Deciding on his own that he was not yet ready to live away from home and his mother, he chose instead to go to the local community college, to which he was able to apply online. No specific planning had been made for this option since Peter had initially rejected it. The local community college offered a basic academic assistance program, but it was not specific to students with ASD. Peter chose not to enroll in it because of his firm belief that the community college would be "a piece of cake" compared with the 4-year college he had initially selected. Unlike some community colleges, there was a counseling center on campus, but it was closed during the summer. Peter and his home providers were unable to connect with the student disability center during the sparsely staffed summer months to learn what other supports and services might be available to him.

Additionally, his mother made the decision (against the advice of the treatment team) to offer much less supervision and support than she had provided while he was in high school. She felt it was "time to let him fly on his own," perhaps reflecting some of her own frustration and disappointment with Peter's "last minute" decision to stay at home and commute to the community college. All of this was further complicated by Peter no longer having access to his high school counselor to help coordinate the transition of services from the high school to the college system and the unfortunate timing of his therapist being out on maternity leave through the last month of the summer.

Without the same level of support at home and college that he had relied upon during high school, Peter quickly floundered. He did not seek academic or counseling supports. He was anxious about having classes in multiple buildings and could not keep track of assignments. Outside of the classroom, he found social interactions fast paced and confusing. Rather than stay at school after classes to study or take part in social activities, he would go home and play video games. Without his mom insisting on a consistent schedule, he stayed up late at night, playing on the computer, and slept late the next day. He began to miss classes and appointments, as well as doses of his medication, which added to his stress and anxiety. His grades were poor from the beginning and Peter withdrew from the community college before the end of the first semester.

Eventually, Peter was able to work with his therapist and CAP on accepting his diagnosis and the need for support. After deciding to return to the local community college, he made independent visits to the student counseling and disability centers to line up services prior to resuming classes. He and his mom agreed on what each of their responsibilities would be at home. Peter granted consent for his mom and home treatment team to be able to communicate with his college counselor and disability services coordinator and gave his mom access to his online school account that provided information on class schedules and grades. He completed a 2-year associate's degree and then successfully transitioned to a 4-year residential college with a program specifically geared for students with ASD, where he is currently working toward a degree in computer science.

Analysis of Transition

There were several aspects of this case predictive of a positive transition outcome. Peter had solid intellectual abilities. He had strong support from both his high school and parent, as well as a trusted and consistent treatment team. Peter understood the importance of, and made an effort to comply with, his medication regimen. Both the therapist and CAP attempted to prepare Peter for the social challenges he would face in the college environment. Also, a clear and thorough plan was in place for continuity of care at his original college of choice. But there were also several features of this case predictive of a negative transition outcome. Peter was not fully accepting of his ASD diagnosis, and this would make it difficult for him to buy into the need for supports on campus and to advocate for himself. None of the extensive organizational and learning supports he had in high school were established at the community college. He was inflexible and routine driven and was not able to change his routines to fit his college schedule and demands. Peter's level of independence in daily life skills and in managing his illness had not been adequately developed given Mom's extensive caregiving, and when she withdrew support she did so abruptly. Likewise, though improved, Peter's social skills had not been tested outside of his immediate school and home environment. Lastly, Peter had a comorbid anxiety disorder.

Initially, Peter was not able to make a successful transition to college. He struggled academically and socially and subsequently withdrew from college. He was unable to advocate for himself or make use of available resources. In retrospect, there were several things that could have been done differently to improve Peter's transition outcome.

Peter was overly dependent on his mother and the supports that had been provided to him in high school, more so than his treatment team realized. Peter's readiness for the transition in key domains of functioning had not been fully assessed. Both Mom and the school team required additional guidance around fostering the development of the life skills needed to function independently and for self-advocacy. He was not put into enough situations that would enable him to develop these skills. For Peter and his mom, a college readiness checklist, reviewed with his mental health providers, may have served as a guide to what Peter should have practiced and been able to do prior to leaving for college. Tasks which foster independence include: getting yourself up and ready in the morning, cleaning up after yourself, having a part-time job, using public transportation and/or learning to drive, navigating relationships independently, and managing a multi-step school project. In regard to school, if Peter's therapist and CAP had been consulted, they could have ensured that the mandated transition plan portion of Peter's IEP was designed to maximize his independent academic and executive function skills. It is important that in an effort to protect them, families and providers not do too much for their children/patients/students at the cost of sacrificing their opportunity to learn how to do for themselves. Mistakes and failures are important opportunities for learning and are likely to be less harmful when they are made while still at home.

Peter was not prepared for the complexity of the college social milieu. Students with ASD should visit their chosen college as many times as possible prior to matriculation. Though he changed his mind late in the summer, Peter might have benefited from visits to the community college's cafeteria, student center, and classroom buildings. If he had followed through on his original residential college plan, an overnight stay on campus coordinated with the college's admissions office could have given him a true "taste" of college life.

Peter's resistance to accepting the ASD diagnosis and not wanting to be "different" complicated transition planning and limited his ability to advocate for himself. Being able to identify and declare one's disabilities and how they impact function in various settings is a necessary step in obtaining services and Peter was not able to do this initially at the community college. Mental health providers, in collaboration with the school team, should make consistent efforts to educate young people (and their families) about their illness and their specialized needs and facilitate the practice of self-advocacy skills. Given the complexities and challenges in doing this with some patients, it is important to start this work early. Strategies to promote self-advocacy can include having the young person meet one-to-one with providers for some office visits to provide status updates and explain any acute issues themselves. Also, patients can benefit from a careful review of any testing reports and joint preparation of a psychiatric treatment summary. Students attending and actively participating in their IEP meetings provides an opportunity to clarify what impact their ASD diagnosis has on them in the school setting and allows them to contribute to the identification of necessary and appropriate supports and services. While doing our best to foster competence, confidence, and self-advocacy, it is important to openly discuss the wishful thinking common among transition age youth that going to college and having a "fresh start" will magically fix things, including mental health issues. This can be countered by helping patients realistically identify their strengths and vulnerabilities and take on the challenges that come with having an ASD.

More attention should have been paid to Peter's mother's response to his transition. She was not adequately coached and supported around how to effectively promote autonomy while continuing to provide necessary support. Parents can also be subject to overly wishful thinking. Seeing their child receive a high school diploma can contribute to the unrealistic belief that it confers and equates to readiness for the next step. Parents cannot be faulted for being tired and worn down by the effort required to fight the many battles needed to get their child with an ASD to this point. So, it is important to help them understand that their job is ongoing and to provide them with the support they need to continue.

Additionally, parents are often making a tremendous financial commitment to their son or daughter in paying for their college education. It is reasonable to support parents in placing clear expectations on their child regarding: attending classes, maintaining a minimum GPA, living within an agreed upon budget, accepting emotional support, granting permission for communication with care providers, registering with student disability, and utilizing the supports and services offered. These kinds of expectations typically begin in high school and carry over into the college setting.

Ensuring college readiness in this especially vulnerable but rising college population requires active involvement of the student, family, clinicians, and schools on both ends (high school and college). Students and their families should be educated on their specific needs for college and how to advocate for themselves and where to access services. Clinicians may be helpful by fostering realistic expectations and challenging unrealistic ones, as well as by being supportive while still promoting autonomy and helping both patients and their families work on readiness.

Clinical Pearls

- Start early! Given the developmental challenges associated with ASD, begin to assess general transition readiness early in middle school or grade 9 and then focus efforts on transition to college as soon as the goal of postsecondary school is identified.
- Challenge the stigma! Help your patients accept, understand, and take ownership of their diagnosis and normalize the need for getting help. It will take a unified effort, time, and even a few false starts to overcome the inherent cognitive rigidity that can prove to be an obstacle in youth with ASD.
- Work as a team to maximize the development of social, organizational, time management, self-advocacy, and other life skills. The patient, CAP, therapist, the high school special education team, the parents, and the receiving providers are all key stakeholders in a successful transition. Many students with ASD will likely need ongoing comprehensive services for college success with progression toward independence as a goal.
- Be involved in your patient's planning. Beyond providing support around finding the "right" college, ensure that patients and families take diagnosis and mental health needs into consideration when looking at the resources available on/near different campuses.
- Make sure that patients and their families consider alternative postsecondary options even with the ultimate goal of independence and college success. A "fifth year of high school" which includes taking a college level course locally, a structured gap year combining part-time work/school/volunteer work, a year commuting to a local college before living on campus, may be options that they have not considered on their own.
- Take an especially close look at programs that offer social and academic support specifically for students with ASD either as a summer bridge to college or incorporated into the student's college curriculum and residential life. Check out the *Autism Speaks* website.
- Students with ASD are particularly vulnerable to being taken advantage of socially. Role playing many different college social situations (in dormitories, dining halls, sporting events, classrooms, parties) with explicit feedback and coaching can be especially helpful for these students who typically find it challenging to generalize strategies to novel situations. In vivo experiences may be particularly helpful.
- Be real! Provide developmentally appropriate sexual education counseling on how to interact with others in the college milieu, including those they find attractive. Address boundaries, appropriate vs. inappropriate things to say or do,

respecting the privacy of others, handling intimacy and relationships. Establish no question as being off-limits.

- Encourage patients and their families to connect with local Autism support and social groups. Many community Autism organizations offer education and resources specifically related to students with ASD making the transition to college.
- Provide resources for your patients and their family. Readiness tools, transition to college websites, and transition "tool kits" can be extremely helpful and some are geared specifically for students with ASD.
- Establish a clear plan for continuation or transfer of care and ideally have it in place before your patient heads off to college. Be prepared to stay involved until the hand-off is completed and confirmed by communication with the team on the other end. Identify expectations for appointments, managing care on school breaks, and how prescription refills will be coordinated. A sample College Transition Care Plan and Agreement is included in the chapter's Helpful Resources section.
- Active student and parent participation in IEP meetings, including the establishment of transition goals, can be a key step in learning self-advocacy skills.
- Offer coaching and support to parents around setting reasonable and appropriate academic and continuing care expectations of their transitioning college student with ASD.

Brief Literature Review

Knowing how best to assist students on the autistic spectrum to make a successful transition to college is becoming increasingly important as the number of these students continues to increase. This is a trend that should continue as the number of children diagnosed with an autism spectrum disorder continues to grow. Based on surveys conducted by the CDC [1], rates of ASD in children in the U.S. have increased from 1 in 150 to 1 in 68 between 2002 and 2012. A large number of these children have at least average intellectual abilities, giving them the potential to meet academic criteria for admission to postsecondary education institutions. Combined with the implementation of services and supports in secondary education settings federally mandated through the Individuals with Disabilities Education Act of 2004 and under Section 504 of the Rehabilitation Act of 1973 and the Americans with Disabilities Act of 1990, it follows that many children with high functioning autism spectrum disorder (HFASD) will have the desire, capabilities, and success in their secondary school programs necessary to gain acceptance to postsecondary schools.

The literature indicates that increasing numbers of students with HFASD are matriculating to college [2]. This has led to additional efforts to identify and plan for meeting the needs of this growing population [3]. Attempts have been made to identify what allows some HFASD students to be successful in negotiating the transition to a postsecondary school when faced with increased risk for social and academic failure in college even when compared to student groups with other disabilities [4]. VanBergeijk and Volkmar [5] proposed many thoughtful interventions in the areas of counseling support, classroom modifications, academic evaluation and testing, social functioning, and mental health care to support this transition. There is a growing body of literature on which programs, supports, and accommodations are proving beneficial in successfully aiding the transition and the adjustment of HFASD students once at school [6]. Further support for transitioning students can come in the form of a bridge program. Currently, bridge programs exist ranging from a summer to multiple years in length and can be either institution based or unaffiliated though cost may limit accessibility for many students. And many postsecondary schools are now offering specialized programs for students with an ASD [7].

For the CAP in private practice, interventions to aid the transition of HFASD patients that choose to go to college should address three broad areas: (1) the biological—the complexities of psychopharmacological treatment of maladaptive behavior and psychiatric comorbidities in a group that has both lower rates of medication response and higher rates of medication side effects; (2) the academic—the need for developing study, time management, and organizational skills [8] in a group that commonly suffers from executive function deficits; and (3) the social—preparing for the increased complexity and diversity of social interactions in college through the use of modalities such as video modeling [9] and mobile technology [10].

Helpful Resources

- American Academy of Child & Adolescent Psychiatry Resource Centers https://www.aacap.org/AACAP/Families_and_Youth/Resource_Centers/Autism_Resource_Center/Home.aspx
     https://www.aacap.org/AACAP/Families_and_Youth/Resource_Centers/Moving_Into_Adulthood_Resource_Center/Moving_Into_Adulthood_Resource_Center.aspx
- Jed Foundation's Transition Year website: "Your roadmap to emotional health and wellness at college starts here."—http://www.transitionyear.org
- Autism Speaks Postsecondary Educational Opportunities Guide and Transition Tool Kit—https://www.autismspeaks.org/family-services/tool-kits
- Autism Speaks information on Bridge Programs—https://www.autismspeaks.org/sites/default/files/docs/postsecondary_resources.pdf
- List of 2- and 4-year college programs for students with ASD—http://www.collegeautismspectrum.com/collegeprograms.html
- Tips for Teaching High-Functioning People with Autism—https://www.iidc.indiana.edu/pages/Tips-for-Teaching-High-Functioning-People-with-Autism
- TRAQ: the Transition Readiness Assessment Questionnaire—http://www.etsu.edu/com/pediatrics/traq/registration.php
- Brown, J., Wolf, L., King, L., & Bork, G. (2012). *The Parent's Guide to College for Students on the Autism Spectrum.* Shawnee Mission, KS: Autism Asperger Publishing Co.
- Wolf, L. E., Thierfeld Brown, J., & Bork, G. R. K. (2009). *Students with Asperger syndrome: A guide for college personnel.* Shawnee Mission, KS: Autism Asperger Publishing Co.

Office-Based Tool

COLLEGE TRANSITION CARE PLAN AND AGREEMENT

Student Name: _____   Date of Birth: _____

The following are my standard care plans and expectations for patients who will be going to college out of state or more than 1 hour's distance from home but wish to continue treatment with me. A copy of this plan/agreement should be shared with the clinicians who will be providing any of your care when you are at school.

1. While you are away at college, the plan for ongoing mental health treatment is: Medication management: _____
    Therapy: _____

2. If requested I will provide you with a Portable Medical/Psychiatric Summary to share with your providers at college.

3. I will be available to consult with your providers at college as needed and they can contact me by phone at (XXX) XXX-XXXX, extension XXX, or by fax at (XXX) XXX-XXXX.

4. If requested, I may be able to continue to provide your psychiatric care, provided we agree on (and you comply with) the following:
    A) You will keep at least 1 appointment with me during winter break and at least 1 appointment with me during summer break. This is a minimum requirement and additional appointments may be required depending on the situation and your needs.
    B) You will consent to communication between your college and myself if requested.
    C) You will consent to communication between your parent(s)/guardian(s) and myself.
    <u>Failure to meet these requirements will result in your case being closed</u> and I will be unable to see you or provide additional treatment or medication prescriptions.
    I strongly recommend that you schedule your winter break appointment in the summer or fall beforehand as spaces can fill quickly during the winter break period and not being able to get an appointment will not be an acceptable excuse.

5. If you develop any problems or things destabilize while you are away at school, you must be able to come to my office to be evaluated. If this is not possible, then you should go to the student health or counseling centers for help. I can collaborate with them to determine an appropriate treatment plan. But I cannot evaluate or treat you over the phone.

6. If you are receiving treatment at your college or in the local community during the academic year, I will attempt to notify your providers at college of any changes in your treatment plan that take place when you are at home and will expect them to attempt to notify me of any changes in your treatment plan that take place when you are at school.

7. You will request recommendations from your providers at college or the student counseling center for the best course of action to take in an emergency and keep emergency numbers on your cell phone. In the case of a psychiatric emergency while you are away at college, you will attempt to contact your providers at school or utilize the college's crisis service or go to the local hospital emergency room in the surrounding community for help.

Student Signature _____   Date _____

Provider Signature _____   Date _____

References

1. Autism and Developmental Disabilities Monitoring Network Surveillance Year 2008 Principal Investigators; Centers for Disease Control and Prevention. Prevalence of autism spectrum disorders—Autism and Developmental Disabilities Monitoring Network, 14 sites, United States, 2008. MMWR Surveill Summ. 2012;61:1–19.
2. Wei X, Wagner M, Hudson L, Yu J, Javitz H. The effect of transition planning participation and goal-setting on college enrollment among youth with autism spectrum disorders. Remedial Spec Educ. 2016;37(1):3–14.
3. White S, et al. Students with autism spectrum disorder in college: results from a preliminary mixed methods needs analysis. Res Dev Disabil. 2016;56:29–40.
4. Shogren K, Plotner A. Transition planning for students with intellectual disability, autism, or other disabilities: data from the national longitudinal transition study-2. Intellect Dev Disabil. 2011;50(1):16–30.
5. VanBergeijk E, Klin A, Volkmar F. Supporting more able students on the autism spectrum: college and beyond. J Autism Dev Disord. 2008;38:1359–70.
6. Pinder-Amaker S. Identifying the unmet needs of college students on the autism spectrum. Harv Rev Psychiatry. 2014;22(2):125–37.
7. Brown J, Wolf L, King L, Bork G. The parent's guide to college for students on the autism spectrum. Shawnee Mission: Autism Asperger Publishing Co.; 2012.
8. Zeedyk S, Tipton L, Blacher J. Educational supports for high functioning youth with ASD: the postsecondary pathway to college. Focus Autism Other Dev Disabil. 2014;31(1):37–48.
9. Hume K, et al. Increasing independence in autism spectrum disorders: a review of three focused interventions. J Autism Dev Disord. 2009;39:1329–38.
10. Mintz J, et al. Key factors mediating the use of a mobile technology tool designed to develop social and life skills in children with autistic spectrum disorders. Comput Educ. 2012;58(1):53–62.

"Time Is Not on My Side": A College Student with ADHD and a Reading Disability

A.L. Rostain

Case History

Charlie is a 19-year-old Caucasian male college student who is currently on medical leave after failing to complete his freshman year at a private top-tier university in the Northeastern US. He is the younger of two children born to his parents, having a 22-year-old sister who is a senior in college. His parents are both employed in professional positions, and the family lives in the suburbs of Philadelphia.

Charlie was formally diagnosed with a reading disorder in 3rd grade for which he received educational assistance via an IEP (i.e., intensive tutoring plus extra time on assignments and exams). Through middle school, he was no longer designated as a special education student, and he performed well under a 504 plan. He began to have academic difficulties in high school despite continuation of his accommodations. In 10th grade, after repeat psychoeducational testing revealed "slow processing speed," Charlie was referred to a child and adolescent psychiatrist (CAP) for evaluation and was diagnosed with ADHD predominantly inattentive presentation. He was started on extended release methylphenidate with excellent results. His grades quickly improved and he remained consistently in the top 5% of his class throughout the rest of high school. He also performed extremely well on the SATs with extended time. Described by his teachers as likable but inattentive, he was gifted in computer science, math, and physics, and he excelled in music, playing percussion in the school's jazz band, and writing and performing original music for a rock band he had formed with friends. He showed no signs of depression, anxiety, or substance abuse and was generally viewed as well adjusted and highly motivated to perform.

A.L. Rostain, M.D., M.A
Perelman School of Medicine, University of Pennsylvania Health System,
Philadelphia, PA, USA
e-mail: rostain@pennmedicine.upenn.edu

© Springer International Publishing AG, part of Springer Nature 2018
A. Martel et al. (eds.), *Promoting Safe and Effective Transitions to College for Youth with Mental Health Conditions*, https://doi.org/10.1007/978-3-319-68894-7_8

    In the spring of his junior year, Charlie and his parents began visiting colleges throughout the Northeast. In the summer before his senior year, he spent a month at one of his favorites, taking classes in computer science and philosophy and participating in a music ensemble. He found the campus to be very congenial and decided on his own that this was the right school for him. During the fall, several family sessions were held to review the college selection process and to assess Charlie's readiness for going away to school. He and his parents agreed that he should go to a school with a strong academic program and with ample resources for students with ADHD and learning problems which were available at his top choice school. There was some disagreement about his ability to manage time efficiently and to get started on assignments without procrastinating. According to his parents, Charlie would often wait until the last minute to get started on writing assignments which would lead to late nights completing papers. But for the most part, there were no red flags to suggest that Charlie would have trouble adapting to college life away from home. In fact, he was very responsible in taking medication on his own, in working on his college applications and in undertaking several music projects. He applied early decision to his top choice and was accepted there in early December.

    During the spring of his senior year, Charlie was less motivated to stay on top of his schoolwork and required a great deal of parental prompting to get up in the morning in time for school. Parents reported no problems with his mood and his deportment at school was unchanged. In monthly sessions to review his readiness for college, he admitted that he was routinely staying up late to play World of Warcraft (WOW) and that he was spending much of his creative energy playing music rather than studying. When he was challenged about how these tendencies might influence his ability to succeed in college, Charlie verbally acknowledged they might pose some challenges but he did not seem too concerned. "Everybody in my class has senioritis," Charlie reported, "and as long as I don't blow any classes, my parents are okay with me taking it easy this semester."

    During a late spring visit to his campus, Charlie and his parents met with the disability services officer and presented his testing reports and a letter from his treating psychiatrist. He qualified for academic accommodations (extended time for assignments and tests and access to special document reading software) and learned more about the school's resource center. As he prepared to leave for school in late August, Charlie requested to continue working with his home-based psychiatrist for medication management, preferring to remain with someone who knew him well. His provider agreed to do this with the stipulation that Charlie present for follow-up appointments every 2–3 months. He also encouraged Charlie to utilize the academic support resources available to him. At his final visit prior to departing, Charlie described his intentions to take his medications as prescribed, to meet with his professors to get accommodations in place, to work with a counselor at the learning center on a weekly basis, and to limit his online gaming activity.

    During his fall mid-semester break, Charlie reported a good adjustment to campus life. He made friends, played in a jazz-rock ensemble, went to most of his classes, turned in most of his assignments on time, avoided use of alcohol and drugs, and reportedly took his medication. When he came home for the winter break, however, it was clear that he had miscalculated the time required to do well in his courses, finishing the semester with a 2.3 GPA including a "D" in his college writing class (for which he had handed in his assignments consistently late). During a follow-up appointment to review his first semester and his ongoing medication needs, Charlie reluctantly acknowledged that he had gotten back into playing WOW, staying up late, missing his early morning writing class, and falling behind in a couple of other subjects. He also admitted that he had stopped going to the learning center and that he was taking methylphenidate in the late evening to stay awake. The consequences of these decisions were thoroughly discussed, and Charlie expressed a strong desire to avoid repeating this pattern in the coming semester. In a family session, these issues were discussed openly and a plan of action was discussed. This included keeping to a strict bedtime (midnight), limiting online gaming, meeting with a study coach at the learning center, and taking his medication as prescribed.

Unfortunately, despite the best of intentions, spring semester turned out badly for Charlie. After a few weeks of "toeing the line" and complying with the game plan, he slipped back into his old patterns of avoiding class, procrastinating about completing his assignments, misusing his medication, and staying up late playing music or WOW. When he came home for spring break, he was hopelessly behind in all his classes and was virtually certain to fail two of them. When asked why things had come to this point, he replied "I guess time wasn't on my side." A family session was held to review the situation, and after considering the option of remaining in school to complete two or three courses, it was agreed he should withdraw from school prior to the end of the semester. Charlie reluctantly agreed that he needed to leave the campus environment to get a handle on his problems. A letter requesting a medical leave was prepared, and Charlie agreed to begin weekly Cognitive Behavioral Therapy (CBT) to address the underlying executive function deficits that interfered with his ability to succeed in college. His academic dean and the disability center director explained that he could return to school with a letter from his treating mental health provider documenting productive participation in the recommended treatment plan.

Charlie is back from college a second time having tried unsuccessfully to return there the prior semester. He continues with intensive CBT and medication management for his EF difficulties. Charlie is coming to the realization that he will need to seriously limit his WOW and his music, given his learning issues, in order to succeed in school. He is still trying to figure out what the next step should be. In the meantime, he is working steadily as a music instructor, writing/making music with his band, and even making some money as an online gaming expert.

Analysis of Transition

In retrospect, it's obvious that Charlie's intelligence, creativity, motivation to succeed, cooperation with treatment, acceptance of his need for accommodations and his family's support were positive factors that concealed his lack of readiness to tackle the demands of college life. Indeed, it was the failure to address negative factors (e.g., procrastination, poor time management, excessive online gaming, learning challenges posed by the combination of ADHD and reading disorder) that makes this case a valuable illustration of the concept of establishing "effective scaffolding" in the college setting.

Several indicators of executive function difficulty were evident in high school but these did not appear to signal serious problems with adjustment to college. After Charlie experienced setbacks during the first semester of his freshman year, his willingness to accept responsibility for these made it seem as if he had "learned his lesson" and was prepared to adjust his behaviors accordingly. What was missing was an ability to turn his intentions into actions.

This case is a typical example of how college students with ADHD can run into trouble. Despite knowing the "formula" for success in college, being highly motivated to do well, having access to services and accommodations and taking an effective medication, patients like this tend to overestimate their abilities (positive attributional bias), underestimate the amount of academic work required, and minimize the consequences of staying up too late, missing class, misusing medications, etc. They also underutilize campus resources and mistakenly believe they can "catch up" on assignments at the last minute. Gifted students with ADHD and learning disabilities who over-rely on intellectual prowess and "last minute" cramming, instead of on health lifestyle and disciplined study habits, all-too-frequently discover their attempts at altering the college success formula are ill fated.

Several steps might have been taken that could have improved the outcome in this case. During high school, Charlie might have benefitted from CBT-informed coaching to help him work on his EF deficits and to demonstrate his mastery of procrastination and of time management. Prior to leaving for college, a behavioral contract could have been established stipulating clear expectations that he attend classes, keep regular appointments with an academic coach and/or therapist, maintain a healthy sleep schedule and take his medications as prescribed. Communication between these on-campus helpers and the CAP, authorized with a signed release by Charlie, may have improved compliance. More frequent and regular contact with his CAP (either by phone or skype) and ongoing education about the impact of ADHD and reading LD on college student success might have also benefited this patient.

Clinical Pearls

- Readiness for college needs to be assessed on multiple dimensions beyond those of academic preparation, social competence, and motivation. Executive functioning (EF) skills are critical predictors of college success and should be evaluated prior to the search for college. EF skills should be practiced as much as possible prior to high school graduation and immediately after starting college.
- Trouble with following through on treatment recommendations can cause college students with ADHD to underutilize helping resources, miscalculate time demands of academic work, and employ ineffective coping strategies when

encountering difficulties. This has been referred to as the "implementation problem" of ADHD [1].

- Getting college-bound patients with ADHD to prepare for being on their own involves engaging them in an honest self-examination of the following key constituents of EF:
- *Conscientiousness*: Are you ready to take responsibility for the consequences of your actions?
- *Self-Management*: Are you ready to take over the routine tasks of everyday life in the relatively unstructured environment of college?
- *Self-Control*: Are you ready to set limits on the time spent watching TV or interacting on the Internet whether through virtual reality games, social media, or web surfing that can lead to insufficient sleep, and disruptions in self-care, and studying, among others?
- *Distress Tolerance/"Grit"*: Are you ready to cope with frustration, disappointment, and failure, and persist in the face of setbacks and obstacles?
- *Open Mindset/Help-Seeking*: Are you ready to ask for help when things are not going well for you?
- A "gap year" prior to the start of college is often a good way for students with ADHD and learning disabilities to practice self-management skills and to prepare for living on their own. There are no shortcuts to learning these skills; the sooner they are mastered, the better.
- Never underestimate the addictive power of social media, online gaming, YouTube videos, etc. The ability to resist the temptations of this technology is a critical measure of self-control and should be assessed as thoroughly as alcohol and substance use.
- When difficulties arise in the transition to college, a weekly monitoring plan should be implemented to increase the likelihood the patient remains adherent to treatment goals. This is best achieved through the creation of a behavioral contract. For students experiencing serious academic setbacks, it may make sense to transfer care to providers on or near campus to facilitate more frequent contact.
- Medication adherence is a critical issue that demands close monitoring by prescribing clinicians. The high risk of stimulant misuse and stimulant diversion among college students with ADHD has led some schools to restrict or eliminate stimulant prescribing by campus health services providers and by raising the evidentiary requirements for establishing the diagnosis of ADHD (via neuropsychological testing). In such instances, options for ongoing medication management may be limited to the home provider or a community provider near the college.

Brief Literature Review

Clinicians treating college-aged youth are often asked to ascertain the diagnosis of ADHD in students experiencing academic difficulties, many of whom are convinced this is primary cause of their problems. The assessment of ADHD in this population includes a comprehensive review of symptoms, impairments and co-existing conditions (via interview, questionnaires/self-report scales, and collateral information) as well as screening for malingering (see [2]).

College students with ADHD are more likely than their peers to encounter problems adjusting to school including utilizing less effective coping skills to meet the academic and social demands of higher education, experiencing more distraction, reporting higher rates of internal restlessness and depressive symptoms, achieving lower GPAs, and being more likely to be placed on probation [3–6]. While they are *not* at greater risk for psychiatric diagnoses and they perform as well on intelligence tests as their age-matched peers, they often report mild mood or anxiety symptoms, substance use, and self-esteem issues.

Academic accommodations are recommended for students with ADHD who demonstrate learning impairments. These accommodations include "formal" modifications of the standard teaching and testing approaches environmental adjustments, the use of assistive technology, and focused educational support from learning specialists. Furthermore, there are many "informal" accommodations of coping strategies that can be instituted by students including study groups, tutoring sessions, and coaching sessions. ADHD coaching has been shown to be an effective intervention for this population [7]. These coaches help individuals identify and develop action-oriented approaches for completing personally valued tasks and goals by providing encouragement, frequent reminders, and problem-solving tips for getting through the more difficult aspects of college life.

Relatively little is known regarding the effectiveness of medications for college and university students with ADHD, or about the impact that taking medication has on academic success. Rabiner et al. [5] found no correlation between treatment status and college adjustment including academic concerns, depressive symptoms, social satisfaction, and alcohol/drug use. In a follow-up study with a larger sample, Blasé et al. [3] reported that adjustment to college was unrelated to treatment status. Advokat et al. [8] reported no medication treatment-related differences in the GPA of college students with ADHD. These results may reflect a combination of poor adherence, poor study skills, and the presence of major distractions on campus without concomitant limits. Given reports of stimulant diversion rates of up to 30%, prescribing medications for college students with ADHD is fraught with risk, and great care must be taken to educate about proper usage (including safe storage and prevention of diversion) and to monitor adherence.

Among evidence-based psychosocial interventions for adults with ADHD, CBT approaches have shown the most promise [9, 10]. These treatments emphasize the implementation of coping skills to address common EF deficits, and focus on planning, time management, organization, and dealing with procrastination. They also target rationalizations and motivational deficits that can undo effective coping. While less is known regarding the effectiveness of CBT specifically for college students with ADHD, four recent small N studies found that it is moderately helpful in improving inattentive symptoms and in reducing impairments (see summary in [11]).

To summarize, academic accommodations, ADHD coaching and psychosocial interventions have been shown to help improve academic functioning and adjustment to college life. ADHD medication is also recommended, but there is less evidence to support its use. Whatever interventions are used, patients need to take an active role in learning and practicing implementation strategies to daily life.

Helpful Resources

Organizations and Websites

- Attention Deficit Disorder Association (ADDA)—www.add.org/
- ADDISS—www.addiss.co.uk/
- ADD Resources—www.addresources.org/
- Association on Higher Education and Disability (AHEAD)—www.ahead.org/
- ADD Warehouse www.addwarehouse.com
- American College Health Association www.acha.org
- Canadian ADHD Resource Alliance (CADDRA)—www.caddra.ca/
- Children and Adults with Attention Deficit/Hyperactivity Disorder (CHADD) www.chadd.org
- Edge Foundation www.edgefoundation.org
- Learning Disabilities Association of America National Resources Center on ADHD www.ldanatl.org
- National Attention Deficit Disorder Association (ADDA) www.add.org
- National Resource Center on ADHD www.help4adhd.org
- Parents' Medication Guide (APA and AACAP)—http://www.parentsmedguide.org/
- Totally ADD—http://totallyadd.com/

Professional Scientific Information

- ADHD in Adults (AHRQ sponsored website)—http://adhdinadults.com/
- ADHD Self Report scale (ASRS)—http://psychology-tools.com/adult-adhd-self-report-scale/ http://www.uvm.edu/medicine/ahec/documents/Adult_ADHD_Self_Report_Scale.pdf
- American Association of ADHD and Related Disorders (APSARD)—www.apsard.org/
- Centers for Disease Control (CDC)—www.cdc.gov/ncbddd/adhd/
- National Institute of Mental Health (NIMH):
- http://www.nimh.nih.gov/topics/topic-page-adhd.shtml
- http://www.nimh.nih.gov/news/science-news/science-news-about-attention-deficit-hyperactivity-disorder-adhd.shtml
- http://www.nimh.nih.gov/health/topics/attention-deficit-hyperactivity-disorder-adhd/index.shtml

Clinical Tools

https://transitioncoalition.org/blog/assessment-review/a-guide-to-assessing-college-readiness/

- Conners' Adult ADHD Rating Scale (CAARS)
- Barkley Current and Childhood Symptom Scales (includes self and "other" measures)
- Barkley Adult ADHD Rating Scale—IV (BAARS-IV)
- ADHD Rating Scale IV with Adult Prompts (ADHD-RS-IV)
- Brown Attention Deficit Disorder Scale (BADDS)
- Barkley Disorder of Executive Functioning Scale (DEFS)
- Behavior Rating Inventory of Executive Function (BRIEF)
- Weiss Functional Impairment Rating Scale (WFIRS)

References

1. Ramsay JR, Rostain AL. Adult attention-deficit/hyperactivity disorder as an implementation problem: clinical significance, underlying mechanisms, and psychosocial treatment. Pract Innov. 2016;1:36–52.
2. Ramsay JR, Rostain AL. College students with ADHD. In: Adler LA, Spencer TJ, Wilens TE, editors. Attention-deficit hyperactivity disorder in adults and children. Cambridge: Cambridge University Press; 2015. p. 366–77.
3. Blase SL, Gilbert AN, Anastopoulos AD, Costello EJ, Hoyle RH, Swartwelder HS, Rabiner D. Self-reported ADHD and adjustment to college: cross-sectional and longitudinal findings. J Atten Disord. 2009;13:297–309.
4. Norwalk K, Norvilitis JM, MacLean MG. ADHD symptomatology and its relationship to factors associated with college adjustment. J Atten Disord. 2009;13:251–8.
5. Rabiner DL, Anastopoulos AD, Costello J, Hoyle RH, Swartzwelder HS. Adjustment to college in students with ADHD. J Atten Disord. 2008;11:689–99.
6. Weyandt LL, DuPaul G. ADHD in college students. J Atten Disord. 2006;10:9–19.
7. Prevatt F. Coaching for College Students with ADHD. Curr Psychiatry Rep. 2016;18(12):110.
8. Advokat C, Lane SM, Luo C. College students with and without ADHD: comparison of self-report of medication usage, study habits, and academic achievement. J Atten Disord. 2011;15:656–66.
9. Safren SA, Sprich S, Mimiaga MJ, Surman C, Knouse L, Groves M, et al. Cognitive behavioral therapy vs relaxation with educational support for medication-treated adults with ADHD and persistent symptoms: a randomized controlled trial. JAMA. 2010;304:875–80.
10. Solanto MV, Marks DJ, Wasserstein J, Mitchell KJ, Abikoff H, Alvir JMJ, et al. Efficacy of meta-cognitive therapy for adult ADHD. Am J Psychiatry. 2010;167(8):958–968. Advance online publication. https://doi.org/10.1176/appi.ajp.2009.09081123.
11. Knouse LE. Cognitive-behavioral therapy for ADHD in college: recommendations "hot off the press". ADHD Rep. 2015;23:8–15.

Rob's World: Evolving Psychosis and the Transition to College

Daniel Kirsch and Ashley Holland

Case History

Rob is a 19-year-old, Caucasian, cis-gender identifying male. He was diagnosed with anxiety and depression when he transitioned to high school and later showed signs of the at-risk mental state (ARMS) for developing psychosis. He was diagnosed with schizophrenia in the second semester of his freshman year in college. He is the middle of three male children from an intact middle class family. Both parents are professionals. His family is religious and regularly attends services at their place of worship. He grew up in a suburban neighborhood of a large city and attended public school without any educational support.

Rob showed no signs of illness until high school. He was an A/B student through middle school, was involved in sports, spent time after school with friends, and enjoyed spending time with his family. In ninth grade he had trouble settling in to high school and showed signs of social anxiety. He was hospitalized for 3 days after he told his parents he had smoked cannabis a few times to diminish his anxiety. The cannabis made his anxiety worse and harder for him to differentiate reality from drug effect in a way that he found disorienting. He began to cut himself superficially and the cutting simply hurt. The admission evaluation found no other substance use and no suicidal ideation or intent. He was diagnosed with "anxiety and depression", started on venlafaxine (VFN), received drug and alcohol counseling, and was

D. Kirsch, M.D. (✉)
Department of Psychiatry, University of Massachusetts School of Medicine,
Worcester, MA, USA
e-mail: Daniel.Kirsch@umassmemorial.org

A. Holland, D.O.
Department of Child Psychiatry, University of Massachusetts Medical Center,
Worcester, MA, USA
e-mail: Ashley.Holland@umassmemorial.org

© Springer International Publishing AG, part of Springer Nature 2018
A. Martel et al. (eds.), *Promoting Safe and Effective Transitions to College for Youth with Mental Health Conditions*, https://doi.org/10.1007/978-3-319-68894-7_9

referred to outpatient providers, a therapist and a child and adolescent psychiatrist (CAP). The VFN was too stimulating and was stopped. As he was improved, and it was his preference, his CAP adopted a "watchful waiting" approach to medication. He did not use cannabis or any illicit drugs or alcohol again. Therapy helped him sort out his worries about the transition to high school and his anxiety diminished.

Rob's grades returned to their previous level, he resumed his usual activities, and his parents felt, "Rob was back." As his first year in high school wound down and Rob maintained his functioning, treatment frequency decreased by mutual agreement. By the start of sophomore year, he was no longer in treatment. Rob did well until the beginning of junior year, when he became anxious again. His studies fueled his interest in individual rights and personal privacy, which would later influence his college choice, but his parents, concerned it had become an obsession, contacted Rob's former CAP. Though very anxious again, Rob denied self-injurious behaviors. He was deeply concerned about privacy and how much information governments could collect on their citizens. He understood that everything we did online was retrievable and was uneasy that people and organizations know so much about us. His doctor, musing that not that long ago that kind of talk would be labelled psychotic, began to listen more closely for other soft signs of psychotic thinking. He asked more about family history and discovered a maternal aunt had schizophrenia. He had Rob fill out a Prodromal Questionnaire-16 (PQ-16), and was surprised by the score of 16, indicating a high risk state. Rob commented, "Wow, no one's ever asked me about this stuff before. Does it mean anything?"

Rob and his parents were involved in shared decision making (SDM) around his diagnosis and treatment. Rob agreed with a jointly crafted plan: to continue in treatment, monitor his mental state, abstain from cannabis, and start omega-3 fatty acids. He also agreed to treat other psychiatric conditions that might arise, including anxiety and depression. Rob and his family responded well to this intervention and felt even more inclined to trust the CAP. Rob returned to his usual function. He maintained his A/B academic work, was able to take several AP courses, and volunteered in political campaigns. With exposure to like-minded peers and adults, Rob's interest in personal privacy and individual rights blossomed into a passion and political activism. Rob decided he wanted to double major in computer science and political science at a college with an activist community.

Rob, his family, and his doctor came to refer to themselves as "Team Rob" or simply "the team". There were times the team felt Rob couldn't "shut it off". He would be preoccupied with an issue, stay up late working on it, and pay less attention to his grooming and eating. This might last up to 3 days. The team called it retreating to "Rob Island", but also hypo-mania. His doctor wondered about a bipolar disorder and they continued to watch together, work on self-care, and help Rob recognize his limits. Countering his concerns, the CAP recognized that Rob maintained his academic functioning and was developing a clear sense of self. He had a close-knit group of friends who shared his activism and he was becoming close with a young woman in the group. In the middle of his senior year, while on "Rob Island", Rob's concerns with privacy crossed into delusion. He felt there was "a force or being or something of greater intelligence watching and controlling us". He heard murmurs of voices that could be aliens communicating telepathically. He denied command hallucinations to harm himself or others. He was prescribed aripiprazole 5 mg and the delusional thinking, hallucinations, and sleeplessness resolved within days. However, the medication made him "woozy" and fatigued, diminished his concentration, and interfered with studying. The side effects did not improve, so given symptom resolution, the medication was discontinued after 3 weeks but the team remained vigilant for psychotic thinking and signs of mania and depression.

The CAP shared the diagnostic uncertainty with Rob and his family and discussed the differential diagnosis, including bipolar disorder and schizophrenia spectrum disorders. He stressed the opposing risks of premature diagnosis and failing to diagnose and treat early. He underscored the importance of the ARMS as a therapeutically useful concept and stressed SDM as an evidence-based treatment. He supplied psychoeducation, encouraged the family to ask questions, and ensured treatment decisions were consistent with Rob's and his parents' values and wishes.

Rob was accepted to his first-choice college, a small, private university with a cohesive student body, a reputation for community activism, and good computer and political science departments. The school was a 5-h drive from home so Rob would have to change his treatment team. Added to the usual stresses associated with going away to college, Rob was diagnosed as being in an ARMS and there was strong evidence he had something—either a bipolar disorder or schizophrenia spectrum disorder. Would Rob be able to manage a new city, a less structured environment, increased academic competition, easy availability of drugs and alcohol, surrounded by strangers and away from his important supports when he was at risk of a serious mental condition?

The CAP appreciated the complexity that the diagnostic uncertainty added to the planning and recommended focusing on Rob's competencies. Rob was capable of self-directed academic work, had good study habits, and maintained good grades through high school. He was motivated by his passion for individual rights and had a carefully thought out plan for a double major. He had a solid understanding of his condition, was an active participant in his treatment, and showed good judgment by avoiding illicit substances. Rob independently managed daily activities such as waking up on time, maintaining good hygiene, managing his allowance, and driving to and from school—with the important exception of his "hypomanic" periods. He had close friendships within his interest group and was developing a romantic relationship with a girl. In almost every way, Rob was ready to head off to college. Rob felt strongly that neither came close to satisfying his academic needs and that he would be deeply disappointed to fall out of step with his friends, one of whom was going to Rob's first choice school. The adults all counseled Rob on the side of caution and staying local but Rob persisted in his desire to go away to college and in so doing demonstrated a capacity to advocate for himself.

The team then evaluated treatment options in the new city, both on and nearby campus. A call between Rob's doctor, the school's consulting psychiatrist, and the counseling center director clarified available resources. The private practice community was saturated and most of those practitioners were fee-for-service and did not accept insurance. There was an academic medical center two miles away but outpatient services there were limited to referrals from within their system. The school had a well-respected counseling center and consulting psychiatrist. In addition to their clinical services, they were tasked with outreach, educational programming, and screening of at risk students, and could provide only limited therapeutic interventions before referring students out to community providers. Their policy was six therapy visits per semester, but this could be flexed for special circumstances. Plus, the center had a training program and trainees were encouraged to see clients more frequently than the proscribed six sessions.

Given Rob's history, the counseling center director said that, at a minimum, he would be seen twice per month. The center's education and outreach activities with resident life, academics, athletics, campus police, chaplain, and administration had built a network throughout the campus community to help identify students at risk. If Rob were to experience a crisis, someone was likely to pick up on it. The consulting psychiatrist opined that while the on-campus services were not ideal they seemed to accommodate Rob's needs and schedule. She thought there was value to an on-site treatment team familiar with the nuances of the school's environment and connected with internal resources. She recommended that Rob maintain contact with his home treatment team. It did not appear that Rob would require academic accommodations.

Rob moved to school and met his new therapist during the second week of classes. Rob was assigned to a bright but inexperienced psychology intern for therapy and the consulting psychiatrist. Rob and his therapist had evaluation meetings over three consecutive weeks, during which time the therapist consulted with the home CAP with Rob's written authorization. The therapist presented the case at a clinical staff meeting. She found Rob engaging, motivated to be in treatment, and capable of sharing his inner world. As part of her report, she described the following risk assessment. Rob reported only one episode of cutting and that was in ninth grade. He had never been suicidal or homicidal or had command hallucinations to harm himself or others. He had no history of aggression or other antisocial behaviors or trouble with the law. He had no access to guns or other firearms at home or on campus. When he used cannabis in ninth grade, he became anxious and felt disconnected but not paranoid, and had abstained from cannabis and alcohol use since that time. All of this was confirmed by the home psychiatrist. The senior staff present recognized Rob was at risk for developing a serious mental disorder and needed to be monitored. They discussed balancing Rob's needs and the need to maintain access for the rest of the campus community. They recommended a plan for Rob to meet with his therapist every 2 weeks and with the psychiatrist monthly. Although Rob was not taking medications, direct contact with an experienced psychiatrist who could intervene quickly was felt to be clinically appropriate and a wise investment. The therapist discussed this with Rob, his parents, and the CAP via phone.

Rob kept all his appointments with his campus providers. He liked the school, loved his classes, formed a close peer group, and started dating. He kept in contact by phone with his parents who visited once each month and he went home for fall break and Thanksgiving. He saw his CAP during those breaks and again during winter break. There were no signs of any problems so they continued to monitor him from afar and encourage him to continue to see his campus therapist.

Rob felt "unsettled" as winter break wound down. He was unsure why but reasoned he was nervous about starting several classes reputed to be difficult. He felt better after the first week of classes and resumed treatment. The week before midterms he felt under pressure. He was studying hard and pulled some all-nighters. He felt like he was back on "Rob Island". He saw his therapist and psychiatrist the week before and was not due to see them for two more weeks. He spoke with his parents but reassured them he was not doing all-nighters back to back. By the next week he thought his friends acted differently with him and believed they were talking about him behind his back. He was having auditory hallucinations and delusional thinking involving aliens communicating with him. He missed an exam and a classmate, knowing this was unusual for Rob, sought him out. He was startled by Rob's appearance and behavior, recognized something was very wrong, and contacted the resident advisor. He in turn followed the school's procedures and contacted the counseling center's on-call therapist who spoke to Rob and arranged for transportation to the emergency room. He was found to be psychotic and admitted to hospital. He did not respond well to treatment, his symptoms did not fully remit, and he withdrew from school. He entered a first-episode psychosis program near his home. A year later he was diagnosed with schizophrenia, is living at home and taking two classes at the local community college.

Analysis of Transition

This case illustrates a carefully planned and executed transition and serves as a reminder that a good plan does not guarantee a good outcome in the face of serious mental illness. Transition planning arose organically out of Rob's treatment. His doctor engaged Rob and his family, openly discussed his informed opinion, provided education, and elicited feedback and input from Rob and his family. Rob made clear his preference to go away and the team worked with the school's team to establish a plan. The initial transition went well, but the timing of his first break perfectly caught a 2 week gap in care.

There were numerous indicators associated with a positive transition outcome. Rob had an intact, stable, financially comfortable family. His first-degree relatives were medically and mentally healthy. He had no early history of trauma, abuse, or neglect. The family had private medical insurance, and Rob had excellent medical care, education, and support through his childhood. His parents recognized early behavioral changes and sought help. His single episode of psychotic symptoms was time-limited and treated appropriately. Rob's commitment to abstinence protected him from complications of his ARMS associated with substance use. The possibility of a successful transition to college predicated on competencies and milestones, was evaluated including his ability to advocate for himself. A transfer of care plan was in place. Direct doctor-to-doctor communication supported Rob's choice, provided information exchange, and reassured Rob and his family.

The most important negative predictor was the at-risk mental state (ARMS). Rob was evolving some mental disorder, but it was not diagnosable when he started college. Concerning items in his history included attenuated psychotic symptoms, a brief psychotic episode, and possible hypomanic/paranoid episodes. There was a pattern of symptom escalation during transitions. Rob's parents would not be as available and Rob would not be seeing his CAP, with whom he enjoyed a strong alliance. Lastly, individual treatment options at school were more limited.

Rob's mental status deteriorated in second semester to the point he required inpatient hospitalization. He took a medical leave and then withdrew from his college of choice. What could have been done differently to change this outcome?

Current evidence indicates that nothing would have changed the outcome which appears to be the expression of a set of not fully defined genetic risk factors for schizophrenia. A broader developmental approach, however, that recognizes the number of co-occurring and interrelating processes during the transition to college—neurological, psychological, emotional, interpersonal, cognitive, social, among others—informs a view that growth is itself stressful.

Perhaps Rob's numerous positive qualities disguised the impact of these developmental stresses on an individual in the ARMS and with a history of trouble with adaptation. Schizophrenia spectrum disorders and mood disorders were in the CAP's differential. One wonders, given that Rob struggled at times of transition and he had a psychotic episode mid-senior year, if Rob should have stayed on a neuroleptic. Shortening the duration of untreated psychosis (DUP) is associated with better outcomes in schizophrenia, but data are less clear for individuals in the ARMS. Neuroleptics can be prescribed in the ARMS, although evidence supporting their use is not strong and they confer long-term medical risks. First-line mood stabilizers could have been considered as well.

Furthermore, the stability provided by Rob's family, his familiar environment, and his treatment was underestimated by "Team Rob". Rob transitioned to a new system of care. In high school, he received highly individualized and flexible care. Like at many IHE nationwide, increasing suicide awareness and a focus on prevention broadened campus behavioral health care from an individual to a population-based perspective aimed at caring for the mental health needs of a community. As a result, although all the necessary treatment components were available at his school, Rob was less likely to receive the same kind of individualized care he had before. On the other hand, the broader perspective toward the health of the community had helped craft a richer safety net to proactively identify and respond to students in need. Fortunately, there was a sufficient safety net to catch Rob early and intervene effectively. In retrospect, one wishes Rob had stayed at home for another year with his treatment undisturbed while he transitioned from high school to college.

In retrospect, it may have been helpful for Rob's providers to recommend that he connect, proactively, with the ODS at the start of each semester to understand what accommodations were available to him given his ARMS. If he recognized signs of early decompensation, he may have been able to reduce his course load and decrease his overall stress level. With regard to future planning, neuropsychological testing done during a stable period in high school, would be beneficial. It would establish an objective cognitive baseline, since cognitive deterioration is a core component of many schizophreniform spectrum disorders. It would also identify learning strengths and liabilities to inform academic counseling and study approaches. Finally, testing would be helpful should academic accommodations be required.

Clinical Pearls

- Good transition planning emerges from good care. Approaching diagnosis as a process; soliciting input from multiple sources; respecting personal, family, and cultural values; all serve to shift diagnosis into treatment.
- Future orientation is a critical component of TAY treatment, which takes place in the conditional present. The early signs of psychotic disorders are disturbing, but non-specific. Treating adult illnesses that begin in TAY calls for treatment that addresses current distress where neither the illness nor the host individual are fully formed. It challenges the treater to be attentive to the present moment while looking into the future.
- With serious mental illness, treatment comes first, everything else second. Treatment primacy rises with increasing potential of SMI. Care transfers (hand-offs) impart medical risk and are to be minimized. When risk of SMI is high and extant care is good, it is best not to transfer care. This informs a transition to college care plan that incorporates present treatment providers.
- Deal with diagnostic uncertainty directly. Psychotic symptoms, however transient or attenuated, are scary, but accurate diagnosis may not be possible until the mid- to late-20s. Until then, deescalate anxiety, fear, and distortion with psychoeducation, openness, optimism, and reassurance.
- It is a good thing not to be able to make a definitive diagnosis of schizophrenia. Office-based instruments like the PQ-16 are easy to administer and many patients respond to positive responses by saying, "No one's ever asked me about these things", thus opening a door for further exploration.
- Assess functional competencies, particularly cognition, insight, self-care skills, self-advocacy skills, and social skills.
- Harm reduction and risk avoidance are important. Be neuroprotective. "It's hard to make things better, easy to make things worse." Adopt a layered approach from less to more regarding treatment intrusiveness, complexity, toxicity, and expense. Counsel about substance misuse, including tobacco. Use neuroleptics cautiously. Try to avoid stimulants; if cognitive decline is present, it will be difficult.
- Teach wellness and positive behaviors. Diet, exercise, sleep hygiene, stress management, recreation, socialization.
- Use neuro-psychological testing to delineate cognitive strengths and vulnerabilities. Cognitive decline is a core symptom of schizophrenia. Testing supports application for accommodations and establishes a baseline of cognitive capacity. Testing also delineates cognitive strengths and vulnerabilities and these data can be used to inform a more effective learning approach.

- SDM is essential in the TAY population. SDM is an evidence-based treatment in which the clinical expert shares expertise, opinions, and recommendations, along with the reasoning behind them and solicits the patient's (and/or family's) input, values, experiences, and preferences. There follows a process of active dialogue to formulate the best plan for the individual at this time.
- Watchful waiting is a treatment option. "I'm not sure just what to do. We can consider keeping an eye on things and re-evaluating after some interval."

Brief Literature Review

Psychotic syndrome disorders are associated with increasing morbidity and mortality over the lifetime of an individual. Contributions from mental health clinicians, public health authorities, and health services researchers agree that any transfer of care—from a prescription changing hands, through shift changes in hospitals, to aging up from child and adolescent to adult mental health services—increases risk of negative outcomes. The last imparts significant risk to young persons with serious mental illness when they reach the age of majority [1]. Disruption in these patients' mental health care coupled with poorer outcomes for transition age youth with mental illness contribute to adverse health outcomes [2]. Graduating from college confers social, financial, employment, psychological, and health advantages to young adults, but psychotic syndrome disorders (PSDs) diminish the likelihood of success in college [3]. The risk of first onset of psychotic illness is most common during later adolescence and young adulthood [4, 5]. Important core features of PSDs diminish cognitive function and socialization—critical competencies necessary for successful transition to, and success in college. Disordered, strange, or frankly delusional thinking, and associated bizarre behaviors impede socialization, which facilitates more withdrawal, isolation, and paranoid projections. Cognitive decline may make completion of college level work impossible.

Individuals suffering from prodromal symptoms of psychosis most commonly have low rates of graduation and high rates of school dropout [3]. It is important to note that of prodromal symptomatic patients, not all go on to develop long term psychotic disorders, and of those cases that develop long term psychotic symptoms only half go on to develop diagnosable schizophrenia [6–8]. Most of the current evidence based programs for early intervention in psychosis involve family therapy, individual therapy, and very mild medication management such as omega-3 fatty acids and CBT for Psychosis (CBT-P) [9].

There are few data to guide decision making about college for high school students with prodromal symptoms. Prodromal students who succeed in college have been shown to possess qualities that facilitate adapting to the academic rigor and social challenges of college that differentiate them from unaffected individuals. Those who succeed are more motivated and have clear personal goals, they have more support—family and systemic supports like housing. They typically manage developmental tasks with a more singular focus, utilizing adaptive skills focused on one task rather than several—they take it one step at a time. They use strategies to improve chances of succeeding like taking classes or programs that require fewer social interactions or aim for a passing grade only. In contrast, non-affected individuals rely more on cognitive and social skills, derive support from peers, and have a higher perceived ability to manage multiple developmental tasks at a time despite perceived stress [10]. These are early data, but support accepted clinical principles of individualized assessment and treatment, evaluating the need for supports and ensuring they are in place, and assessing and providing accommodations through disability and academic services.

Helpful Resources

- Prodromal Questionnaire PQ-16 Loewy, R.L., Bearden, C.E., Johnson, J.K., Raine, A., & Cannon, T.D. (2005). The prodromal questionnaire (PQ): preliminary validation of a self-report screening measure for prodromal and psychotic syndromes. Schizophrenia Research 79(1): 117–125.
- **headspace** is the Australian National Youth Mental Health Fdn. providing early intervention mental health services to 12–25 year olds. https://www.headspace.org.au/resource-library/
- NAMI: https://www.nami.org/earlypsychosis and https://www.nami.org/getattachment/Learn-More/Mental-Health-Conditions/Early-Psychosis-and-Psychosis/NAMI-Early-Psychosis.pdf
- Shared decision making for mental health—what is the evidence? https://headspace.org.au/assets/Uploads/Resource-library/Health-professionals/sdm-evidence-summary.pdf

References

1. Hower H, Case B, Hoeppner B, Yen S, Goldstein T, Birmaher B, Weinstock L, Topor D, Hunt J, Strober M, Neal R, Axelson D, Gill M, Keller M. Use of mental health services in transition age youth with bipolar disorder. J Psychiatr Pract. 2013;19(6):464–76.
2. Vander Stoep A, Beresford S, Weiss N, et al. Community-based study of the transition to adulthood for adolescents with psychiatric disorder. Am J Epidemiol. 2000;152(4):352–62.
3. Goulding S, Chien V, Compton M. Prevalence and correlates of school drop-out prior to initial treatment of nonaffective psychosis: further evidence suggesting a need for supported education. Schizophr Res. 2010;116:228–33.
4. Kessler R, Angermeyer M, Anthony J, et al. lifetime prevalence and age-of-onset distributions of mental disorders in the World Health Organization's World Mental Health Survey Initiative. World Psychiatry. 2007;6(3):168–76.
5. Merikangas K, He J, Burstein M, et al. Lifetime prevalence of mental disorders in US adolescents: results from the National Comorbidity Survey Replication—Adolescent Supplement. J Am Acad Child Adolesc Psychiatry. 2010;49(10):980–9.
6. Cannon TD, Cadenhead K, Cornblatt B, Woods SW, Addington J, Walker E, Seidman LJ, Perkins D, Tsuang M, McGlashan T, Heinssen R. Prediction of psychosis in youth at high clinical risk: a multisite longitudinal study in North America. Arch Gen Psychiatry. 2008;65(1):28–37.

7. Larson MK, Walker EF, Compton MT. Early signs, diagnosis and therapeutics of the prodromal phase of schizophrenia and related psychotic disorders. Expert Rev Neurother. 2010;10(8):1347–59. https://doi.org/10.1586/ern.10.93.
8. McGorry PD, Nelson B, Amminger GP, et al. Intervention in individuals at ultra-high risk for psychosis: a review and future directions. J Clin Psychiatry. 2009;70:1206–12.
9. McFarlane W. Prevention of the first episode of psychosis. Psychiatr Clin North Am. 2011;34(1):95–107.
10. Roy L, Rousseau J, Fortier P, Mottard J. Postsecondary academic achievement and first-episode psychosis: a mixed-methods study. Can J Occup Ther. 2016;83(1):42–52.

Coping with Highs and Lows: A Student with Bipolar Disorder Goes to College

Adelaide Robb

Case History

Brie is an 18-year-old European American female with bipolar disorder. She is a middle child with an older sister and twin younger brothers. She lives in a suburban area on the East Coast. She had been attending a local public high school with an IEP for emotional disturbance. Her primary diagnoses were bipolar I disorder, most recent episode manic, and ADHD combined presentation. Her parents were both college educated, and her older sister was already in college when she was a senior in high school. Family history was significant for a maternal Grandfather who had ECT in the 1930s.

In the first grade, Brie was diagnosed with ADHD and responded to stimulants, prescribed by her child and adolescent psychiatrist (CAP). Brie had a 504 Plan during elementary and middle school, which included tests in a quiet area, preferential seating, and breaks for movement. Neuropsychological testing in grade 5 confirmed ADHD and ruled out comorbid learning disorders. She took summer holidays from her ADHD medication and did well in summer day camps.

The summer before 9th grade, Brie became much more active in sports and other activities. She started staying up late texting friends in the middle of the night and going over to friend's houses on her bike at 1:00 or 2:00 am. Parents noted she was speaking quickly, and she thought she could drive a car although she had no learner's permit. She was seen in the office by her CAP, found to be manic, and was hospitalized. She was stabilized on a combination of lithium and a second-generation anti-psychotic. A long-acting stimulant medication was reintroduced to treat her

A. Robb, M.D.
Psychiatry and Behavioral Sciences, Children's National Health System,
Washington, DC 20010, USA
e-mail: AROBB@childrensnational.org

© Springer International Publishing AG, part of Springer Nature 2018
A. Martel et al. (eds.), *Promoting Safe and Effective Transitions to College for Youth with Mental Health Conditions*, https://doi.org/10.1007/978-3-319-68894-7_10

ADHD. She returned to her public high school where her supports were expanded through an IEP. After the diagnosis of bipolar disorder, she began individual therapy with a community psychologist. She developed a good working relationship with her therapist, and they worked extensively on academic productivity, self-esteem, and recognizing symptoms of mood dysregulation. During her sophomore year, her therapist retired and moved out of state. Despite visits to several other psychotherapists, she failed to make a connection and decided that therapy was not for her.

Through high school she remained fairly stable, requiring minor medication adjustments during her monthly medication management visits. Her grades were primarily A's and B's (B average) and she tended to do better in subjects involving literature and writing papers. She regularly used her high school accommodations which now included a pass to the school nurse as needed for trouble coping, flexible scheduling of exams given mood fluctuations, extended time for classroom and standardized testing, and the ability to ask for extended time on writing assignments given fluctuations in energy. She completed all assignments and standardized testing. She had a small group of close friends in high school but had not dated nor had any serious romantic relationships.

At the time, Brie and her family felt she was ready for college. Her mood had been stable for over 3 years, and she was functioning well in high school with educational supports and monthly monitoring of her mood symptoms. She had mastered independent daily living skills and independent academic functioning. She did her own laundry and hygiene and monitored all her own classroom assignments including planning for long-term projects. She understood her bipolar and ADHD diagnoses and the need for adherence to medical regimens for them.

However, Brie relied on her parents to direct her medical care including facilitating appointments, medication refills, and contact with her prescribing clinician. Brie was uncertain of the dosages of her medications although she knew their names and colors. In the classroom, even though she knew it was important to do so, it was still hard for her to advocate for herself, ask questions, or ask to use accommodations. Her social relationships and psychosocial development appeared to be at the level of an early high school student rather than a graduating senior. Safety issues had not been a concern in over 3 years and safety planning had not been part of her later high school treatment. Because her parents were so attentive to her symptoms, and her psychiatrist was so responsive to concerns, ups and downs were addressed very quickly with medication adjustments, and Brie was only passively involved in the process. Brie was not aware of what to do if her manic symptoms became worse, if she developed a depression, or what lifestyle decisions she would need to make (i.e., protecting her sleep, minimizing drug and alcohol abuse, and managing stress) to help minimize her risks for relapse.

With the advice of her psychiatrist and parents, Brie restricted college applications to a limited number of colleges near home. She ultimately chose a 4-year small state college in the southern part of her home state approximately a 6 h drive from home. The college was located in a small town and was not close to a medical school or hospital. There was a student health center, which included a limited number of on-campus counseling sessions for students struggling with the transition to college or the end of romantic relationships. There were no psychiatrists close to campus and very few psychologists in the community who provided therapy for students. One psychiatrist came every 2 weeks from a medical school across the state to provide emergency consultations. The college had a robust academic support program, which included outreach during orientation week, a strong academic advising program, writing support, and tutoring for any student who asked for help. Academic resources did not include ADHD coaches or other specific illness-related academic supports. On-campus formal psychotherapy, as opposed to supportive counseling, was very limited for those students who sought help.

In planning for the transition to college, Brie decided to register for a minimal course load the first semester, continue her current medication treatment, and request a single room to minimize sleep disruption due to having a roommate. Her home psychiatrist wrote a letter on Brie's behalf documenting the need for a single room. She completed repeat psychoeducational testing with adult norms and a copy was sent to the college. It was strongly recommended that she find a therapist on staff or close to campus, but she continued to refuse.

Brie's parents had been involved in transition preparation and planning in the following ways. They accompanied her to all visits with her clinician. They took her on college visits and supported her decision to attend a 4-year college. They, too, supported the concept of a single room, low course burden, and selection of an in-state college. They would have preferred that Brie resume psychotherapy, but were not willing to push on that issue. They supported her decision to continue medication management with her home-based clinician. They committed to having her return every 8 weeks for medication management during the academic year.

Brie arrived on campus, moved into a single room, and participated in all of the freshman orientation activities. The academic support team, having seen her testing report, met with her during orientation to explain the range of services available and reminded her that she should discuss her learning needs with her advisor and professors and advocate for accommodations. She continued to take all her psychotherapeutic medications as prescribed and had regular contact with her family. She had several quizzes and did not do well, which caused her to worry and have trouble sleeping and eating properly. She initially wondered if she felt low because she was stressed out by the academic demands in the absence of an IEP and her high school guidance team. She also began to stay up late studying precipitated by fears about failing another quiz, which led to oversleeping and missing her morning classes. Brie was reluctant to ask for help from academic support and her professors, wanting to appear as if she had everything under control. She remained in her room, withdrew from peers, stopped showering or washing her hair, wandered the dorm in her pajamas, and ate only breakfast cereal and regular coke. She refused to go to class, missed three quizzes and one paper, and had incompletes in all four subjects at the end of 6 weeks on campus. In the middle of the night, she called her parents sobbing uncontrollably and told them she was overwhelmingly depressed and asked to withdraw from college.

It is now several years after her start in college. Brie spent the first year home fine-tuning her medication and assuming more responsibility for her medical care. She still was not interested in seeking therapy, with the excuse that she wanted to focus on her academics. She did not want the pressure of a job, so she volunteered at a local animal shelter and started Zumba classes to add some structure and routine to her day. She began taking introductory level classes at the local community college. Academic supports included note-taking services, extended deadlines for writing assignments, and flexible exam scheduling to avoid sleep deprivation during finals week. She made straight A's and rapidly earned her Associate's degree in 2 years while living at home and continuing to see her outpatient clinician. She transferred to a local 4-year college, commuted for one semester, and then moved on to campus. She was successful in her course work. She learned to better advocate for herself regarding academic accommodations and explaining her needs to professors. She learned to problem-solve with her roommate. She graduated with a degree in social sciences and moved to the Midwest. She is now working for a large company, manages her medications, and resumed psychotherapy.

Analysis of Transition

The aspects of Brie's case that were predictors of a successful transition to college included her excellent performance in high school with challenging academic classes. Useful accommodations had been developed by her team under an IEP. She was shy socially but was able to initiate and maintain friendships with peers. She was also aware of her medications and the need to continue taking them regularly, and would continue with her long-term psychiatric care provider. Brie showed some insight into her needs, choosing a college close to home, a minimal course load, and a single room. Finally, she had not been hospitalized or had a clinical destabilization of her bipolar disorder in more than 4 years. She had not been suicidal at all over the same time period.

Several predictors of a negative outcome were also present in Brie's case. Her insistence that no therapist would ever replace her first one made it extremely difficult for her to seek therapy during the transition to college. She had not practiced all the necessary skills to manage her illness independently. The high school accommodations she utilized may not all easily translate to the college setting, and she was an inconsistent self-advocate in regard to her learning needs. The positive impact of a single room on her sleep and work habits were counterbalanced by the negatives of social isolation and the loss of accountability that comes with having roommates. Brie's concerning behaviors were not being noticed by anyone nor reported to campus authorities. A separate risk factor was the comorbid diagnosis of ADHD that put her at higher risk of not doing well with the transition to college and of not managing the tasks needed to help keep her emotionally stable (taking medication, tracking moods, sleeping, and eating properly). Finally, she had never been away from home overnight in an educational setting other than a 1-day field trip to New York for one of her English classes.

This case represents a suboptimal or failed transition to college. Brie experienced a significant deterioration in her mood, despite medication compliance, within weeks of matriculation. Her academic function declined, and she did not utilize available resources. She returned home voluntarily during her first semester.

Additional attention to several aspects of transitioning preparation and planning could have improved Brie's transition outcome. It is important for students to understand their diagnosis and the importance of self-care regarding sleep, nutrition, and exercise. They should know the details of their medications, including dosages, indications, and common and serious side effects, and should be aware of the need for medication management and psychotherapy visits during the transition. Brie's parents and providers did address much of this, but parents should have stepped back and empowered her to manage her medical care while she was still living at home. Brie could have learned to use electronic reminders and symptom management tools on her smart phone.

In addition, she could have started with one or two courses at the local community college to identify gaps in academic readiness for college, which could be addressed before starting a full course load. Brie needed a college with good supports for young adults with more serious mental health disorders and on-campus access to both prescribing clinicians and therapists. The home team must coordinate transition of care with on campus prescribing and therapeutic clinicians. Brie may also have benefited from more experience in meeting new peers and friends and living in a communal setting away from home prior to the actual transition. A summer course for high school students would have allowed Brie to spend a week in a college dormitory while taking a college class. High school exchange programs are another option for students to gain experience living in an unfamiliar setting and attending school without the usual supports at home.

From the clinician perspective, there were four main areas needing additional focus: (1) empowering Brie to assume management responsibilities for her mental health care, (2) deeper exploration of her reluctance to engage in therapy. While her resistance seemed to be focused on an idealization of her first therapist, the clinician and parents allowed Brie to direct treatment against the clinician's judgment, (3) identification of clinicians on or near campus to provide both therapy and medication management services during the academic year, even if the patient plans to remain with original providers during college breaks, (4) obtaining written consents for contact between the clinician and parents (if desired) and also between the home clinician and campus clinicians. Ideally, the home clinician sends a summary note of diagnoses, medication trials, key therapy issues, and response to treatment to the campus therapist and psychiatrist.

Finally, campus systems of care can provide another layer of protection. Making resident advisors (RAs) aware of Brie's diagnoses could have helped with her academic and social integration. Training regarding the signs and symptoms of mood and anxiety disorders and suicide prevention is an important part of the preparation that most RAs undergo. A properly trained RA might have noticed that Brie was not going to class and could have served as the first level of a safety net. Strongly encouraging patients with serious psychiatric illness to disclose their illness to select "gatekeepers" on campus, and to have therapy during the first semester could also provide another level of protection and help monitor emotional well-being during the transition.

Clinical Pearls

- Transitioning patients to college is an ongoing discussion between the teenager, the family, and the clinician where multiple factors are considered. These include the student's desire to attend college, career aspirations, and the ability to demonstrate stable mood. Those who can sign themselves up for standardized testing, handle a full course load, and complete college applications are the ones best prepared for independence on campus. Topics for discussion and a sample transition timeline are included in the chapter's Helpful Resources section.
- Individuals with bipolar disorder can be especially sensitive to changes in medication levels. Consistent adherence to time and dosage of medication is a crucial aspect of success in college. Having reminders so that refills do not go unclaimed is an important part of success.
- Having ready access to clinicians on or near campus with expertise in bipolar disorder for both psychotherapy and medication is very important. Encourage patients and families to look for a college with a good psychiatry department, not just a counseling center. It is important to recognize the difference between "counseling" and "psychotherapy." Many counseling centers provide a limited number of sessions for adjustment and relationship concerns but refer more complicated mental health issues to community providers.
- Develop patient-specific lists of early warning signs of impending manic and depressive episodes—signs of altered sleep, energy, and mood rather than at full symptomatic expression-early recognition and intervention may abort a full blown affective episode.
- Consider encouraging the student to disclose their diagnosis to a few key gatekeepers, such as resident advisors, on campus to increase accountability and provide another layer of protection to their safety net.
- Youth with bipolar disorder are at high risk for substance use disorders. Special care should be taken during the transition to college to educate about the perils of experimentation with illicit substances and alcohol. Remind them that partying can lead to mania.
- Youth with bipolar disorder are at high risk for suicide. Review suicide risk factors and monitor for suicidality. Crisis safety plans should be developed for students with significant risk factors and previous suicidal ideation.
- Sleep deprivation and interpersonal conflict are frequently triggers of mood episodes in youth with bipolar disorder. Remind patients that late night cramming can lead to mania.
- Students should continue to work on maintaining stable patterns of sleep, eating, exercise, and adherence to therapy and medication to ensure success in college.

Brief Literature Review

The articles on bipolar disorder fall into three main topic areas, the first of which is managing bipolar on campus. In youth with bipolar who attend college, stigma around disclosure to medical staff, professors, and peers makes adherence and treatment during college difficult [1]. In surveying peers, the authors found that younger students and those unfamiliar with mental illness were even more likely to stigmatize and isolate those with signs and symptoms of mental illness. Since bipolar disorder may begin in college, clinicians need to form a treatment alliance with the young adult [2]. The patient–clinician alliance may focus on lifestyle changes, adaptation to illness, careful use of medications to minimize side effects, and management of fear of relapse. One important aspect of lifestyle is the need to avoid experimenting with alcohol and drugs, which may precipitate mood episodes or make current moods more difficult to treat. Intoxication can also lower the barrier to suicide which is a high-risk outcome in bipolar disorder. Youth who enter college with a bipolar diagnosis may wish to have plans in place should they begin to show signs of a manic or depressive episode. One large university recruited 40 students with serious mental illness in this study to examine the feasibility of using Psychiatric Advanced Directives (PADs) [3]. The positive aspects of PADs include allowing students control over their treatment and negatives included breach of privacy and stigmatizing those with serious mental illnesses. Students with bipolar disorder may wish to have advanced directives in place should a severe episode occur while on campus.

Another topic area includes statistics on illness and college achievement and completion. Findings from several large epidemiological surveys demonstrate the need for intervention and diligence in youth with bipolar disorder as they navigate high school and college to ensure successful high school graduation, matriculation in college, and graduation from college. In a comparison of youth ages 19–25 from a large National Epidemiologic Study on Alcohol and Related Conditions (NESARC), there were several findings on college achievement and completion. Almost half of college-aged individuals had a psychiatric disorder in the past year and overall rates did not differ between those in college and those not attending college. Less than 25% sought help and bipolar disorder was less common among those in college [4]. In the same NESARC data set looking at the adults 22 and older who had started college, three substance use disorders (amphetamine, cocaine, and marijuana) and bipolar disorder were associated with failure to graduate [5]. The National Comorbidity Survey in 1990–1992 and follow up in 2001–2003 examined people ages 15–54 and found students with bipolar disorder at the initial wave were less likely to graduate from high school and had lower odds of going to college. If the students developed bipolar disorder after the initial survey, they were less likely to graduate from college [6]. Mental disorders accounted for 5.8–11.0% of high school and 3.2–11.4% of college non-completion.

Finally, suicide rates in bipolar disorder remain one of the highest among Axis I disorders with some studies showing rates as high as 15–20%. Two studies examined the risks of suicidal ideation in college students with specific attention paid to bipolar disorder. A large web-based survey of university students between the ages of 18 and 29 examined the associations between non-suicidal self-injury and suicidal thoughts and behaviors [7]. Both bipolar disorder and problematic substance use were positively associated with the risk for suicide attempt. Another large web survey from over 1500 predominantly US colleges/universities examined risk factors for suicidal ideation [8]. Most notably, suicidal ideation (SI) occurred in 47.1% of students, with women evidencing somewhat stronger findings than men. SI was seen more commonly in substance, bipolar and panic disorders than in depressive disorders. The authors suggested examining emotional volatility and psychiatric disorders beyond depression as risk factors for suicidal ideation among college students.

Helpful Resources

A variety of transition resources are available for youth with bipolar disorder.

- Illness-centered publications and websites such as BP magazine (www.bphope. com/) and Jed Foundation (https://www.jedfoundation.org/) have a variety of online resources
- Campus organizations that provide peer outreach and support MINDHAND-HEART initiative at MIT is one such example.
- National organizations such as National Alliance for the Mentally Ill (www. nami.org) and Depression and Bipolar Support Alliance (www.dbsalliance.org)

A variety of patient level medication and mood tracking applications are available for phones.

- Smart phone resources for iPhones or android include a variety of mood screening/monitoring T2 Mood tracker, iMoodJournal, InFlow: Mood Diary, Moodlytics, Moodtrack Diary, DBT Diary Card and Skills CoachMood Tracker and Mood Tracker Pro.
- Medication reminder applications include Medisafe Medication Reminder

Office-Based Tools

- SAMSHA has a screening tool website and the direct link for bipolar screening tools is (www.integration.samhsa.gov/clinical-practice/screening-tools#bipolar). They use the Mood Disorder Questionnaire as the primary screening instrument and the STABLE (standards for bipolar excellence) as a resource toolkit for practitioners.
- Sample Transition Timeline (next page).

Transition to College—Topics for Discussion and Timeline

Multiple factors are involved in the decision about attending college: Future educational opportunities, career choices, treatment needs, and family involvement. Below is a list of things that may be involved in this ongoing discussion.

- Teen's desire to attend college
- Overall academic performance during middle school and high school in the classroom and on standardized testing
- Learning disability or other Axis I and II disorders that impact the teen's ability to learn
- Family's emphasis on the importance of education
- Family resources and the ability to provide for postsecondary education
- Career aspirations for the teenager and for the family and mismatch between them (parents want teen to be neurosurgeon and he prefers English literature courses)
- Treatment needs including therapy and medication management
- Role of the parents and extended family in treatment
- Independence of the teenager in managing their mental health care needs; insisting on stopping all medication and therapy, the summer before college does not signal independence
- Proximity of school to mental health care facilities

As early as middle school, encourage patients to consider options at the end of high school for next steps. Explore life after high school before high school even starts. This timeline can be broken down by developmental stages.

- In middle school, focus on independence and timely completion of work. Visit local colleges and try to have short-term overnight visits away from home where the adolescent must manage medication, sleep, and eating.
- In 9th and 10th grade work on time management, assuming responsibility for their own medical care, and planning out courses over the next 4 years.
- In 11th grade, the focus is preparation, academic success, and stress management. Identifying appropriate school choices and use of college counselors are other areas of focus.
- In 12th grade teens who can sign themselves up for standardized testing, handle a full course load and complete college applications are the ones best prepared for independence in campus life. If the year has not demonstrated independence and a stable mood, the teen and family might consider whether a gap year might be helpful after admission decisions arrive.
- In the spring of senior year after admission decisions arrive from the colleges, the work focuses on identifying the best option for the teenager. Attending the accepted student weekends and speaking with student health and the counseling centers clarifies the supports available on campus. Clinicians can also work through AACAP and APA to identify clinicians able to see the student near campus.
- Final steps include a transfer of care letter for the receiving clinical team, and a release of information to ensure communication between teams, consider whether parents are included on the HIPPA form so that the college mental health care team may communicate with families especially in the event of an emergency.

References

1. Feeg VD, Prager LS, et al. Predictors of mental illness stigma and attitudes among college students: using vignettes from a campus common reading program. Issues Ment Health Nurs. 2014;35(9):694–703.
2. Lejeune SM. Special considerations in the treatment of college students with bipolar disorder. J Am Coll Heal. 2011;59(7):666–9.
3. Scheyett AM, Rooks A. University students' views on the utility of psychiatric advance directives. J Am Coll Heal. 2012;60(1):90–3.
4. Blanco C, Okuda M, et al. Mental health of college students and their non-college-attending peers: results from the National Epidemiologic Study on Alcohol and Related Conditions. Arch Gen Psychiatry. 2008;65(12):1429–37.
5. Hunt J, Eisenberg D, et al. Consequences of receipt of a psychiatric diagnosis for completion of college. Psychiatr Serv. 2010;61(4):399–404.
6. Mojtabai R, Stuart EA, et al. Long-term effects of mental disorders on educational attainment in the National Comorbidity Survey ten-year follow-up. Soc Psychiatry Psychiatr Epidemiol. 2015;50(10):1577–91.
7. Paul E, Tsypes A, et al. Frequency and functions of non-suicidal self-injury: associations with suicidal thoughts and behaviors. Psychiatry Res. 2015;225(3):276–82.
8. Tupler LA, Hong JY, et al. Suicidal ideation and sex differences in relation to 18 major psychiatric disorders in college and university students: anonymous web-based assessment. J Nerv Ment Dis. 2015;203(4):269–78.

Driven to Depression: Overachieving College Student with Recurrent Depressive Episodes

Christina G. Weston

Case History

Colin is a 17-year-old Caucasian male who lives in an affluent suburb of a medium-sized Midwestern city. He is the older of two children with a sister 3 years his junior. He lives with his parents, both high achieving professionals with advanced degrees from prestigious universities. He is in the top 1–2% of his high school class and was diagnosed with Major Depressive Disorder before he transitioned to college.

Colin first sought mental health treatment when he was age 17 in the winter of his junior year in high school. His mother became concerned after he took her car keys and gave her the impression he was going to start the car in the garage to die from carbon monoxide poisoning. He described symptoms of depression which were related to his desire to be valedictorian of his high school class and the intense pressure he felt from himself and from his parents to succeed. Given his heavy course load, he often stayed up late at night to complete schoolwork; on those nights when he did not have classwork to complete he had difficulty falling asleep. He found little enjoyment in activities; and, although he had friends in school, he did not see them outside of school. He was tired most of the day and felt as if his body movements were slowed.

He admitted to occasional thoughts of suicide but none currently. The suicidal ideation and plan that prompted him to seek treatment occurred when he was afraid that he would be accused of cheating by a teacher on a test when he in fact hadn't done anything wrong. He also reported having some anxiety in social situations, but

---

C.G. Weston, M.D.
Department of Psychiatry, Wright State University, Boonshoft School of Medicine, Dayton, OH, USA
e-mail: Christina.weston@wright.edu

© Springer International Publishing AG, part of Springer Nature 2018
A. Martel et al. (eds.), *Promoting Safe and Effective Transitions to College for Youth with Mental Health Conditions*, https://doi.org/10.1007/978-3-319-68894-7_11

he did not meet criteria for Social Anxiety Disorder. He and his parents denied symptoms or history of mania or psychosis. He denied the use of alcohol and drugs and his medical history was non-contributory.

This is the first time he had been depressed. His mother had a history of recurrent depression and had a manic episode after the birth of his younger sister. She has been successfully maintained on bupropion hydrochloride and lithium without recurrence. His mother still receives medication refills from a psychiatrist in another state whom she established care with after the onset of her mania. She has not had any recurrences of mood symptoms since starting medication. His paternal grand-mother had difficulty with depression requiring electroconvulsive therapy.

Colin had some difficulty fitting in with his more politically conservative peers. He ran cross country when younger but gave it up to have more time to complete schoolwork. He had a rigorous course schedule, taking one AP class as a sophomore and five as a junior as they are weighted and he needed to enhance his GPA to be valedictorian. He enjoyed volunteering 3–4 days a week at several local charities although he initially did it at the urging of his parents to enhance his resume for college.

He was initially diagnosed with Major Depressive Disorder, Single, Moderate and was started on bupropion hydrochloride since his mother had responded well to it. Given the family history, Colin and his parents were cautioned to observe for symptoms of hypomania and mania. He was seen by his CAP every other week or monthly for supportive therapy in addition to medication management. After 4 weeks on bupropion hydrochloride, he showed some initial improvement; how-ever, despite 4 months of compliant treatment, his depressed mood and suicidal ideation recurred when he received a poor grade. He was switched to fluoxetine. In therapy, he discussed his relief to not be in contention for class valedictorian after he received a B in an AP class. He also discussed difficulty managing his school work, his ongoing pattern of staying up late to complete work, then oversleeping, and calling in sick to school. The addition of sleep aids including trazodone or mela-tonin were unsuccessful as Colin deliberately did not take them on nights he had work to do. During this time, he also applied to a prestigious selective writing com-petition which involved a summer program, and was nervous about his acceptance. In light of his continued depression, fluoxetine was increased and the school agreed to decrease his academic load at an informal meeting attended by his parents and his psychiatrist. He did not have an IEP or 504 plan.

Colin developed intolerable gastrointestinal side effects as well as sedation. So, after 2 months, and concurrent with the end of the academic year, fluoxetine was stopped and he was switched to sertraline. His mood improved with the addition of a new medication and the absence of schoolwork. He was accepted to the summer writing program and spent several weeks away over the summer. He had some mild symptoms of depression and anxiety when he forgot to take his medication for 4 days but was able to make new friends who shared his values.

During senior year of high school Colin took a full academic load and although he would occasionally stay up late to complete school work he did very well aca-demically and socially. He was compliant with medication and remained euthymic.

He started dating a classmate who became his girlfriend. After the start of school, he stopped coming regularly for therapy and was seen in early spring of his senior year for a medication refill visit. At that visit, Colin informed his CAP that he anticipated acceptance and a scholarship to a very small, prestigious, 2-year school focusing on music and creative writing in the West. Though ready for college in many ways, particularly in the realm of independent academic functioning (tracked due dates, completed work on time, studied for tests), the CAP hoped to work with Colin in conjunction with his parents on independent daily living skills (such as waking up in the morning, doing laundry, and managing money) and more independent management of his illness (making appointments, refilling prescriptions). The plan was to meet during the summer, once Colin finalized his college choice, to discuss the risks of recurrence of depression with the transition to college and to develop a transfer of care plan including a crisis management plan. Neither Colin nor his parents came to the next session and, despite a reminder phone call, did not reschedule.

Colin's parents called for medication refills after he left for the college out West. They mentioned the remote location of the college, the lack of formal mental health services on campus and in the nearby community, and their desire/need to have Colin's medications managed by his home psychiatrist. There was one community psychiatrist a 1 1/2 h drive from campus which was not practical and who did not accept the family's insurance. He did emergency consultations at the college. Subsequent to this conversation, the home psychiatrist spoke with Colin to check in and agreed to prescribe remotely and see Colin on school breaks and via phone sessions as needed. Though not ideal, it was important for Colin to remain on his medication.

Colin was seen twice over the Christmas break after his first semester. His parents had some concerns about depression after his girlfriend broke up with him; they were at different colleges and could not see each other. He discussed the breakup as a mutual decision. Colin appeared to be doing well, his depression was still in full remission, and he was taking his medication. He felt comfortable with his college peers and denied use of alcohol and other substances. He presented the same during spring break and spent the summer at school. No contact occurred until the fall of his sophomore year, when he had a recurrence of his depression and suicidal ideation. He was found by a classmate in a remote area of the school with a rope attempting to hang himself.

Colin was seen urgently by the consulting psychiatrist who called the hometown provider. He recommended that Colin get hospitalized back at home so that he could be near his family. He had determined that Colin was safe to travel alone so school staff took Colin to the airport and observed him get on the plane. He had a brief psychiatric admission and was diagnosed with Major Depressive Disorder, Recurrent, Severe. Lithium was added to augment the sertraline. He remained at home for about 2 weeks while he stabilized and saw his home outpatient provider. He identified two triggers for his depression, the stress of applying to transfer to 4 year colleges and pressure from a parent to retake the SAT to get a perfect score (he had very high scores when he took them in high school). His return to college was discussed with parents and advisors at the school who felt that Colin could be safely monitored in his small school community. The school agreed to arrange transportation, at parents' cost, to see the community psychiatrist for medication management twice per semester. Initially, he was also going to have phone psychotherapy sessions with his hometown provider however the logistics of that were difficult as there were no secure phone connections. Colin was seen by his hometown psychiatrist when he was available on school breaks. Colin's mood remained stable and he successfully completed the 2-year college program. He planned to transfer as a junior to a small selective liberal arts college on the East Coast.

Colin met with his home provider a few times to discuss the transition to his second college. He made a plan for how he would try to fit in and make friends at a school where there are few other transfer students and minimal orientation activities specifically designed for transfer students. He had not experienced peer pressure in high school or at his previous college to use alcohol or drugs and he identified ways to deal with those situations when they occurred. Colin, his parents, and psychiatrist had a frank discussion about the triggers for his past depressive episodes and his/ their pattern of not reaching out until he was found in crisis. There were more mental health services available at this college and he was encouraged to connect with a therapist and he tentatively agreed to do so. Both he and his family were reluctant to initiate a relationship with a new psychiatrist as they felt that his history and issues were well understood by his hometown psychiatrist, so it was decided that he would continue to get medication refills from his CAP as he would be back frequently. He agreed to communicate weekly with his parents via phone or Skype. He was seen over fall break and was doing well, making intentional efforts to socialize. He was bothered by the drug and alcohol use on campus but remained in good spirits without any recurrence of depressive symptoms. He had not followed through with the recommendation to see a counselor.

About 3 weeks after fall break, his father called with concerns about Colin. He was making odd, paranoid statements about his peers, saying they were making fun of him. He appeared thinner to them on Skype. He admitted to isolating in his room and some suicidal thinking. His parents called the dean of students to have him evaluated. Colin was accompanied to the student mental health service by his resident advisor and a member of the security staff. The results of the evaluation were not fully shared with his parents because of strict interpretation of college privacy rules. He was felt to be safe and in need of additional treatment. Parents were encouraged to come to school, pick him up, and have him seen by his psychiatrist. They also requested that Colin be seen at the campus counseling center upon his return. On interview, he was cooperative and made good eye contact. His speech was rambling and thought process tangential. He heard voices making derogatory comments about him. He felt that his depression had returned. His affect was of full range though predominantly sad and appropriate. He had no symptoms of mania and his psychotic symptoms had occurred within the context of the depressive episode. His diagnosis was changed to Recurrent Major Depressive Disorder with Mood-Congruent Psychotic Features. Colin exhibited improvement with the addition of lurasidone to his medication regimen and returned to school 2 weeks later.

Colin and his family were again cautioned to monitor for hypomania/mania given that he was at risk for Bipolar Disorder.

Over Christmas break, he reported that he met with a therapist at the campus counseling center a few times and planned to continue during second semester. He met once with the consulting psychiatrist at the campus mental health clinic, as requested by the home CAP, for Colin and the campus psychiatrist to develop some familiarity with each other and as a safety net in the event of a worsening of Colin's symptoms. Despite a release, the therapist shared little information with the home provider. The home CAP was relieved that Colin was monitored at school and continued as the primary prescriber.

Colin was not seen again until July while he was home on summer break. He was successful academically with a 3.7 GPA. Except for a 1 week recurrence of depression and paranoia which resolved quickly his mood had been stable. He asked to do some CBT work that summer to address his negative cognitive style as a follow-up to some work he had done on campus. He came for a few psychotherapy sessions but then reverted to medication visits only. He remains resilient and uses the experience to reflect on his life leading him to take a year off from college to work on music composition. He spent time volunteering and teaching math at a private school in his hometown. He had in-person visits with his CAP every 3–4 months for medication refills. He has been in remission for a full year and anticipates returning to school next year to complete his bachelor's degree and then go on to graduate school.

Analysis of Transition

At the time Colin left for college, his depression had been in remission for a year and it was hoped that being in a more intellectually rigorous academic environment surrounded by other like-minded individuals would help continue his recovery. He accepted his illness and was compliant with his medication and was able to engage in therapy when it was needed. These were all aspects that would predict a successful transition to college. He also was very bright and had no difficulty completing academic work, as long as his mood remained stable, another factor that would allow him to be successful in college. His last year of high school he made social gains by having a girlfriend and had made friends while away from home for several weeks in the summer.

At the same time, there were several aspects of this case predictive of a negative transition outcome. First was the patient's and family's repeated habit of not attending regular psychiatric appointments when he was doing well. He and his parents only came when he had an exacerbation of his symptoms and until he had stabilized with medication interventions. He required multiple antidepressant medication trials before remission occurred suggesting that his depression would be more difficult to treat. The most significant negative predictive factor was the avoidance of planning for continued mental health care at both colleges he attended. His first college was remote with extremely limited, accessible services. And, he and his parents were reluctant to engage in the significant mental health services available at his second college, on or off campus. His near suicide attempts in high school and college seemed to come with little warning suggesting the need for clear oversight and vigilance. Another possible factor contributing to a negative outcome was the decision to choose a 2-year college, requiring a transfer to complete his bachelor's degree. His anxiety over transfer in as a junior could have contributed to the recurrence of his depression. With a recurrence of his depression at the first college, relapse at his second college was predictable.

Colin had two suboptimal transitions. He experienced two recurrences of his depression, both in the fall of his first year at each school, one requiring hospitalization and one with psychotic features. Resources available at his first college were inadequate for his needs and at the second school, Colin did not take full advantage of the available services. Fortunately, Colin had supports who intervened during his suicide attempts and he responded quickly to medication so he was able to successfully complete his coursework without needing to withdraw from classes or suffer any academic failures. He may have avoided a worsening of his illness, a hospitalization, unneeded disruptions in schooling, and may have not taken a voluntary leave if supports and monitoring had been put in place.

In this case, there were several aspects of transition preparation and planning that could have been approached differently and improved Colin's transition outcome. Colin and his family had an expectation, perhaps related to his mother's own mental health treatment process, that Colin's psychiatrist would remain with him through several geographic and life transitions, would essentially be available to manage crises, and would work remotely. Given Mom's professional success despite a serious mental illness and Colin's productive and safe senior year of high school while on medication, it is understandable that, as in many cases, the family, patient, and provider want to continue with a successful treatment relationship.

The treating provider could have been more forceful in insisting that some sessions be held to address transition preparation and transfer of care planning. These sessions could have focused on several topics: (1) the family's seeming lack of appreciation of the seriousness of Colin's illness particularly in the context of his vulnerable developmental stage; (2) the patient's and family's avoidance of investigating mental health treatment options at the colleges he was interested in during the college application and selection process; (3) the known triggers for Colin's depressed mood and suicidal ideation and how to manage them, including both self-induced and parental pressure to succeed; (4) how depression may interface with college academic and social demands; and (5) how to enhance Colin's daily living skills and independent health management skills before he heads off to school. The provider could also have insisted on more proactive, clear, and thorough transfer of care planning with measures of accountability built in. At the first college, this would have meant regular phone contact as well as planning in advance to schedule visits when he returned home on college breaks. At the second college, this would have meant the provider maintaining the importance of securing on/near campus care to substitute for or augment the care by the CAP and perhaps taking a more active role in establishing connections with new providers. With a treatment team at the second college, Colin may have been more successful in finding a comfortable peer group, would not have had a second mental health crisis, and perhaps would not have decided to take a leave of absence.

With regard to the IHE themselves, given the lack of easily accessible psychiatric services at the first college, it would make sense for the institution to provide a list of local pediatricians, internists, or family practitioners willing to share medication management possibilities with home providers. And, being remote, the college needs to have plans for managing a suicidal student and getting the student safely to a distant hospital or home. As in this case, hospitalization is often necessary when depressed patients become suicidal. Ideally, colleges develop relationships with local psychiatric hospitals to refer students when necessary. For both institutions, although Colin was not placed on formal medical leave status, it would be prudent to have return to school guidelines, particularly after a suicide attempt.

Clinical Pearls

- Depression is often a recurrent illness. When it occurs young in life not only is there more time for other depressive episodes to occur, but the depressive illness may evolve into other illnesses such as bipolar disorder or schizophrenia. It is important to remind parents and patients of this, monitor for recurrence, and develop a plan for how to address recurrences when they occur.
- Do not be afraid to help patients consider how a college's distance from home may affect a student's mental health. Some students might find being a distance away from family healthy and others, particularly those with chronic or recurrent mental illness, need to be closer to family in order to have a support system to remain stable.
- Many young adults find transitions difficult others thrive on change. For those that have difficulty making friends and finding a peer group choosing a college path that requires transfers (i.e., community college with transfer to a 4-year institution) may make them more susceptible to having a recurrence of their illness
- Encourage families to consider more than academics and selectivity when choosing a college. Finding a school with the best fit social environment as well as resources and supports for students with mental illness is often the best path. A selective college will not help with a student's career goals if they are unable to finish due to an exacerbation of their mental illness.
- Do not be afraid to express objection when you feel that a patient's college choice and transfer of care plan is inadequate. A psychoanalytic silent stance is not needed here. Your opinions need to be expressed. It is acceptable to discuss your standard of patient care and, in extreme cases, to responsibly and ethically discuss and execute termination of care for non-compliance.
- If medication management from afar is being considered for stable patients when they leave for college, discuss your and their expectations beforehand to prevent misunderstandings and poor outcomes later. How frequently will you meet?

How will phone sessions be handled and paid for? How will emergencies be handled? How much medication will be made available at any one time and how many refills will be authorized between patient encounters?

- When high school students are in their senior year encourage their families to let them become more responsible for managing their mental health care such as taking their medications, ensuring that medications are refilled, and scheduling/keeping appointments. This can provide an indication of how responsible they will become when they are away at college.

- In most cases, parents know their children the best and can serve as a part of a safety net by establishing a regular communication plan with their transitioning child via phone, and/or some sort of video-conferencing, and regular (perhaps spontaneous) visits to campus.

- Given the increased demands placed on youth with mental illness who are transitioning to college, it is often necessary for the CAP to take a more active role in helping them establish follow-up care.

Brief Literature Review

In a recent literature review of studies of depression in university students, the mean prevalence of depression was found to be 30.6% with prevalence rates ranging from 10 to 85% [1]. The authors note that this is higher than the general U.S. depression prevalence of 9%. In a survey of students across 26 college campuses, the overall incidence of any form of depression was 17.3% and women had a slightly higher prevalence of major depression than men (10% vs. 7.5%; $p < 0.01$) [2]. The authors also found that Asian, Hispanic, and African American students had slightly higher rates of depression when compared to white students. Iarovici [3] notes that African American college students are at increased risk for depression and that they under-utilize campus counseling services. She also cautions that other diverse students may minimize mood symptoms and may avoid seeking help for various reasons.

The stressors of college and transition from family to independence are a susceptible period for the development of depression. Young adulthood is also a vulnerable time for the new onset of mental health disorders. It is also widely known that suicide is the second leading cause of death in college students. Still, there may be an advantage to being in the college environment and having easier access to treatment options and other supports leading to prevention of actual suicide attempts [4]. A recent study found that college students had lower rates of suicide attempts when compared to part-time and non-college attending young adults [5].

When evaluating college students with depression it can be difficult to distinguish the effect of substance use disorders on depressive symptoms as few college students abstain from use of alcohol. Alcohol and drug abuse can contribute to dysphoria making diagnosis difficult [3]. The decision to prescribe antidepressants to depressed college students who are abusing substances is a difficult one. Tolliver [6] summarizes the current evidence for treating mood disorders in the context of substance abuse. Other confounders in diagnosing depression in college students include the ebb and flow of mood which can come with the changes in stress over the course of the academic year [3] and seasonal changes in weather, especially for those students who move from geographic locations without marked seasons.

In a recent survey of college students, it was found that the top three concerns were academic performance, pressure to succeed and post-graduation plans. Relevant to this case, the most stressed, anxious, and depressed students were found to be transfer students and upperclassmen [7]. Many adolescents have significant difficulties developing a regular sleep schedule in high school, often staying up late to finish projects and study, a pattern that initially continues into college. In a study looking at sleep deprivation among college students, it was found it was linked to lower grade point average, impaired mood, increased risk of academic failure, and a higher rate of motor vehicle crashes [8].

Treatment of depression should consider evidence-based medications and therapies. Many therapy types such as cognitive behavioral, psychodynamic, interpersonal, and mindfulness can be used with college students although the evidence-base remains preliminary [3, 9]. A meta-analysis found that various psychological treatments were equally helpful in college students as in other adult populations [10]. Treatment selection should be based on the unique clinical needs of each individual patient and a provider's clinical judgement.

Helpful Resources

- Patient Health Questionnaire-9. http://www.phqscreeners.com/sites/g/files/g10016261/f/201412/PHQ-9_English.pdf

References

1. Ibrahim AK, Kelly SJ, Adams CE, Glazebrook C. A systematic review of studies of depression prevalence in university students. J Psychiatr Res. 2013;47(3):391–400.
2. Eisenberg D, Hunt J, Speer N. Mental health in American colleges and universities: variation across student subgroups and across campuses. J Nerv Ment Dis. 2013;201(1):60–7.
3. Iarovici D. Mental health issues and the university student. Baltimore: JHU Press; 2014. p. 140–51. Depression and other mood problems.
4. Drum DJ, Brownson C, Burton Denmark A, Smith SE. New data on the nature of suicidal crises in college students: shifting the paradigm. Prof Psychol Res Pr. 2009;40(3):213–22.
5. Han B, Compton WM, Eisenberg D, Milazzo-Sayre L, McKeon R, Hughes A. Prevalence and mental health treatment of suicidal ideation and behavior among college students aged 18–25 years and their non-college-attending peers in the United States. J Clin Psychiatry. 2016;77(6):815–24.
6. Tolliver BK, Anton RF. Assessment and treatment of mood disorders in the context of substance abuse. Dialogues Clin Neurosci. 2015;17(2):181.
7. Beiter R, Nash R, McCrady M, Rhoades D, Linscomb M, Clarahan M, Sammut S. The prevalence and correlates of depression, anxiety, and stress in a sample of college students. J Affect Disord. 2015;173:90–6.

8. Hershner SD, Chervin RD. Causes and consequences of sleepiness among college students. Nat Sci Sleep. 2014;6:73–84.

9. McIndoo CC, File AA, Preddy T, Clark CG, Hopko DR. Mindfulness-based therapy and behavioral activation: a randomized controlled trial with depressed college students. Behav Res Ther. 2016;77:118–28.

10. Cuijpers P, Cristea IA, Ebert DD, Koot HM, Auerbach RP, Bruffaerts R, Kessler RC. Psychological treatment of depression in college students: a metaanalysis. Depress Anxiety. 2016;33(5):400–14.

"There's No Place Like Home": The Challenge of Going to College with Separation Anxiety Disorder

Dara Sakolsky

Case History

Sarah is an 18-year-old Caucasian female who presents to the college counseling center due to increased anxiety and panic attacks. She reports that panic attacks began 3 weeks prior to the start of college. Panic attack symptoms include shortness of breath, increased heart rate, diaphoresis, shaking, dizziness, nausea, and emesis. She reports 4–5 panic attacks per day since moving into the dormitory. She was seen at the local emergency room two nights ago due to panic symptoms and dehydration. In the emergency room, she was given intravenous fluids, lorazepam, ondansetron, and discharged to home with recommendation to follow-up with her primary care physician. Sarah admits excessive worries about change and separation from her mom and boyfriend. She denies anxiety about academics, finances, health, or judgement by others. She denies untriggered panic attacks. She reports increased irritability, low mood, anhedonia, hypersomnia, anergia, decreased appetite, and hopelessness over the past 2 weeks. She denies passive or active suicidal ideation. She denies symptoms of mania, psychosis, posttraumatic stress disorder, eating disorder, or substance use disorder. Sarah has a family history of depression and has been diagnosed with exercise-induced asthma and celiac disease.

Sarah is the youngest of three siblings. Her parents were divorced when she was young and she was raised primarily by her mom. After the divorce, Sarah continued to have contact with her dad every other weekend until 4th grade when he moved out of state. Sarah continues to see her dad a few times of year on holidays or summer vacations. She has maintained a close group of friends since middle school and

D. Sakolsky, M.D., Ph.D.
Department of Psychiatry, University of Pittsburgh, School of Medicine, Pittsburgh, PA, USA

Western Psychiatric Institute and Clinic, University of Pittsburgh Medical Center, Pittsburgh, PA, USA
e-mail: sakolskydj@upmc.edu

© Springer International Publishing AG, part of Springer Nature 2018
A. Martel et al. (eds.), *Promoting Safe and Effective Transitions to College for Youth with Mental Health Conditions*, https://doi.org/10.1007/978-3-319-68894-7_12

has been dating her boyfriend for 2 years. She graduated in the top 50% of her class from a competitive public high school. She is a freshman in communications at a small, suburban, mid-Atlantic university.

Sarah was diagnosed at age 8 with separation anxiety disorder and treated with psychotherapy for 1 year. With improved coping skills, she was able to sleep alone by age 9. Since symptoms improved with therapy alone, medication was not recommended. Sarah continued to avoid sleepovers in middle and high school except with her best friend. She was able to participate in band trips throughout high school since Mom traveled with the band as a chaperone. During her freshman year of high school, Sarah reported 6 months of depressed mood with loss of interest, hypersomnia, weight loss, and low energy, but did not seek treatment. During her junior year of high school, she was evaluated by a child and adolescent psychiatrist after her mom canceled vacation plans with friends because Sarah was feeling "too anxious" to stay with her aunt and uncle while her mom traveled. Although cognitive behavior therapy (CBT) was recommended, Sarah and her mom did not feel that her separation anxiety disorder symptoms were problematic enough to restart therapy. The child and adolescent psychiatrist discussed that separation anxiety disorder may interfere with Sarah's future plans to attend college. Sarah remarked that she was planning to apply only to schools within a short drive from home and that she would be able to manage. Mom supported this plan since she described Sarah as independent in other ways that would help her in college. Sarah kept track of her school assignments, completed homework, did chores around the house, and had a consistent group of friends. The child and adolescent psychiatrist also recommended that Sarah attempt several separations from Mom (e.g., weekend trip with friends, overnight summer camp, or weeklong summer enrichment program on a local college campus) to determine how she will cope with extended separations from her mom.

Sarah chose to attend a small, suburban university approximately 30 min from her home and made plans to room with a friend from high school. Sarah did well academically in her senior year and had no difficulty with anxiety since she did not engage in any extended separation from her mom and boyfriend. In the summer before starting college, she attended a weekend freshman orientation program at her college with her friend, managed the experience with much anxiety, but felt hopeful for her upcoming transition to living on campus. Given that Sarah was not in active treatment, no formal transfer of care plans were made. The family continued to make adjustments to their schedule and activities to help with Sarah's anxiety.

One week after starting school, Sarah was accompanied by her mom for the initial assessment at the counseling center with a licensed professional counselor. She was scheduled to see the psychiatrist the following day given the severity of anxiety symptoms and recent emergency room visit. Sarah was diagnosed with separation anxiety disorder with panic attacks and major depressive disorder, recurrent episode, moderate. On examination, she appeared dehydrated and vital signs revealed orthostatic hypotension and tachycardia. She also endorsed dizziness with standing. With Sarah's consent, Mom was brought into the appointment and collateral history was obtained to confirm the diagnoses. It was recommended that she return to emergency department for additional medical treatment (i.e., more intravenous fluids) since Sarah continued show signs of significant dehydration. Effective treatments for separation anxiety disorder including CBT, selective serotonin reuptake inhibitors (SSRIs), and their combination were discussed. Initial treatment recommendation involved commuting to campus for the initial weeks of school to temporarily reduce anxiety while medication was started, skills were learned, and gradual exposures performed. Sarah's mom requested a prescription for a benzodiazepine since the lorazepam given in the emergency room was "very effective" at reducing Sarah's anxiety. Given that hypotension and dizziness are common side effects of benzodiazepines and that Sarah was currently experiencing these problems, the psychiatrist explained that a benzodiazepine would likely result in more harm than benefit at this time. The psychiatrist recommended starting fluoxetine once Sarah was medically stable.

Sarah began weekly CBT sessions with a therapist at college counseling center. She was sleeping in her dormitory room Sunday through Thursday and returning home on weekends. At her follow-up appointment 10 days later with the college counseling center's psychiatrist, Sarah reported continued worries about being apart from family and difficulty making new friends. She denied full symptom panic attacks, but reported episodes of nausea and shakiness when worrying. She also described worsening mood with low motivation, hopelessness, and social isolation. She denied suicidal ideation, plan, or intent. She had not started fluoxetine due to concern about side effects, but was taking alprazolam 0.5 mg, 3–4 times per week when feeling acutely anxious and ondansetron 4 mg, 2–3 time per week for acute nausea. Both medications were prescribed by the emergency room physician whom she saw after her initial appointment with the psychiatrist. Risks, benefits, and side effects of fluoxetine and alprazolam were discussed in detail. The psychiatrist recommended stopping alprazolam and starting fluoxetine to target separation anxiety disorder and depression. Additional recommendations included commuting to school for the next month to reduce anxiety while engaging in planned overnight exposures to campus life with support of therapist.

Despite weekly therapy and taking fluoxetine 20 mg daily for 1 month, Sarah's separation anxiety and depressive symptoms persisted. She began losing weight and her concentration became problematic. Sarah started to have difficulty attending class. Given her worsening condition, a higher level of care was recommended. She was referred to a transitional age intensive outpatient program (IOP) and her dose of fluoxetine was increased to 40 mg daily. Sarah initially declined the recommendation for IOP; however, after performing poorly on midterm exams, she accepted a referral to the transitional age IOP, dropped two classes, and began living at home full time. For the rest of the semester, she commuted to campus 2 days per week and traveled to IOP at a nearby academic medical center 3 days per week. By the start of her spring semester, Sarah's depression had remitted and anxiety was lowered by fluoxetine 80 mg daily and effective use of CBT skills. Sarah worked with her therapist at the college counseling center on gradually spending more time on campus and sleeping more nights in her dorm room. By the end of the spring semester, Sarah was able to live on campus full time.

Analysis of Transition

Several factors indicated that Sarah might have a successful transition to college. First, Sarah was fortunate to select a college with excellent mental health resources. The university counseling center had walk-in crisis appointments, therapists who provide evidence-based treatments, no limits on the number of therapy sessions, and a psychiatrist on staff who worked closely with the other treatment providers. Second, Sarah had intelligently chosen a university that was located close enough to home, so she could commute if her separation anxiety symptoms began to impair her functioning at school. Third, Sarah had chosen to room with a friend from high school that she already had a positive relationship. This allowed Sarah to avoid the additional stress of living with an unfamiliar person during the start of college. Fourth, Sarah quickly identified her need for mental health treatment and sought help through her university counseling center early in the academic year. Lastly, Sarah demonstrated college readiness in several domains of functioning. She was a solid student academically with good organizational and time management skills. She also had experience with daily living skills (e.g., laundry, cooking, and managing money). Thus, several positive factors signaled that Sarah might have a smooth transition to college.

Other factors suggested that Sarah might have a more difficult time transitioning to college. Since Sarah was not actively engaged in treatment during her senior year of high school, she and her family did not develop a specific transfer of care plan. Additionally, both Sarah and her mom failed to recognize the importance of adequately treating her separation anxiety disorder prior to starting college. Many of the symptoms and much of the functional impairment caused by separation anxiety disorder can be masked by parental accommodations while children and adolescents are living at home. For example, Sarah was able to participate in developmentally appropriate activities such as band trips without enduring separation from her primary attachment figure since her mom attended these trips as a chaperone. Likewise, parents of adolescents who have separation anxiety disorder become active with their child's sports or academic team and travel regularly with the group. In summary, Sarah and her family's limited insight into the severity of her anxiety disorder, modest treatment prior to college, and no specific transfer of care plan contributed to her difficult transition to college.

This case exemplifies a failed transition to college since the patient experienced a dramatic increase in her anxiety symptoms at the start of college which precipitated a major depressive episode and eventually lead to a reduction in her academic course load, returning home to live and IOP level of care. If several aspects of the transition preparation were carried out differently, a better outcome may have been achieved.

Adolescents with separation anxiety disorder may tolerate day long separations from parents without difficulty and only develop symptoms during separations of greater length. To realistically assess college readiness in youth with history of separation anxiety disorder, separations of adequate duration and distance are needed. Because the opportunity for this type of experience occurs infrequently, it is important to start the process early. Students in middle school should be encouraged to attend overnight school trips and sleepover summer camp experiences. High school students should participate in week long trips of greater distances (e.g., French club trip to Montreal, band trip to Disney World, or youth group trip with their church or synagogue). If youth with history of separation anxiety disorder are able to complete these types of experiences in middle school and high school, parents and clinicians can be more confident in their college readiness. If youth experience significant anxiety during extended separations or need to return home early, then additional treatment including systematic desensitization with an experienced CBT therapist is indicated to help prepare for college.

Clinical Pearls

- Symptoms of separation anxiety may not be observable in older teens and young adults unless they engage in separations of extended duration and/or distance. If youth are unable to complete extended separations, treatment with CBT, an SSRI, or their combination (CBT and SSRI) should be recommended.
- If separation anxiety disorder persists during the senior year of high school, youth should consider education options close to home (e.g., branch campus of a large university or community college) for at least their first year. It is often difficult to transfer credits among traditional four colleges, so advanced information gathering is needed to make a good choice if the student plans to transfer after the first year or two.
- Parental accommodation can mask symptoms of separation anxiety disorder and contribute to the maintenance of the disorder. Child and adolescent psychiatrists have a role in assessing for parental accommodation, educating parents that their well-meaning behaviors can have unintended negative consequences, and promoting change in family behavior.
- Youth with separation anxiety disorder are likely to experience exacerbation of comorbid disorders (e.g., major depressive disorder, generalized anxiety disorder, or social anxiety disorder) during the transition to college. Thus, transition planning is very important in this group of patients.
- If young adults experience impairing separation anxiety symptoms during their first weeks of college, commuting to school for the first month to reduce anxiety while engaging in treatment may be necessary in order to promote academic success.
- If anxiety symptoms lead to significant academic impairment despite appropriate treatment, a reduction in course load and referral to high level of care (e.g., transitional age IOP) may help to avoid medical withdrawal from school.

Brief Literature Review

The epidemiology of separation anxiety disorder has been well studied in youth, but until recently much less was known about separation anxiety disorder in adults. Cross sectional data from the National Comorbidity Survey Replication found lifetime prevalence of childhood and adult separation anxiety disorder are 4.1% and 6.6%, respectively [1]. In the National Comorbidity Survey Replication, 36% of childhood cases persist into adulthood while 77% of adult cases have first onset in adulthood. According to the National Comorbidity Survey Replication, the majority of childhood onset cases began in early or middle childhood and the majority of adult onset cases began in late teens or early 20s. Cross-sectional data from the World Mental Health Survey found lifetime prevalence of separation anxiety disorder averaged 4.8% across countries, with 43.1% of onsets occurring after the age 18 [2]. In the World Mental Health Survey, 12-month prevalence rates were considerably lower than lifetime prevalence rates (1% vs. 4.8%) and median persistence of the disorder was 4–8 years. In contrast, longitudinal data from the Great Smoky Mountains Study showed that separation anxiety disorder affects 4% of 9–10 year olds, 1% of 11–12 year olds, <1% of those 13–14, 15–16, 19, 21, and 24–26 years old with cumulative rate of 5% by age 26 [3]. Consistent among these studies is a relatively common (5–7%) lifetime prevalence of separation anxiety disorder. Adult cross sectional data suggest that a large percent of adults with separation anxiety develop the onset of their disorder after age 18. Given the distorting influence of recall bias and differing results between cross sectional and longitudinal studies, it remains possible that most cases of adult separation anxiety disorder are reemergence of symptoms from childhood. Additional longitudinal data is needed to further clarify this matter.

Only two studies have systematically examined separation anxiety disorder in college students. Ollendick and colleagues [4] used questionnaires to identify first semester college students who reported symptoms consistent with the diagnostic criteria for separation anxiety (*separation anxiety group*, $n = 20$), students without separation anxiety disorder but similar history of childhood mood and anxiety disorders (diagnostic control group, $n = 20$), and students without current separation anxiety disorder or past mood and anxiety disorders (normal control group, $n = 20$). The separation anxiety group reported higher levels of trait anxiety, anxiety sensitivity, and depressive symptoms than the diagnostic or normal control groups. The separation anxiety disorder group also reported more difficulty in adapting to college in social, personal-emotional, and institutional attachment domains when compared to diagnostic or normal control groups. Seligman and Wuyek [5] used questionnaires to collect information on symptoms of separation anxiety, educational decisions, and academic performance in first semester college students ($n = 190$). This study found 21% ($n = 39$) of the students endorsed symptoms meeting diagnostic criteria for separation anxiety disorder. Students who reported higher levels of separation anxiety also endorsed greater childhood separation anxiety symptoms, experienced more panic attacks in the weeks leading up to the start of college, and were attending college closer to home. Both studies found no correlation between levels of separation anxiety and academic performance during the first semester. These preliminary studies show that separation anxiety disorder is common in youth transitioning to college and these young adults are more likely to struggle in adapting to college life.

Helpful Resources

- Anxiety and Depression Association of America www.adaa.org
- Webinar: Back-to-School Anxiety in High School and College presented by Ann Marie Albano http://www.adaa.org/living-with-anxiety/ask-and-learn/webinars#children teens and young adults

References

1. Shear K, Jin R, Ruscio AM, Walters EE, Kessler RC. Prevalence and correlates of estimated DSM-IV child and adult separation anxiety disorder in the national comorbidity survey replication (NCS-R). Am J Psychiatry. 2006;163(6):1074–83.
2. Silove D, Alonso J, Bromet E, Gruber M, Sampson N, Scott K, Andrade L, Benjet C, Caldas de Almeida JM, De Girolamo G, de Jonge P, Demyttenaere K, Fiestas F, Florescu S, Gureje O, He Y, Karam E, Lepine JP, Murphy S, Villa-Posada J, Zarkov Z, Kessler RC. Pediatric-onset and adult-onset separation anxiety disorder across countries in the world mental health survey. Am J Psychiatry. 2015;172(7):647–56.
3. Copeland WE, Angold A, Shanahan L, Costello EJ. Longitudinal patterns of anxiety from childhood to adulthood: the Great Smoky Mountains Study. J Am Acad Child Adolesc Psychiatry. 2014;53(1):21–33.
4. Ollendick TH, Lease CA, Cooper C. Separation anxiety in young adults: a preliminary examination. J Anxiety Disord. 1993;7(4):293–305.
5. Seligman LD, Wuyek LA. Correlates of separation anxiety symptoms among first-semester college students: an exploratory study. J Psychol. 2007;141(2):135–45.

Elisabeth M. Kressley, Adele Martel, and Jennifer Derenne

Case History

Jennifer (Jen) is a 22-year-old Caucasian female, eldest of three siblings, from an intact family. She resides in an urban setting. She was in the top 20% of her public high school class. Both of her parents are college graduates and work full time. She was diagnosed with both Social Anxiety Disorder (SAD) and Major Depressive Disorder, in remission, prior to transitioning to college.

Jen was initially seen in the middle of her Sophomore year of high school, after being referred to a CAP by her therapist for depressed mood, low energy, and ongoing social avoidance. She appeared uncomfortably shy, visibly blushing, and making little eye contact. She spoke softly and with normal prosody. Mannerisms were diminished but appropriate. She quietly requested that Mom remain in the room for the evaluation. Jen endorsed symptoms of depression. Mom reported that since starting high school, Jen had become increasingly anxious in the classroom. She

E.M. Kressley, M.D. (✉)
Child Study Center, Yale School of Medicine, Yale University, New Haven, CT, USA
e-mail: elisemd@sbcglobal.net

A. Martel, M.D., Ph.D.
Division of Child and Adolescent Psychiatry, Department of Psychiatry and Behavioral Sciences, Ann and Robert H. Lurie Children's Hospital of Chicago, Northwestern University Feinberg School of Medicine, Chicago, IL, USA
e-mail: adele.martel@gmail.com

J. Derenne, M.D.
Division of Child and Adolescent Psychiatry, Department of Psychiatry and Behavioral Sciences, Stanford University School of Medicine, Lucile Packard Children's Hospital, Stanford, CA, USA
e-mail: jderenne@stanford.edu

© Springer International Publishing AG, part of Springer Nature 2018
A. Martel et al. (eds.), *Promoting Safe and Effective Transitions to College for Youth with Mental Health Conditions*, https://doi.org/10.1007/978-3-319-68894-7_13

was fearful of being called upon by teachers, rarely volunteered to respond to questions even when she knew the answer, and had refused to give oral presentations. Jen took pride in her schoolwork and had always been an excellent student. Both she and her mom were concerned that her fear of speaking in class had begun to impact her grades. Jen conversed with a few peers at school, who like her, were focused on academics, but did not see them outside of school due to feeling anxious. She did not currently participate in any extracurricular activities though had been in Yearbook Club in junior high. She spoke openly to the CAP about her sexual attraction to females. However, she felt too awkward to talk and engage with others, and this made it difficult for her to begin dating. She denied self-harming behaviors and suicidal thinking. There was no history of trauma and she denied use of alcohol and other illicit substances. Mom described Jen as always being shy and clingy around new people and in novel situations. Family history was notable for Mom with Anxiety Disorder NOS and older brother with OCD. Jen was diagnosed with Major Despressive Disorder, Recurrent, Moderate, and Social Anxiety Disorder.

Per Jen, and confirmed by the referring therapist, Jen first experienced symptoms of depression and anxiety in junior high school. She also had a few incidences of superficial cutting and passive suicidal ideation. With much persistence on the part of her mother and with much reluctance on her part, Jen went to see a therapist. Therapy was supportive in nature and focused on communication patterns in the family and on Jen's sexual identity.

Historically, Jen and her mother had little communication with one another. Her mother had worked when she was younger and Jen had developed greater ease in communicating with her father. Both Jen and her mother yearned for a more open, communicative relationship, but did not know how best to approach it. Jen said she was shy and introverted like her mother, who enjoyed quiet, restorative time, pursuing independent interests. Her mother was fearful of saying the wrong things to Jen. Regarding her sexual preference, Jen worried that her parents might be angry and disappointed in her and reject her. This issue contributed to her anxiety and depressed mood resulting in increased social isolation from peers as she felt she could not be herself around them or her family. When made aware of her sexual orientation, her parents were accepting and supportive. Once these issues were more settled, Jen's mood and anxiety improved and she saw her therapist every 4–6 weeks. At one of these check-up visits, it was apparent that Jen's depression and anxiety had worsened, which precipitated the referral to the psychiatrist.

Jen was started on an SSRI and resumed weekly visits with her therapist, who provided psychoeducation on social anxiety and worked with her on relaxation strategies. Jen was also followed by the school guidance counselor, who advocated with Jen's teachers to allow for oral presentations to be done in a small group of select peers outside of class time. There was no formal IEP or 504 plan put into place, as neither the patient nor her mother wanted more attention drawn to Jen. Over the next few months, Jen's depression improved to full remission. The social anxiety was somewhat improved and more manageable. She spent time with one friend, outside of school, once or twice per month. She reluctantly got a part-time job stocking shelves at a small, local grocery store the summer before junior year and held that job through high school. She made more eye contact, blushed less, and spoke louder in sessions with the CAP. Jen went to all follow-up appointments accompanied by her mom. With much encouragement, Jen met with the CAP alone for 10 min of each half hour monthly medication follow-up session but she continued to mostly depend on her mom for reporting on her status. She refused to join any clubs at school and she avoided participation in drivers' education to get her permit as she felt it would be an awkward situation.

After consultation with each other, the CAP and therapist suggested that Jen see a therapist with expertise in CBT with the hope of further improving her understanding of social anxiety and to develop more advanced skills in managing her symptoms. Jen was fearful of meeting a new therapist. Given that her grades at school remained high, likely due to her intelligence, academic drive, and informal accommodations, Jen's parents did not force the issue. She began to see her therapist less frequently and by the end of her junior year was seeing her on a once per month basis. Both the CAP and therapist offered ongoing support and monitoring, continued to suggest CBT-focused therapy, provided some self-help resources, and began discussions with Jen and her parents about heading to college.

Jen attained high grades in junior year of high school and, other than accommodating her need for an alternative setting for oral presentations and not calling upon her in class, teachers were not aware of any other anxiety issues. She managed her academic work independently. She also took care of her personal hygiene and set her own wake-up alarm. She still needed reminders to take her medication. There were very few expectations of her at home with regard to life skills and chores such as cleaning, doing laundry, and preparing meals.

Jen was accepted to an all-female, small, urban, liberal arts college, quite a distance from her home. She had only applied to three schools and preferred to go to a single sex school. Neither distance nor academic majors/programs offered were factors in her decision-making. She enjoyed learning but had not yet determined her interests or thought about future career options.

While she was applying to schools in the late fall of senior year, Jen's providers let her and her family know that they would need to transition both psychiatric care and therapy to the counseling center on campus. Together, they reviewed the supports she had been utilizing, which included twice per month mental health visits, regular visits with her school guidance counselor, and classroom supports. Jen was likely to have ongoing therapeutic needs that would best be addressed locally, and on-campus providers would have familiarity and knowledge of other resources, such as disabilities services, and how to navigate them. This was reiterated after she made her final decision in the spring.

As advised, the family called the counseling center prior to the end of the college's current school year, and learned that weekly therapy was available but an initial appointment could not be made until freshman orientation. Only after establishing care with a campus therapist would Jen be referred to the college's consulting psychiatrist. Her parents had done most things for her in terms of arranging appointments and advocating for her, so they were unsure of her own independent initiative, and were anxious that she would not attend counseling sessions. Jen reassured them that she would make an appointment once on campus.

Given her diagnosis of SAD, as well as identifying as an introvert who needed alone time to recharge and refresh, Jen and her parents were anxious about the stress of having a roommate. Jen was also concerned about undressing and sleeping next to a female roommate. The family formally requested a single room and the psychiatrist wrote a supporting letter. The college granted the request.

She saw her home psychiatrist and therapist throughout the summer and it was decided that, in addition to seeing new providers on campus, she would see them on breaks from school. The CAP worked with Jen and her family on using a pill box and her cell phone's alarm to take her medications independently. Both providers cautioned Jen about the availability of alcohol and other drugs on campus and how she was vulnerable for misuse given her social anxiety. Jen signed releases of information so that both home providers could communicate with the college counseling center.

Despite these plans, Jen did not make an appointment at the counseling center and so did not establish care with a new psychiatrist. Her mother was concerned and reached out to the home CAP frequently. It was suggested that she assist Jen in setting up an appointment and then facilitate getting her to the first one to establish contact. Mother did this and Jen went to the first appointment, but remained intermittently noncompliant thereafter.

During mid-semester break, both home providers were concerned that Jen was becoming depressed again. She appreciated the academic focus of college. However, her classes were challenging and she avoided going for extra help during her professors' office hours. She did not ask questions in class. Though she talked with a few peers for team-based class projects, she skipped class on the days her group made presentations. She was upset about her C mid-term grades in three of five classes. She was cordial with her hall mates but was socially isolated. She was not involved in any clubs or on-campus activities. She was again strongly encouraged to attend weekly therapy sessions, establish a relationship with a treating psychiatrist at school, and connect with the ODS at school with the help of the school therapist. In response to a phone message from the CAP describing multiple concerns, the school therapist did not feel they could reach out and encourage Jen to attend visits given she was an adult and that their services were voluntary.

Between semesters, Jen reported that she saw the campus therapist more regularly and found him to be a good support. She still had not been referred to a psychiatrist or the ODS and did not question why referrals had not been made. The therapist encouraged Jen to get involved with the LGBTQ student organization on campus and she attended one meeting. Jen also participated in a few dorm events that semester which surprised her CAP. Jen quietly stated that she found if she had a glass of alcohol or a beer before meeting friends she was more comfortable conversing and participating in the group process. The CAP cautioned Jen against this approach and together they decided to increase Jen's SSRI dose. The medication change was small due to the lack of an identified prescriber at college to monitor side effects or efficacy.

Jen and her parents were disappointed in her final grades of Bs and Cs. At their request, the home CAP wrote a letter for second semester requesting that the professors be made aware of the social anxiety and to assist Jen in her self-advocacy skills. While agreeing to do this, the home CAP left a message for the school therapist about Jen's use of alcohol to self-medicate, to ascertain why a referral for accommodations had not been made, and to report the increase in medication.

The therapist finally called the home CAP 6 weeks into the second semester reporting that Jen had been taken to the hospital for alcohol intoxication. Jen's parents were also notified since she was under the age of 21. They made a visit to school to check on her. They accompanied Jen to meetings with the heads of the counseling center, disabilities services office, and the office of student conduct. Jen was given a disciplinary warning and attended a mandatory alcohol education program. She was granted classroom accommodations which helped to some extent but she still had trouble meeting with her professors. She was referred to the campus psychiatrist and met with her only twice before completing the semester with more Bs than Cs this time around. Medication changes were made unilaterally, without communication with the home CAP, despite a release of information and the expectation that the home CAP would see Jen over the summer.

That summer, the CAP firmly told Jen and her family that she needed to maintain a complete treatment team at school that fall, otherwise, medications would no longer be prescribed. If the resources at school were inadequate, then the family was to pursue private providers near school.

Between sophomore and junior years of college, and subsequent to a second alcohol infraction, Jen participated in a young adult IOP program with a focus on social anxiety and substance misuse. Jen ultimately graduated from college with a low B average, below expectations for her IQ. She is living at home and is dating a same sex peer, while working as an aide at a local day care center. She obtained her license during senior year of college. Despite the fact that she is underemployed for her level of education, she is happy with her life and relationships for now. She is still followed by her home doctor and therapist. Her social anxiety, while slightly improved, is still present. The depression is in remission.

Analysis of Transition

In this case, there were several factors that were predictive of a positive outcome. Jen had solid, independent academic and executive functioning skills; she was intelligent and excited about going to college. She was able to form stable relationships with home providers, which suggested that she might be able to do the same in the college setting. She and her parents regularly attended appointments and there was improved communication within the family. Jen was compliant with her medication, including taking them on her own before she left for college. Her depression was responsive to the medication. Jen made some small developmental gains in the last 2 years of high school so she was on a positive trajectory. With the CAP, Jen and her family had proactive, timely and repeated discussions about the need and rationale for transitioning care to campus. They were aware of the resources available on campus and the process to connect to those services. Jen readily signed releases for communication between her home and school teams. She was offered psychoeducation about the risks of alcohol and other substances.

Despite the positives, Jen was at risk for a negative transition outcome for a few reasons. She was socially and emotionally immature and did not seek out normal developmental milestones, such as getting her driver's license, in a timely manner. She was overly dependent on her mother to speak for her and make choices for her so she had little skill or practice with self-advocacy. Jen seemed to have only an elementary understanding of her diagnosis. The school's willingness to provide informal accommodations likely minimized Jen's understanding of their importance. She and her family had declined the recommendation to pursue a course of CBT. In addition, while she had a few friends at high school, these relationships were largely superficial, which did not bode well for making new friends in the college setting. Living in a single room, while more comfortable, may also have inadvertently reinforced her anxiety in social situations. Finally, she seemed nervous about establishing care with a new team, which led to long distance (and therefore less than optimal) psychopharmacologic treatment.

This case represents a suboptimal transition outcome for a number of reasons. Jen was not compliant with the plan to establish care at school, and continued to rely on her parents to advocate for her. She experienced a relapse of depressive symptoms and a resurgence of her social anxiety; Jen turned to alcohol for some relief.

In retrospect, there are a few aspects of transition preparation and planning that could have been approached differently to improve the outcome. First, it is important to assess a patient's readiness for transition in the social domain as well as in the academic domain. It may have been helpful to do more in-session exploration of the family's and Jen's expectations of what college life might look like, and to do a frank assessment of Jen's readiness to assume more independence with regard to social interactions and self-advocacy. In turn, this would have allowed for more specific therapeutic interventions aimed at increasing confidence and practicing these skills prior to matriculation. Perhaps Jen's parents would not have been so easily dismissive of the recommendation for CBT had they viewed college from this perspective. Specific treatment approaches such as exposure and response prevention, systematic desensitization, social pragmatics training, group therapy, and/or role play may have increased Jen's confidence in speaking and advocating for herself.

When there are concerns about readiness, providers should raise the possibility of an alternative postsecondary path with the patient and family. Perhaps a year or two at community college would have exposed Jen to broader social experiences and opportunities for self-advocacy while closer to home and processing with her home treatment team. She may have been better prepared to make her needs known to professors and clinicians on campus. A gap year of travel, volunteer work, or participation in an intensive outpatient program may also have been useful to allow her to develop independence and confidence.

Long-standing family dynamics also likely impacted the transition. Jen's parents often spoke for her and declined some treatment choices based on avoiding discomfort for Jen. After she left for college, they continued to call the CAP with concerns as opposed to having Jen make calls, having three-way calls, or encouraging her to utilize the supports available at school. Their behaviors inadvertently reinforced Jen's social anxiety and needed to be more openly addressed long before college began.

In this case, a transfer of care plan was made, but it was not firmly established given the school's scheduling policies. After Jen failed to make an appointment, it was not clear who was "in charge" of treatment once Jen started college. When worried about Jen, the parents defaulted to calling the home psychiatrist instead of the school. In practice, Jen saw her home providers while at home for breaks. Perhaps a change in the school's policies may have removed one obstacle to continuity of care.

Once Jen's treatment team was more firmly established at the college, neither the therapist nor the prescribing clinician communicated adequately with the home provider. Lack of communication made it impossible for the home psychiatrist to know for certain whether the school treatment team was optimizing Jen's access to on-campus supports and resources. Providers working with college age patients need to recognize that IHE vary greatly in the mental health resources and academic supports that are available on and near campus. There may be limitations on sessions and students may be referred into the nearby community for ongoing treatment. There may be no psychiatrist on campus. Some counseling centers contact students who have missed appointments while others do not. Some counseling centers and the clinicians place high value on communicating with home-based providers. It is important, therefore, for home providers to anticipate challenges and barriers to seeking treatment, and to outline a clear plan for the family to follow in the event that the student relapses.

Clinical Pearls

- When delayed developmental milestones and social and emotional immaturity are present, providers and families may want to consider alternative plans for college such as a gap year or community college.
- Students with inadequately treated SAD may be vulnerable to using alcohol inappropriately in order to comfortably participate in social events. Alcohol is widely available and is part of many campus activities.
- Single rooms may be more comfortable for students with anxiety disorders, but they may also increase the likelihood of avoidant behaviors and may make it difficult for students to integrate fully into the residence hall community.
- Despite the fact that they are adults, students with anxiety disorders who are avoidant may need their *campus* treatment providers to be more active in reaching out to establish contact or reschedule a missed appointment. Likewise, *sending* providers may need to play a more active role in accessing the campus system of care for these transitioning patients.

- It is important to distinguish introversion from anxiety disorders. Being quiet, shy, or preferring time alone is not pathologic. Such personality traits are typically ego-syntonic and do not need to be treated. Symptoms of SAD, on the other hand, are ego-dystonic, distressing, and life-impairing.
- Provide psychoeducation to patients (and families) about their mental health diagnoses, how they may impact functioning in the college environment, and strategies to minimize that impact. This will help students with self-advocacy and navigation of campus resources.
- Mental health resources should be discussed early during college planning. Patients and families should visit counseling centers and explore resources when visiting colleges. Colleges have different mental health and academic support resources, and college-bound patients have different needs.
- When the care plan is going to involve shared treatment between campus and home providers, it is essential for the providers to establish a mutually agreed upon system for regular communication to optimize care of the student/patient.
- It would be helpful for counseling centers to have protocols in place and appropriate staffing so incoming students can schedule appointments in advance of matriculation and be seen within the first 2 weeks of school to avoid gaps in continuity of care.

Brief Literature Review

Social Anxiety Disorder (SAD) has a 12-month prevalence of approximately 7 percent in the U.S. and an average age of onset of about 13 years. In clinical samples, men and women are equally affected or prevalence is slightly higher for males [1] but in the general population females have a higher rate of SAD. For many college students, SAD may be a hidden diagnosis [2], causing significant distress and life impairment. It must be differentiated from temperament and personality constructs of introversion and shyness, which are ego-syntonic and do not require treatment.

Students often experience shame around their peers, as they perceive themselves as less than adequate in comparison. Due to their anxiety, students may avoid classes, thus missing out on information or getting credit for class participation. Or, they may attend, yet not participate for fear of speaking or asking questions. They may have difficulty retaining information due to extreme worry about being called upon. Self-advocacy may be hindered due to their high degree of anxiety and urges to avoid uncomfortable situations [2]. Baptista et al. [3] found that female undergraduates with SAD underachieved academically compared to female controls. Public speaking was the most frequently endorsed fear [3].

SAD is often comorbid with depression, as well as use of alcohol and cannabis. Terlecki et al. noted both an increased risk of alcohol use disorder in those with social anxiety and an increased alcohol consumption in anticipation of interpersonal intimacy and in negative emotion situations [4]. In an analysis of data from the National Epidemiological Survey on Alcohol and Related Conditions [5], SAD was associated with both cannabis abuse and cannabis dependence but more so with dependence.

There are a number of evidence-based psychosocial treatments for SAD [6]. CBT with exposure and response prevention is used to practice mastering anxiety provoking situations as well as challenging unhelpful thinking and addressing misperceptions. Other helpful interventions are individual and group social skills training, CBT delivered in a group setting, systematic desensitization, journaling, and relaxation training. Mindfulness and acceptance based therapies are also beginning to be studied [7]. Of note, the subjects in these studies cover a wide age range, with few done solely with college age youth although this research gap is beginning to be addressed [6, 8]. From a psychopharmacology perspective, there are a few classes of medications to choose from but the SSRIs and serotonin-norepinephrine reuptake inhibitors are the first-line choices for treating SAD [9]. Patients may be vulnerable to misusing benzodiazepines; chronic use should be avoided.

Helpful Resources

- "Social Phobia (Social Anxiety Disorder): Always Embarrassed" https://infocenter.nimh.nih.gov/pubstatic/TR%2013-4678/TR%2013-4678.pdf
- "Depression and College Students" https://www.nimh.nih.gov/health/publications/depression-and-college-students/index.shtml
- Anxiety and Depression Association of America www.adaa.org.
- The Shyness and Social Anxiety Workbook: Proven Step-by-Step Techniques for Overcoming your Fear. Martin M. Antony, Richard Swinson. New Harbinger Publ, (2008).
- Social Anxiety Disorder https://www.adaa.org/sites/default/files/SocialAnxiety Disorder-brochure.pdf
- Frequently Asked Questions for Child, Adolescent, and Adult Psychiatrists and Other Profession-also Working with Transitional Age Youth with Substance Use Disorders http://www.aacap.org/App_Themes/AACAP/Docs/clinical_practice_center/systems_of_care/sud-tay.pdf
- Freedom from Fear (advocacy) http://www.freedomfromfear.org
- Bukstein, Oscar G. (2017) Challenges and Gaps in Understanding Substance Use Problems in Transitional Age Youth. Child and Adolescent Psychiatric Clinics of North America, April 2017, Vol. 26(2), pp. 253–269

References

1. American Psychiatric Association. Diagnostic and statistical manual of mental disorders. 5th ed. Arlington: American Psychiatric Association; 2013.
2. Topham P, Russell G. Social anxiety in higher education. Psychologist. www.thepsychologist. bps.org.uk. 2012;25(4):280–2.
3. Baptista CA, Loureiro SR, de Lima Osorio F, Zuardi AW, Magalhaes PV, Kapczinski F, Filho AS, Freitas-Ferrari MC, Crippa JAS. Social phobia in Brazilian university students: prevalence, under-recognition and academic impairment in women. J Affect Disord. 2007;136(3):857–61.

4. Terlecki MA, Ecker AH, Buckner JD. College drinking problems and social anxiety: the importance of drinking context. Psychol Addict Behav. 2014;28(2):545–52.
5. Buckner JD, Heimberg RG, Schneier FR, Liu SM, Wang S, Blanco C. The relationship between cannabis use disorders and social anxiety disorder in the National Epidemiological Study of Alcohol and Related Conditions (NESARC). Drug Alcohol Depend. 2012;124(1–2):128–34.
6. Baez T. Evidence-based practice for anxiety disorders in college mental health. J College Stud Psychother. 2005;20(1):33–48.
7. Norton AR, Abbott MJ, Norberg MM, Hunt C. A systematic review of mindfulness and acceptance-based treatments for social anxiety disorder. J Clin Psychol. 2015;71(4):283–301.
8. Damer DE, Latimer KM, Porter SH. "Build your social confidence": a social anxiety group for college students. J Spec Group Work. 2010;35(1):7–22.
9. Schneier F. Pharmacotherapy of social anxiety disorder. Expert Opin Pharmacother. 2011; 12(4):615–25.

"Anxiety Galore": Transition to College with Generalized Anxiety Disorder

14

Basheer Lotfi-Fard, Jennifer Derenne, and Adele Martel

Case History

JT is an 18-year-old white male who presented for initial outpatient consultation for help with anxiety the summer between graduating high school and starting college. He was the younger of two children. JT's parents divorced when he was 6 years old. JT and his sister moved to a suburb of a large metropolitan city where he was raised by his mother. His father did not follow them and became estranged from the family. JT developed normally and reached milestones on time. Medical history was significant for hypothyroidism, which was treated and carefully monitored by an endocrinologist. Family history was significant for anxiety and ADHD. He attended a public high school, received average grades, and did not participate in extracurricular activities.

During the first appointment, JT reported problems with anxiety since age 6. At that time, his parents felt that this was due to difficulty coping with their divorce, so

B. Lotfi-Fard, M.D. (✉)
Department of Psychiatry and Behavioral Health, The Ohio State University,
Columbus, OH, USA
e-mail: basheer.lotfi-fard@osumc.edu

J. Derenne, M.D.
Division of Child and Adolescent Psychiatry, Department of Psychiatry and Behavioral
Sciences, Stanford University School of Medicine, Lucile Packard Children's Hospital,
Stanford, CA, USA
e-mail: jderenne@stanford.edu

A. Martel, M.D., Ph.D.
Division of Child and Adolescent Psychiatry, Department of Psychiatry and Behavioral
Sciences, Ann and Robert H. Lurie Children's Hospital of Chicago, Northwestern University
Feinberg School of Medicine, Chicago, IL, USA
e-mail: adele.martel@gmail.com

© Springer International Publishing AG, part of Springer Nature 2018   151
A. Martel et al. (eds.), *Promoting Safe and Effective Transitions to College for Youth
with Mental Health Conditions*, https://doi.org/10.1007/978-3-319-68894-7_14

they did not seek treatment. JT states that although this was one concern, throughout elementary school and middle school he struggled with excessive worries about a variety of issues (e.g., grades, well-being of friends, his competence in academics and gym class compared to his peers, eating healthy foods). He found it hard to control his worries which made it difficult for him to concentrate at school and complete tasks efficiently and this impacted his grades. His worrying also tired him out. Given the family history of ADHD and information from his 6th grade teachers, his pediatrician prescribed a series of stimulant medications over a several month period but none helped with his concentration. His 8th grade teachers, however, noticed that his concentration difficulties were intermittent, across all subjects, and not related to external distractions. JT saw a CAP at the end of 8th grade, close to his 14th birthday, and was diagnosed with Generalized Anxiety Disorder (GAD). Since he and his family had not had therapy targeted to anxiety, the CAP recommended a structured, time-limited, group therapy program which included family psychoeducation sessions. JT developed some skills to assess and manage his anxiety and had some improvement in grades. Given the modest response to CBT and the upcoming transition to high school, the CAP recommended a trial of an SSRI. JT worried that he would not be himself and doubted it would be effective given his experience with stimulants. Instead, JT agreed to continue with CBT-focused individual therapy (with one of the co-leaders of his group therapy program) through the transition to high school. He continued to underperform at school but he had good attendance, good behavior, and a few good friends.

JT's anxiety became significantly worse in the middle of junior year of high school. During this time, JT's biological father contacted the family and informed them that he was moving to be closer to them and wanted to reestablish a relationship. JT was also starting to prepare for his college applications, including taking his ACT and SAT exams. As a result of these stressors, he started feeling restless, irritable, hypersomnic and fatigued. He also had cued panic attacks which included trembling, abdominal distress, fear of losing control, and depersonalization upon awakening and getting ready to attend school. JT began to avoid school due to the significant distress his anxiety caused.

JT's mother, who was also present for the initial appointment, shared her observations. His mother verified that JT's worsening anxiety coincided with his father wanting to return into their lives and attempting to use financial pressure and influence to reestablish a relationship with the family, including assisting with paying for JT's college. Most concerning to his mother was that JT spent most of his day isolated and lying in bed, not wanting to attend school, for the prior 4 weeks. This led to failing grades and he was at risk of not passing classes. At this time, JT's mother was worried about his ability to manage his anxiety. JT's former CAP and CBT therapist were able to see him again. They confirmed the diagnosis of GAD and ruled out other possible concerns including Major Depression and use of alcohol and illicit drugs. JT took clonazepam for 2 weeks while he was titrated to an average dose of an SSRI.

Due to his extended absence, his school developed an IEP to assist with academics and encourage return to school. Accommodations included home instruction, online course work, and extra time to make up incomplete work. Office-based counseling was temporarily changed to home-based counseling and focused on better management of anxiety in the morning so he could attend school. JT attended school on a regular basis throughout senior year and was back on schedule to complete academic requirements and graduate on time. His IEP was modified over time to have extra time for assignments, testing in a quiet area, and extended time on exams. Teachers in all subject areas offered these proactively without JT having to ask. He completed college applications and attended several college interviews.

JT initially aspired to attend the same college as his father and sibling. However, due to poor grades, he was not accepted, and instead planned to attend another university and hoped to transfer after completing freshman year. He chose this university because it was about 2 hours from his home, the cost of tuition and board was reasonable (Father was to pay), and he could easily transfer credits to his desired college. He also felt comfortable knowing that several other students from his high school would attend this college. JT and his family had not considered what his mental health needs might be in making a college choice.

Once he graduated from high school, JT was no longer eligible to be seen in the practice of his original psychiatrist given a strict office policy of ending care at high school completion. This surprised JT and his mother as they anticipated continuing his care into college. Given improvement with anxiety, they needed a new psychiatrist to continue with the SSRI. They obtained a referral from his therapist. At the end of the initial appointment, JT and his mother decided to continue with the new psychiatrist through the summer, and develop a plan for treatment through the transition to college and into the academic year.

During the summer, neither JT nor his mother reported significant difficulty with anxiety. Although JT's mother voiced concern that he spent most of his days lying in bed, he participated in all orientation activities at his college and was making the preparations necessary for starting college. For example, JT knew his future roommate, a classmate from high school, and they were coordinating how best to set up their room. When asked about Mother's concern for excessive time spent in bed, JT said he was using avoidance as a coping tool to get away from negative and stressful interactions with his parents.

The CAP and therapist worked with JT and his mother over the summer on how to best prepare for his upcoming freshman year and plan for ongoing care. The therapist worked on bolstering JT's coping skills and tried to anticipate with him situations on campus which might trigger his anxiety. They discussed the ebb and flow of the academic year and how JT may be fooled into thinking his anxiety was better at times. JT was also able to identify peers who he had a strong relationship with and felt that he could trust for support if needed. The psychiatrist was impressed that JT took his medications independently, along with his thyroid medication. JT was able to identify ways that he had previously dealt with peer pressure regarding underage drinking and drug use.

Regarding ongoing care, JT disagreed with the recommendation that he access counseling services at his college. He stated confidently that being away from his family would decrease stress and allow for better academic performance, and he predicted that he would not need additional counseling. At the insistence of his mother and treatment providers, JT agreed to contact the UCC to schedule an intake appointment once school began, which was when they were going to start taking new referrals. He also agreed to see his home therapist when home on breaks. The UCC did not have a consulting psychiatrist so JT would continue with his home psychiatrist. JT and his mother worked together to plan transportation for routine follow-up visits based on the academic schedule. They were also encouraged to contact the ODS at the university to disclose his previous diagnosis and treatment, including his high school IEP, to ensure that he could receive accommodations, like flexible deadlines, if needed.

JT was seen by his CAP the week before leaving for college and agreed to return for follow-up during Thanksgiving break. He later canceled and rescheduled for winter break. During that appointment, he and his mother reported an initially smooth transition to campus. However, over the course of the semester, as the workload increased and midterms approached, JT's worries became more pronounced and his concentration waned. He worried about fitting in, keeping up with his schoolwork, and not wasting his dad's money. JT felt fatigued. He was having trouble juggling routine tasks like doing laundry, tracking the balance on his student debit card, and getting to the healthy eating alternatives on campus along with managing his academics. He began to miss classes and by the end of the semester was failing two courses. He acknowledged that he did not accurately report the degree and focus of the anxiety he experienced during the summer. He also admitted that, despite having accommodations approved by the university, he was embarrassed to seek assistance from his professors. Due to anxiety and concerns about stigma, JT opted to not seek counseling on campus. Instead, he worked with a therapist his mother found who was initially willing to meet with him using online sessions. However, this therapist soon recommended that he seek treatment in person through the counseling center given the recurrence of anxiety symptoms and panic attacks. JT opted to discontinue all therapy at the time.

Throughout the semester, he remained compliant with medication. He obtained a prescription for more clonazepam from an urgent care clinic after presenting with chest pain that was thought to be secondary to panic. While he found it helpful, he left it sitting on his desk when he went to transfer his laundry into a dryer, and it was stolen by another student. He accessed support through the ODS in time to get incomplete grades for the two classes that he was at risk of failing. He planned to use winter break to make up missed assignments. He was frustrated with himself for not seeking help sooner as the transfer to his desired college would now likely be delayed. After some discussion, JT understood why the psychiatrist was hesitant to prescribe more clonazepam; he did not initially realize that the medication could be considered valuable to his peers. He agreed to a dosage increase of the SSRI. He returned 2 weeks later, at the end of winter break, and was tolerating the medication change.

To ensure that any difficulties would be addressed sooner than in the previous semester, JT contacted the UCC and made an appointment to establish regular therapy on campus and he scheduled a follow-up appointment with the home psychiatrist for over spring break. He signed releases of information authorizing communication between his home and campus providers and his mother.

During spring break, both JT and his Mother noted better control of anxiety. JT attended classes regularly, continued to take his SSRI, and went to weekly therapy at the UCC. He also participated in an on-campus group addressing coping skills for anxiety. JT was earning better grades. He made up missed assignments to pass his incomplete classes from the previous semester. As a result, he had enough credits to seek transfer to his initial college of choice, but would have to wait an additional semester before he would be eligible to apply.

Analysis of Transition

This case was selected due to JT not being able to demonstrate academic performance on par with expectations. He was not attending classes regularly and did not fully utilize the resources that were available. In addition, on-campus psychiatric consultation services were not available.

In reviewing this case, several risk factors were present that may have predicted an unsuccessful transition. As is all too common, JT presented for care to a completely new psychiatrist just a couple of months prior to college transition. Although JT was aware of his diagnosis of GAD, and was compliant with medications and CBT, he seemed to underreport symptoms, which may have led to undertreatment. He and his mother also appeared to lack insight into how GAD might affect his life at college. In retrospect, this can be attributed to denial of the severity of symptoms due to the belief that family dynamics and poor communication within the family were the cause of his school refusal and poor academic performance during high school. JT was not able to see that these dynamics could affect other relationships, and was not interested in working to change them through family therapy. This led to unresolved issues with his father. JT was also not accustomed to asking for help from others, as his high school teachers and treatment providers seemed to provide accommodations automatically. While very helpful, this did not allow him to learn to advocate for himself. He also seemed to have limited preparation in practicing daily living skills and shoring up his executive function. Due to the UCC not accepting a referral prior to beginning classes, there was a significant delay in establishing care. There was no proactive communication by the provider with the UCC on JT's behalf and no communication from JT and his mom about changes in the transfer of care plan.

Positive predictors for transition include the fact that JT established a treatment relationship and maintained psychiatric treatment with the same provider before and after starting college. JT was adherent to treatment in high school, and his symptoms appeared to respond to medications. He was intelligent, able to establish and maintain friendships, and knew a number of other students that would be attending his college. Also, despite her limited ability to advocate for JT, his mother's persistence with reminders about resources available to him and her investment in his improvement were invaluable to preventing an even worse outcome. Another positive predictor was that despite JT's report of long-standing difficulty with anxiety, he had not turned to alcohol or drug use to help him cope, nor was he seeking use of a prescription sedative to help manage his symptoms.

Since psychiatric care was not available on campus and a firm appointment with a therapist could not be made proactively, the home psychiatrist should have insisted on more frequent and regular visits. Having JT sign a release of information ahead of time to allow close and effective communication between all treatment providers may have also helped facilitate a smoother transfer of care. JT did not have a complete understanding of the diagnosis of GAD nor how to manage symptoms other than to be compliant with medication. More time could be spent providing education, especially during the time when he was not reporting significant symptoms. Learning more adaptive coping strategies and wellness behaviors such as leisure activities could have helped him better manage his stress. JT, like many high school students, had been reliant on his mother to advocate for him. He could also have benefited from practicing life skills at home prior to transition and working on relapse prevention to recognize ways that anxiety could return and impact college life. He and his family also needed to work on communication and persistent dynamics that contributed to his emotional difficulties. A good exercise for JT would have been to help him reach out to the ODS and UCC during a session with his psychiatrist to work on communication skills and self-advocacy, and to develop a plan to hold himself accountable to following through on meeting with them when the semester started. It would be ideal for offices like ODS and UCC to be willing to connect with students prior to orientation to optimize transition. Careful consideration of his high school accommodations and a preemptive meeting with ODS may have allowed him to access accommodations earlier, and he may have elected to start with a smaller and more manageable course load in the first semester.

Although JT would be living in campus housing during freshman year, it would still be important to help him develop a daily routine and refine time management skills to encourage adequate sleep, study, and nutrition. He, like many freshmen, would also be facing the unique challenge of developing relationships with peers without parental supervision.

Clinical Pearls

- Healthy sleep and nutrition habits, daily structure to optimize time management, and good self-care are key for managing stress and anxiety.
- Cognitive behavioral therapy with exposure and response prevention can be a helpful tool for resisting avoidance and allowing students to practice managing stressful situations prior to the college transition.
- Students with GAD are at risk for alcohol and other substance use to try to manage their symptoms. Benzodiazepines should be used cautiously in these patients, particularly since diversion is high on college campuses. Anticipatory guidance regarding substance use is particularly important for students with anxiety disorders.

- GAD can present with poor concentration and focus. Symptom overlap makes it important to carefully differentiate from conditions like ADHD and depression, which would require a different treatment approach. Stimulant medications would be likely to worsen anxiety symptoms and would not effectively treat the focus and concentration difficulties.

- Periods of low symptoms and relative stability might be good times to work on psychoeducation, transition readiness, anticipatory guidance, and developing a transition care plan. Students with GAD may benefit from education about the ebb and flow of the academic calendar, so that they do not get completely overwhelmed at exam time.

- Parents and schools can be effectively involved in transition planning by identifying the ways that they provide structure and support for the student, and helping the student practice gradually taking on more responsibility for academics, illness management, self-care, and life skills. Schools and parents may inadvertently hinder the development of independence and self-advocacy by automatically providing assistance without allowing the student to struggle and learn to ask for help.

- Students and parents may have difficulty fully understanding symptoms and appreciating the severity of illness. While it is important to validate the wish that symptoms will dissipate with a "fresh start" or being away from stressful family dynamics, clinicians need to challenge patients to be prepared for recurrences or exacerbations of illness.

- It is also important for families to be aware of the role that stigma may play in preventing follow-through with important resources like counseling and ODS.

- It is not unusual for students to present for treatment with a new provider in the 2 or 3 months prior to college matriculation. Providers must work with the student and family to understand the diagnosis and to develop a shared treatment plan, including relapse prevention, safety planning, and a transfer of care plan.

Brief Literature Review

Anxiety complaints are common among students seeking treatment at college mental health centers [1]. According to the ACHA-NCHA II c Fall 2016 Executive Summary, 61.9% of college students felt overwhelming anxiety at some time within the past 12 months and 19.7% had been diagnosed or treated for an anxiety disorder during this same time [2]. However, only a small percentage of students (approximately 16%) [1] seek active treatment. While not specific to anxiety disorders, there appear to be several reasons for this, including stigma (both self and public) [3], a belief that symptoms will go away on their own, and difficulty recognizing symptoms when not under parental supervision. Anxiety may contribute to avoidance in the therapeutic relationship as well. When there is a disagreement with treatment recommendations, young people are more likely to stop attending sessions rather than working to resolve conflict with the current provider [4].

Adjusting to the ups and downs of the college schedule is a unique challenge for many students, who have never previously managed their own academic responsibilities and social lives. While there are times in the academic year that feel manageable, spikes of activity around exams, events, and projects can seem to throw the entire campus into chaos. Students with GAD may need increased therapeutic contacts and help keeping their schedules in check during busy times. When things are calm and manageable, they may require extra encouragement to continue taking psychotropic medications. Consistent with the ebbs and flows of college stress, there is considerable variability in college counseling center referrals over the course of the year. Referrals tend to be higher at mid-semester and towards end of the semester and final exams. Timing can significantly impact treatment recommendations. For example, both patients and providers may be hesitant to start psychotropic medication during exams due to concern that adverse side effects may negatively affect academic performance [5]. However, untreated, severe anxiety is also likely to impact grades.

Despite barriers to treatment, there are strategies to engage students and optimize adherence [4]. Use of current technology such as text message reminders for appointments, apps for managing prescription refills, and referring students to social media sites that emphasize the importance of treating mental health disorders may be effective [1]. Early treatment of anxiety can mitigate functional impairment and prevent the development of additional psychiatric comorbidities in later adulthood [6]. As with separation anxiety and social anxiety disorders, SSRIs and CBT are the standards of care for GAD. Data suggests that combined treatment is superior to either medication or psychotherapy alone [7]. Misuse of drugs and alcohol is very common in college students, whether anxiety is present or not. According to the 2015 College Prescription Drug Study [8], 8.9% of undergraduate students reported using sedatives for nonmedical reasons. 44.2% of undergraduates reported it was easy or very easy to obtain sedatives, with the majority (60.4%) obtaining them from friends. The most common reason undergraduates gave for wanting to use sedatives was for insomnia (56.1%) or to relieve anxiety (48.8%), but a large percentage also admitted using them to get high (38.9%). For this reason, prescribers need to be vigilant about using benzodiazepines in the college population and must have firm and consistent policies about handling refill requests for lost or stolen medications.

Helpful Resources

Office-Based Tools

- Screen for Child Anxiety Related Disorders (SCARED), Child and Parent versions, Ages 8–18 http://www.psychiatry.pitt.edu/sites/default/files/Documents/assessments/SCARED%20Child.pdf; http://www.psychiatry.pitt.edu/sites/default/files/Documents/assessments/SCARED%20Parent.pdf
- Beck Anxiety Inventory Ages 17–80 https://www.brandeis.edu/roybal/docs/BAI_website_PDF.pdf

Resources for Patients and Families

- Brochures from Anxiety and Depression Association of America: https://www. adaa.org/sites/default/files/ADAA_GeneralAnxietyDisorderBrochure.pdf; https://www.adaa.org/sites/default/files/GotAnxiety-2014.pdf
- Facts for Families on *School Refusal* and *Stress Management and Teens* www. AACAP.org
- CBT Referee is an iPhone and Android app to help with Cognitive Behavioral Therapy
- Deep Breathing Apps: http://www.t2health.org/apps/tactical-breather; http:// www.t2health.org/apps/breathe2relax

References

1. Pedrelli P, Nyer M, Yeung A, Zulauf C, Wilens T. College students: mental health problems and treatment considerations. Acad Psychiatry. 2015;39(5):503–11.
2. American College Health Association. American College Health Association-National College Health Assessment II: Undergraduate Student Reference Group Executive Summary Fall 2016. Hanover, MD: American College Health Association; 2017.
3. Eisenberg D, Hunt J, Speer N. Help seeking for mental health on college campuses: review of evidence and next steps for research and practice. Harv Rev Psychiatry. 2012;20:222–32.
4. Skehan B, Davis M. Aligning mental health treatments with the developmental stage and needs of late adolescents and young adults. Child Adolesc Psychiatr Clin N Am. 2017;26(2):177–90.
5. Garrick M. The calendar; complementarity, pacing, and service delivery in the college mental health setting. Acad Psychiatry. 2015;39(5):517–9.
6. Copeland WE, Angold A, Shanahan L, Costello EJ. Longitudinal patterns of anxiety from childhood to adulthood: the Great Smoky Mountains Study. J Am Acad Child Adolesc Psychiatry. 2014;53(1):21–33.
7. Mohatt J, Bennett SM, Walkup JT. Treatment of separation, generalized, and social anxiety disorders in youths. Am J Psychiatry. 2014;171(7):741–8.
8. Higher Education Center for Alcohol and Drug Misuse Prevention and Recovery. College Prescription Drug Study. 2015. http://hecaod.osu.edu/wp-content/uploads/2015/10/CPDS-Key-Findings-Report-1.pdf. Accessed 20 Jun 17.

"Just Right": Transitioning to College with Obsessive-Compulsive Disorder

15

Dorothy E. Grice

Case History

Chloe is a 19-year-old college freshman who presented for a consultation after her first semester. Chloe grew up with her parents and older sister, 5 years her senior, in the New York tristate area. She graduated from public high school in the top 10% of her class. At her college transition, she was not in treatment although she had been misdiagnosed with generalized anxiety disorder (GAD) and separation anxiety disorder (SAD) early in high school.

Chloe described herself as having been prone to anxiety from a young age. For example, if a parent was late to pick her up from grade school, she would become tearful and distraught—fearful that there had been a car accident or other catastrophic event involving her loved ones. In middle school, she developed superstitious behaviors. She had to rewrite and reread her homework and arrange the blankets and stuffed animals on her bed until everything looked and felt "just right." These rituals, diagnostic of her emergent obsessive-compulsive disorder (OCD), served to temporarily neutralize her worries; if performed correctly, she believed that they would keep her family safe.

Chloe was a bright student and in middle school she functioned at her expected level, both academically and socially. However, at home, she was anxious and often sought reassurance from her parents. Unrecognized OCD symptoms continued. She performed her rituals, but largely in secret or without explanation of their meaning. During her sophomore year in high school, her harm-related obsessions increased and her need to reread, rewrite, and check heightened. She repeatedly asked her parents if they were okay and, if her parents went out for the evening, she had great

D.E. Grice, M.D.
Department of Psychiatry, Icahn School of Medicine at Mount Sinai, New York, NY, USA
e-mail: Dorothy.grice@mssm.edu

© Springer International Publishing AG, part of Springer Nature 2018
A. Martel et al. (eds.), *Promoting Safe and Effective Transitions to College for Youth with Mental Health Conditions*, https://doi.org/10.1007/978-3-319-68894-7_15

difficulty being home alone. At night, her worries and rituals related to her bed and bedtime kept her up late. It was difficult for her to complete chores around the house, or participate in school extracurricular activities, because she spent so much time checking homework and performing rituals. The idea of dating was overwhelming to her, as she did not want to have to explain her compulsions.

Chloe's parents brought her to a therapist who understood the symptoms as GAD and SAD. Unfortunately, the true diagnosis of OCD was missed. Chloe did not explain her obsessional thoughts, the depth of her worries, nor the meaning behind the arranging, rereading, and rewriting compulsions that she needed to perform "just right" to keep her loved ones safe. The therapist offered supportive psychotherapy and worked with Chloe to improve her sleep hygiene, use approaches like progressive muscle relaxation, and Chloe was encouraged to exercise daily. Chloe's parents were coached to set firm limits regarding bedtime and to limit her repeated calls if they went out. Because Chloe's grades were very good, her parents and therapist did not inform Chloe's school about her treatment and formal academic accommodations were not pursued. In addition, Chloe did not like her therapist and once summer came, she refused to go. Her OCD symptoms were less prominent after school was out and her final grades were high; her parents felt they could not force her into treatment. However, through the remainder of high school they allowed Chloe to take frequent "mental health days" when she got behind in her work and teachers often flexed deadlines.

Chloe was accepted to a large university in New York City about an hour from her suburban home. She was excited to start college and told herself that her worries and rituals would be left behind when she moved onto a residential campus. Because Chloe had generally compensated for her OCD-related anxiety and hidden many of her OCD symptoms during high school, her parents were optimistic about her upcoming college transition. Academic accommodations were not sought when she entered college. No one recognized how much Chloe had relied on her informal high school accommodations.

At the start of her freshman year, Chloe got along fairly well with her roommates and enjoyed her classes. However, she was unprepared for the inflexibility and lack of individualized support at a large university. She was continually assessing her performance and was very anxious when she felt she had not performed perfectly. She was spending significant time rereading, rewriting, and checking her work. She had to perform keystrokes "just right" and she couldn't send an email or submit a paper without scouring it for errors. Her compulsions were driven by fears that harm would come to her family and she would be responsible. Chloe began to avoid showering because drying off and getting dressed according to the "just right" rules would result in over an hour of struggle. Her compulsions took up more and more time. Her intrusive thoughts and images that her family would be hurt escalated. She stopped wearing any red clothing because red, to her, represented blood and death and would put her family at risk. She checked her clothing for traces of red and repeatedly reassured herself that she and her family were safe. She was missing breakfast, often late to class and staying up late to complete her rituals.

Her roommates noticed she was particular about her homework, belongings, and bedtime routines, but saw her as a "perfectionist" with quirky behaviors. The roommates frequently commiserated about how stressed they all were but no one noticed the extent of Chloe's struggles, as many students went to class with unkempt hair, wearing yoga gear and flip-flops. However, Chloe continued to deteriorate and began to fall behind in her studies. In early November, after encouragement from a concerned roommate, Chloe sought consultation from the university mental health services. She complained of fatigue and feeling "overwhelmed" but did not reveal the details or depth of her OCD symptoms. She was embarrassed by her rituals and the content of her obsessive thoughts. She emphasized that she was an extreme worrier and perfectionist, rather than explaining her intrusive thoughts, compulsions, and feared consequences. The health center referred her to a support group for anxious students who were struggling to adjust to college. Chloe completed the term with barely passing grades and she was exhausted and relieved to go home for winter break.

At home, her parents noted that her hygiene was off and that she was isolating herself in her room. Her intrusive thoughts about harm continued and as did her drive to perform her rituals and her avoidance of triggers. The more she engaged in her rituals, the more she became convinced that they kept her and her family safe. Her family initially attributed her withdrawal and avoidance of showering and dressing to exhaustion after a challenging fall semester. However, when she did not recover as vacation progressed, her parents brought her to see a psychiatrist.

Chloe opened the session with: "I can't even get dressed anymore and I'm scared something really bad is going to happen." In the assessment, Chloe was able to discuss the roots of her anxiety and behaviors. With appropriate probes, she revealed her obsessions related to harm and perfectionism, her feared consequences, and the associated compulsions. It was important to understand her poor hygiene, social withdrawal, and the meaning and motivation behind her atypical behaviors. She wanted to shower but she could not bear to get caught up in the compulsions. She recognized that her doubts and fears were extreme. There was no paranoia nor psychotic thought process. Her particular hand and arm movements (touching the keyboard, placing items "just right") were voluntary compulsions, not complex motor tics. She had no symptoms of social anxiety or body dysmorphic disorder and did not meet criteria for major depressive disorder. She did not use alcohol or substances. Psychoeducation regarding OCD, its manifestations and treatments were provided to Chloe and her parents. The Yale-Brown Obsessive Compulsive Scale (YBOCS) was completed at Chloe's initial assessment, and re-administered about every 6 weeks to monitor her response to treatment.

Fortuitously, Chloe's parents had chosen a psychiatrist in New York City who was within commuting distance from home, allowing Chloe to come to treatment independently and for her parents to join, as needed. A treatment plan was mapped out with Chloe, her parents, a psychologist who specialized in exposure and response prevention (ExRP—a specific CBT for OCD), and the psychiatrist who would provide pharmacological treatment. Given the severity of symptoms, the team recommended that Chloe take a medical leave from spring semester, and engage in focused treatments for OCD. Chloe was reluctant. Her parents held firm that Chloe needed to tackle the OCD without having the pressure and responsibilities of school.

The treatment team used motivational interviewing approaches to help Chloe engage in treatment and ask for medical leave.

Given her symptom severity, treatment started with titration of a selective serotonin reuptake inhibitor (SSRI). Chloe saw her psychiatrist weekly and the daily fluoxetine dose was increased by 10 mg each week. During session time, supportive psychotherapy and psychoeducation about OCD was provided, helping to set the stage for next steps in therapy. Baseline anxiety and intensity of intrusive thoughts moderated sufficiently at fluoxetine 40 mg per day and Chloe felt ready to engage in active ExRP therapy. ExRP began, according to standard protocols—psychoeducation about OCD and ExRP, symptom monitoring, development of a treatment hierarchy, and then active exposure and ritual/response prevention. Chloe attended therapy twice a week and saw her psychiatrist every 3–4 weeks. Chloe's initial successes in ExRP gave her confidence that she could learn skills and approaches to control her OCD. Her motivation improved. In family and parent meetings, the team discussed how parental accommodation and reassurances had the unintended consequence of reinforcing the OCD fears and rituals. They devised alternate ways for the parents to support and cheerlead Chloe. Chloe worked her way up the exposure hierarchy, mastering ExRP in, and outside of, session. By June Chloe was ready for alternate week sessions. The intensity of her intrusive thoughts had lessened dramatically and she was better able to resist or ignore them. She tolerated the remaining OCD-related doubts with minimal distress and embraced the power of ExRP exposures. She no longer avoided showering, was able to change clothes, wear red, and rereading and checking rituals diminished greatly.

The treatment team recommended that Chloe enroll in summer session at her university and take a partial course load. Her team also noted that Chloe's anxiety made completion of timed tasks very difficult, since she had a tendency become very anxious and reread and rewrite in these circumstances. A neuropsychologist performed a formal assessment which substantiated Chloe's functional academic impairments from her anxiety and OCD symptoms. This formed the basis for Chloe's request to the office of disabilities for academic accommodations which then granted extended time and low distraction settings for tests and exams. And, while she wanted a single room on campus, she was able to see that living alone might make it easier for OCD to sneak back into her life.

The incremental transition to summer school allowed Chloe to build her confidence to manage her residual intrusive thoughts and compulsions, respond to OCD symptom exacerbations, and maintain support from her treatment team while also being challenged academically and expanding her social life. Chloe did well in this circumstance and felt ready to return as a full-time student for fall semester. Her treatment team was a subway ride from her university and she planned to see them monthly for booster sessions and medication monitoring. University health services were updated about Chloe's condition but her ongoing care was provided by her OCD treatment team. In addition, there was concern that adding a concurrent supportive clinician could be confusing and increase the risk of mixed messages (e.g., the supportive clinician inadvertently reassuring OCD doubts).

Analysis of Transition

There are several aspects of Chloe's history that suggested she was at risk for a difficult transition to college. Chloe's childhood symptoms are fairly typical for anxiety-based disorders in youth and while they do not necessarily predict an OCD diagnosis, this pattern is often seen in those who eventually present with OCD. That Chloe was initially misdiagnosed is not uncommon. OCD symptoms are often embarrassing and difficult to discuss. Anxious, regressed, and demanding behaviors are not specific to OCD. In addition, "just right" OCD symptoms are less well-known than, for example, contamination-based OCD. For Chloe, by high school, many of her OCD thoughts and behaviors were ingrained and she minimized and hid her symptoms. Ongoing reassurance from her parents reinforced that the OCD worries were legitimate, and the informal accommodations did not help Chloe to confront her fears and compulsions but instead implicitly accepted them as status quo. Lastly, the general CBT she received in high school was not specifically "anti-OCD" treatment, although there was some generic benefit. In retrospect, the course of Chloe's illness was much clearer but this is not to minimize the complexity of her symptoms and the challenges of providing an accurate diagnosis and treatment for youth affected by OCD. Chloe also had several positive predictors. She was a talented and motivated student who took responsibility for her academics. She maintained good relationships with peers. She responded to motivational approaches and developed good insight into her OCD. In addition, Chloe's parents supported her and accepted a therapeutic diversion from the typical 4-year college path.

In hindsight, Chloe's initial transition to college seemed destined to be suboptimal. Because she was a bright and successful student, her family and teachers overlooked her areas of vulnerability and did not see many of her expressed difficulties as clinical in nature. In addition, the lack of diagnostic clarity in her first mental health visit meant that neither Chloe nor her parents had sufficient knowledge about OCD nor the state-of-the-art treatments. The second college transition to summer session and beyond was optimal. If a college-bound student has active and impairing OCD symptoms, treatment teams often recommend a gap year or at least semester leave to accomplish the goals seen in Chloe's treatment. This investment is usually time well-spent. Students can engage in more intensive treatment, unencumbered by school obligations. OCD historically has been deemed "the doubting disorder." Above and beyond the impairments that arise from obsessions and compulsions, the toll OCD can take on self-confidence and sense of self-efficacy can be quite high. Sensitivity to these secondary issues is also an important aspect of treatment.

Chloe's transition to college could have been improved in several ways. Because she refused ongoing therapy in high school, her parents, high school, and university were unaware of the depth of her mental health challenges so she lacked an external support system. At her college transition, Chloe did not yet understand OCD, how the performance of her compulsions reinforced the power and "truth" of her obsessions, nor how avoidance of triggers served to strengthen the grip of OCD on her day-to-day life. For Chloe, the performance of compulsions temporarily decreased the distress from her obsessions yet they inevitably returned, the classic OCD cycle. Under the stressors of her freshman year, her partially compensated state was insufficient to handle the escalation of OCD symptoms. More awareness and skillful questioning may have helped Chloe's earlier clinicians to elucidate the OCD diagnosis.

Clinical Pearls

- OCD that onsets in childhood is often missed or misdiagnosed even after years of active symptoms. The prodrome of OCD can be nonspecific and OCD itself can be mistaken for separation anxiety, generalized anxiety disorder, social anxiety, phobias, depression, psychosis, Tourette disorder, and even disruptive behavior disorders.
- Colleges and universities have a variable understanding of OCD, its manifestations, and best treatment practices. Even with an accurate diagnosis, psychiatrists experienced in treating OCD and qualified ERP providers can be challenging to find in many areas, college campuses included. Start early in the search for an appropriate OCD treatment team.
- The content of the obsessions and nature of compulsions may be very embarrassing and run counter to an individual's true values (e.g., intrusive thoughts of hurting loved ones, unwanted sexual thoughts or images, extensive personal washing, highly ritualized checking). Patients may be reluctant to reveal thoughts and behaviors unless specific queries are used.
- Helpful probes for OCD symptoms include "Do you ever have thoughts or fears that won't go away?"; or "Some people have worries that they know are extreme or out of character and yet the worries are so upsetting they seem like they might be real"; or "Are there habits that you have to do over and over again even though they don't always make sense?"
- The best clinical tool in the treatment of OCD is knowledge of the disorder and associated best treatment practices. Accurate diagnosis is the first step of good treatment.
- To evaluate the range and severity of OCD symptoms, the YBOCS is a valuable supplement to the clinical interview. The YBOCS aids in severity classification, which in turn guides treatment.
- Those affected by OCD are not immune from other psychiatric disorders. As with all patients, it is important to screen for depression and suicidal or homicidal thoughts and distinguish these from OCD-related fears of harming oneself or others. Co-occurring bipolar disorder and family history thereof is relevant given the risk of precipitating hypomania or mania with SSRIs.
- Inadequately treated OCD in college youth may manifest as academic decline, deterioration in self-care, social isolation, decreased self-confidence, a lowered sense of self-efficacy, or withdrawal from campus activities. Careful, skilled questioning is essential to differentiate OCD from other psychiatric illness or adjustment issues.

- Motivational interviewing can be an important strategy to allow the transitional age youth an opportunity to articulate their values and goals for treatment within a conversational and respectful approach. This is especially important if there is reluctance to engage in treatment or if tensions exist between the young person's stated wishes and the treatment team's recommendations.
- The academic impacts of anxiety in general, and OCD more specifically, can be documented clinically, but some schools require formal neuropsychological testing for the student to qualify for accommodations. Once your patient has decided where to matriculate, investigate that school's specific requirements and begin work to provide the appropriate documentation well in advance of arrival on campus.
- If there is active and impairing OCD as a patient approaches college, do not hesitate to recommend other postsecondary options which would allow the student to devote more time and energy to intensive treatment. Deferring matriculation, taking a more structured gap year, starting with a reduced course load, or living at home and attending community college for a year, each with an OCD treatment team in place, are reasonable strategies.

Brief Literature Review

OCD symptoms often begin in childhood but diagnosis may be delayed until symptom severity is high [1]. Prevalence estimates for OCD are 2–3% but this may be an underestimate due to the inherent diagnostic challenges and that milder OCD cases may be missed. In recognition of the overlapping symptomatology, OCD, body dysmorphic disorder, trichotillomania, excoriation disorder, and hoarding disorder are categorized together in DSM-5, separate from anxiety disorders [2]. Given the common co-occurrence of persistent tic disorders and OCD in childhood, tic-related OCD is a new DSM-5 specifier.

Optimal treatment for OCD often involves both medication and CBT-based treatments [3–5]. ExRP and serotonin reuptake inhibitors (SRIs) are recommended as safe and effective first-line treatments for OCD. Of the CBT therapies, ExRP has the best evidence-based support and is a first-line approach. Whether to provide combined treatment or start with medication or ExRP is individually determined. Factors affecting decision-making include symptom severity, motivation to engage in either treatment, tolerance of pharmacotherapy, and presence of co-occurring conditions that may impact treatment. Too often, ExRP is considered only for patients who have moderate-severe symptoms or for those who refuse, do not respond to, or cannot tolerate SSRI treatment. ExRP therapy and learning associated skills and strategies to fight OCD, whether mild, moderate or extreme, and to actively manage residual OCD symptoms, is empowering to patients.

The efficacy of SSRIs in the treatment of adults and youth with OCD has been demonstrated in blinded, placebo-controlled studies and SSRIs are considered first-line pharmacological treatment for OCD [5–7]. Clomipramine, a nonspecific SRI, also has a good evidence base; however the side effect profile typically relegates it to a second-tier choice. The college-age population is unique in that it spans the traditional adult transition point, 18 years of age. Thus, clinical guidance can be gleaned from research literature on adolescents and adults. Research in both populations indicates that different SSRIs are equally effective in treating OCD. The particular SSRI chosen depends on adherence to FDA guidelines, side effect tolerance, and patient and clinician preferences. SSRI dosages for optimal control of OCD are often higher than dosages used to treat depression but this does not mean that all patients with OCD must be at the maximum dose. Clinical judgment should guide medication dosing.

Helpful Resources

- The YBOCS [8] is a clinician-administered semi-structured assessment instrument that provides a measure of OCD severity. The YBOCS identifies the range of OCD symptoms and assesses their impact on function.
- The International OCD Foundation (https://iocdf.org) provides information, for families and clinicians, about OCD and related disorders. The IOCDF sponsors an annual meeting designed for families affected by OCD, clinicians, and researchers.

References

1. Goodman WK, Grice DE, Lapidus KA, Coffey BJ. Obsessive compulsive disorder. Psychiatr Clin North Am. 2014;37:257–67.
2. American Psychiatric Association. Diagnostic and statistical manual of mental disorders. 5th ed. Arlington: American Psychiatric Association; 2013.
3. American Psychiatric Association. Guideline watch: practice guideline for the treatment of patients with obsessive-compulsive disorder. Washington: American Psychiatric Association; 2013. http://psychiatryonline.org/guidelines
4. Geller DA, March J. Practice parameter for the assessment and treatment of children and adolescents with OCD. J Am Acad Child Adolesc Psychiatry. 2012;51(1):98–113.
5. Koran LM, Hanna GL, Hollander E, Nestadt G, Simpson HB, American Psychiatric Association. Practice guideline for the treatment of patients with obsessive-compulsive disorder. Am J Psychiatry. 2007;164(7 Suppl):5–53.
6. Practice parameter for the assessment and treatment of children and adolescents with obsessive-compulsive disorder. J Am Acad Child Adolesc Psychiatry. 2012;51(1):98–113.
7. Pittenger C, Bloch MH. Pharmacological treatment of obsessive-compulsive disorder. Psychiatr Clin North Am. 2014;37(3):375–91.
8. Goodman WK, Price LH, Rasmussen SA, et al. The Yale-Brown obsessive compulsive scale. Arch Gen Psychiatry. 1989;46:1006–11.

"My Nightmares Aren't Just About Calculus 101": Transitioning to College with PTSD

16

Zhanna Elberg

Case History

Samantha is a 19-year-old Caucasian female, who at the time of the transition to college, was diagnosed with PTSD, chronic type and Major Depressive Disorder, recurrent, in partial remission. She had never received special education services and was at the top 85th percentile of her high school graduating class. She is the youngest of three children and was born and raised in an urban mid-sized city in Upstate New York. Her parents were married until she was 4 years old, at which point her father disclosed to her mother that he was having an affair and wanted to end the marriage. Her mother, who suffered from postpartum depression after Samantha's birth, became progressively more depressed after the divorce. Samantha resided with her mother but every other weekend, she and her brothers would stay overnight with their father. Visitation ended at age 11 at Samantha's request. She essentially stopped playing the piano despite being a talented musician who previously played for hours each day. She also endorsed having passive suicidal ideations but never attempted suicide. She did exhibit some traits of Borderline Personality Disorder but did not meet full criteria.

Samantha began to struggle with depressed mood at age 12 and started cutting herself superficially as a way to cope with her distress. At age 16, she experienced her first depressive episode and asked her mother for help with finding treatment. She was linked with a child and adolescent psychiatry community mental health clinic where she began seeing a therapist (LCSW) and a child psychiatrist within a split treatment setting. The depressive episode was thought to

Z. Elberg, M.D.
Department of Psychiatry, Jacobs School of Medicine and Biomedical Sciences,
University of Buffalo, Buffalo, NY, USA
e-mail: zelberg@buffalo.edu

© Springer International Publishing AG, part of Springer Nature 2018
A. Martel et al. (eds.), *Promoting Safe and Effective Transitions to College for Youth with Mental Health Conditions*, https://doi.org/10.1007/978-3-319-68894-7_16

be precipitated by a friend disclosing sexual trauma to Samantha, who never previously revealed her own history of significant sexual abuse perpetrated by her father from the age of 4 till age 11. Samantha also endorsed nightmares, flashbacks, symptoms of hyperarousal, and was experiencing dissociative symptoms on an almost daily basis. This was the first time she disclosed sexual abuse to anyone but insisted that her mother not be told of the abuse at the beginning of treatment. Samantha was doing well academically prior to experiencing worsening psychiatric symptoms. She began to struggle with motivation to complete schoolwork, had difficulty concentrating in class, endorsed having low appetite, and had difficulty falling and staying asleep. She started isolating from her friends and essentially stopped playing the piano despite being a talented musician who previously played for hours each day. She also endorsed having passive suicidal ideations but never attempted suicide.

Samantha was started on escitalopram for Major Depressive Disorder and although depressive symptoms did improve with treatment, the PTSD symptoms persisted. She began to also see a counselor at her high school for emotional support but did not need any other interventions in school. Academically, her grades improved and she returned to her previous level of functioning in school. Socially, she still felt disconnected with her friends but returned to socializing more often. Samantha and her mother were wary of adding any other medications and most of the treatment focused on psychotherapy, with emphasis on expression of feelings, improving distress tolerance and emotional regulation. The long-term plan was to start trauma work. Eventually, Samantha was able to tell her mother about the abuse but worried more about managing Mom's anxiety over the disclosure.

In some ways, Samantha was ready for the transition to college. She appeared to understand her own mental health needs. She initiated linkage with treatment, kept track of her appointments, picked up her medication from the pharmacy, and would initiate her own medication refill requests. However, she would also isolate and periodically disengage from treatment during times of stress. This was usually in the context of her problems in her social relationships, which would then also affect her academics. She would only reach out to providers when in extreme distress. This was addressed in her treatment and although she appeared receptive to this being a problem during the transition to college, there was no discernible change in her behavior. Samantha functioned fairly well independently. She arranged her own transportation and had a part time job. She never required parental help with regard to academics and when it was time to apply to college, she helped her mother fill out the FAFSA form. If anything, she was encouraged to reach out more and utilize available resources especially during times of stress when she tended to have more difficulty with self-advocacy. Samantha struggled the most in her social relationships. She had difficulty with setting boundaries in her platonic and romantic relationships and often felt overwhelmed by not being able to recognize or advocate for her own needs in relationships. There were a few concerning safety issues including experimentation with drugs and alcohol, managing distress with self-injurious behaviors and tolerating unwanted sexual contact in her romantic relationships.

Samantha identified a goal of attending a 4-year university. She was fairly certain; she wanted to pursue a science-related major and was aware of her own interests and limitations academically. Samantha applied to schools locally and all over the country. Her only hesitation about leaving home was related to the distress it might cause her mother. Transition planning was mostly done around self-advocacy issues during times of stress and managing ongoing mental health needs while at college. Additionally, Samantha, her mom, and her providers discussed the pros and cons of different college settings, their proximity to home, and availability of mental health resources. Samantha's mother was peripherally involved in her treatment in the clinic and with planning for transition to college. Samantha would ask providers to not involve her mother more than necessary because she worried about her mother being "stressed." Mom appeared to expect Samantha to manage independently and attempts to engage Mom were superficially received.

Samantha ultimately decided to attend a 4-year state university located in a suburban setting about 1 h from home. She received an academic scholarship (with requirement to keep her GPA above a 2.8), which was the main reason for choosing this school. The school offered psychiatry services (provided by a nurse practitioner) and counseling services at their student health center. However, the treatment team felt that Samantha needed more mental health support than what was available at the student health center. The team also discussed other follow-up options such as community mental health agencies closer to the school or private providers. Unfortunately, Samantha's insurance precluded linkage with private practitioners and Samantha was unwilling to consider other community-based services that were closer to the university. Samantha indicated an interest in continuing care with the clinic given its (relative) proximity to the university and no alternative plan was developed. She was planning to continue monthly psychiatry appointments along with bi-weekly therapy appointments. Samantha's schedule would allow for more frequent visits if needed.

Although she initially had good class attendance, Samantha began to fall behind due to the demands of her rigorous course load, her part time job, and difficulty managing her social relationships. Her high school boyfriend broke up with her half way through the semester leading to a week of not attending any classes and falling behind. She was also having difficulty adjusting to living in co-ed dorms, which was likely related to her history of sexual trauma. She felt uncomfortable with sharing bathroom facilities with male students and found herself attending to hygiene needs at odd hours to avoid being seen. She never shared her concerns or her trauma history with her resident advisor. Samantha got along well with her roommate but was also triggered by her roommate bringing home random males after nights of partying. Samantha often went home on weekends to avoid overhearing and often seeing her roommate have sex in their dorm room. What was actually more triggering for Samantha was hearing her roommate describe not remembering some of her sexual encounters while drunk and only realizing she had sex after waking up naked the next day with a used condom in the trash can. Samantha's treatment adherence declined significantly as well and she barely attended any therapy sessions and only went to a few psychiatry appointments. She cited transportation and scheduling issues as major barriers to attendance and advocated for transferring her care to the student-counseling center.

At this point she was feeling more depressed, experiencing worsening PTSD symptoms and was engaging in more self-injurious behaviors. Samantha did eventually contact the counseling center and saw a counselor but the psychiatry provider had no availability that worked with her schedule until the following semester. The clinic sent all available information to the counseling center in order to facilitate this late and impromptu transfer of care. However, no provider-to-provider communication occurred despite several attempts by the clinic psychiatrist to reach providers at the counseling center. Samantha finished her first semester with a 3.0 GPA. Spring semester had a similar beginning as the fall. She was initially able to keep up with activities but things fell apart by midterms. Samantha also started binge drinking on the weekends and began smoking marijuana. Self-injurious behaviors also increased and worsened during episodes of binge drinking. At the time care was fully transitioned to the counseling center, Samantha was failing two classes.

Samantha failed the spring semester of her freshman year and took a leave of absence due to worsening depression and concern about her academic performance. She moved into an apartment with a female friend and continued to work. She relinked with her previous psychiatrist in a private practice setting and was receiving evidence-based psychotherapy services in an adult outpatient clinic specializing in trauma. She was able to return to school and back to campus for a brief period of time but had a significant recurrence of PTSD symptoms with worsening in suicidal ideations, requiring partial hospitalization. Graduating from college remained Samantha's top goal. She transferred to a smaller local state college with closer proximity to her mental health providers and was more engaged in treatment. She had to take two more medical leaves of absence due to worsening mental health symptoms that interfered with her ability to do academic work but was able to eventually graduate with a Bachelor's degree.

Analysis of Transition

There are several predictors of positive outcome in this case. Samantha exhibited independent daily living skills and demonstrated a lot of maturity from her first presentation to the clinic. She was independent, responsible, and self-sufficient. She had a part time job and was able to budget her money in order to save for college. She knew how to cook for herself and do laundry and helped her mother with household chores on a routine basis. Samantha was highly intelligent and driven and never needed special education services during secondary education. She was able to set goals and attending college was very important to Samantha. She researched colleges on her own, initiated her own queries into different scholarships and financial aid. She was self-referred to treatment and appeared to have an understanding of her own mental health needs and need for further treatment while in college.

Despite these positive factors, there were negative aspects that were predictive of a poor outcome during the transition to college. During times of stress, Samantha's ability to advocate for herself or recognize need to seek help diminished. She had difficulty recognizing her triggers. This tendency to withdraw put her at risk for a failed transition. Samantha's mother was also minimally involved and would often not intervene or recognize the need to intervene when Samantha was struggling. This was evident when Samantha would go home for the weekends; Samantha worried about upsetting her mother and would not discuss her difficulties in school. The treatment team also could not rely on Mom as a support during the transition to college. Samantha had more difficulty prioritizing her needs or being able to problem solve effectively during times of stress leading to poor decision-making and compromised safety. The above-referred stress was usually in the context of struggles in her social relationships. She had difficulty setting boundaries and would often sacrifice her own needs to please others. She also had deficits with emotion regulation and would engage in self-injurious behaviors at times of stress. During these periods of stress, she was unable to balance academic demands in the face of social crises. Lastly, her history of early sexual trauma had not been fully addressed in therapy and was likely a major contributor to her relational patterns.

There were several transition planning deficits in this case, which may have been predictors of a more negative outcome, including lack of preparation for campus life. Additionally, the transfer of care plan was limited to continuing current care and no back-up or emergency plan was established. By the time an alternative transfer of care plan needed to be established, Samantha was already struggling in college.

This case demonstrates a failed transition to college. The patient did not follow up with outpatient services as initially planned and was not linked with disability services from the onset of starting college. She became overwhelmed by academic and social demands and did not have adequate supports in place to compensate. As a result, she had to take several leaves of absence in order to address her mental health causing an interruption and delay in her college education.

Transition planning and preparation in this case had several deficits. It certainly should have begun earlier but time was limited given that Samantha did not link with the clinic until she was a junior in high school and was already in the midst of college planning. On initial presentation, the clinical focus was on the treatment and management of acute psychiatric symptoms and preparation for the transition to college often took a back seat until her symptoms were more stable. Additionally, in a split treatment model, the question of who takes the lead on transition of care planning can arise requiring careful coordination. Starting transition planning and emphasizing its importance should have occurred very early on in treatment by both psychotherapy and psychiatry treatment providers.

Transition planning in this case was limited to ensuring ongoing care but even this was not optimally done. The referring provider did not anticipate the impact of exposure to sexual activity and lack of structure as triggers for a patient with PTSD and history of sexual trauma. These issues were never addressed with the patient during transition preparation and planning. There were no discussions about how many credits to take during first semester of college or weighing the pros and cons of continuing a part time job. Even planning the type of residential setting would have been useful given that Samantha had difficulty adjusting to living on campus.

Campus life can be a highly sexualized environment and exposure to this without adequate preparation likely contributed to Samantha's worsening PTSD symptoms. Her roommate's reports of not remembering her sexual encounters and thus bringing up the question of consent was the most difficult for Samantha and likely contributed worsening of PTSD symptoms. Her first depressive episode was triggered by her friend recalling sexual trauma and in light of Samantha's own early sexual trauma, she was more vulnerable to the triggers found on campus.

Additionally, no linkage with disability services was established, as Samantha had not previously needed academic supports. However, linkage with disability services could have been useful during times Samantha experienced more difficulty balancing academic and psychosocial demands or began to experience more psychiatric symptoms. Although unclear how much it contributed to a negative outcome, the treatment team also never addressed risk of alcohol abuse in this patient and did not appreciate the increased risk in this patient population.

The transition care plan in this case was not comprehensive or realistic because the initial plan did not account for scheduling conflicts or provide alternative resources. There was a delay in coordinating on-campus university services with a lack of response from the counseling service during attempts to transfer care and lack of available psychiatry resources on campus. The university resources could have served as a back-up plan if this linkage was established earlier in the process. Additionally, referring providers should have evaluated benefits and limitations of available on-campus services. For example, weekly sessions with therapists are often not feasible given that total visits at this university-counseling center are limited. In light of Samantha's struggles with emotional regulation and functional impairment during times of stress, she likely needed a more intense level of care than what is usually offered on college campuses. The referring psychiatrist did not look into off-campus resources such as community programs that specialize in trauma and DBT. Samantha's independent living skills and the ability to self-advocate during periods of wellness may have allowed her provider and her mother to underestimate her significant difficulties during times of stress and this needed to be the focus of transition planning as well. In light of this, considering a local college or university at least initially, in close proximity of adequate mental health supports, could have been prioritized during the preparation and planning process and may have contributed to a more successful outcome.

Clinical Pearls

- Patients with PTSD especially due to sexual trauma are at a higher risk for reactivation of their symptoms while on campus. Identifying and preparing for potential triggers that may bring on flashbacks, nightmares, panic attacks, or dissociation episodes can be key in facilitating a successful transition for patients with a history of trauma or PTSD.
- Potential triggers of worsening PTSD include living in co-ed dorms and being exposed to a sexualized living environment. Patients can also be

triggered by certain class/lecture materials, Take Back the Night Rallies, or other sexual assault awareness programs. Reports of sexual assault or witnessing partner violence on campus can reactivate symptoms. Dating itself can be triggering for patients with PTSD. Being aware of other environmental triggers or specific anniversary dates can help patients and providers plan accordingly.

- Sexual assaults on campus have been a focus of much discussion on college campuses. Title IX legislation has tried to ensure that institutions of higher education work towards addressing and preventing risk of sexual assault. Bystander training has also been implemented on campuses
- The living environment on campus needs to be carefully assessed prior to the transition. Ideally, patients with PTSD would have their own bedroom but reside in a suite to prevent isolation. Consideration might be given to living in a single sex dormitory or one that practices "healthy living."
- Alcohol and drug use can be problematic on college campuses. Screening for excessive alcohol and drug use is imperative since patients may use drugs and alcohol to deal with emerging PTSD or trauma-related symptoms. Additionally, alcohol use can be a risk factor for both victims and perpetrators of sexual assault.
- Discouraging an alcohol-centric social life on campus and in fraternities and sororities can decrease alcohol-related assaults and misbehavior. Giving inservices on "consent" in physical and sexual encounters can help establish campuswide expectations about "safe dating."
- The college selection process should reflect the mental health needs of the patient. Depending on the severity of PTSD symptoms and risk of reactivation of symptoms, campus-based services may not be adequate for patients with PTSD due to limitation of available visits in college-counseling centers. Providers who have experience with trauma patients or have expertise in trauma-focused CBT or DBT would be best suited for this patient population.
- Easily accessible off-campus services and back-up linkage with on-campus mental health services is often needed. Additionally, availability (should it be needed) of higher levels of care such as inpatient or partial hospitalization should be assessed. Colleges that lack availability of these resources may not be able to meet the needs of patients with PTSD. Referring providers should also consider whether linkage with disability services would be helpful to support students who may have academic struggles due to their symptoms.
- Providers must aim to promote safety and encourage activities that improve self-esteem and healthy pastimes. Similarly to reasons for alcohol use, patients with PTSD may engage in self-injurious behaviors as a way to deal with their symptoms. Thus, treatment should also aim at screening for self-injurious behaviors and suicidal ideation.
- In cases where treatment is split between a therapist and prescriber, clinicians must work together to present consistent messages to the family about developing a transition care plan. Treatment team members should be in close communication to determine roles in transition care planning, and to be clear on the recommendations and timing of any interventions.

Brief Literature Review

Transitioning to college with a history of trauma or PTSD can be a challenging endeavor. Rates of PTSD among newly matriculated college students is estimated to be around 9%, which is similar to rates found in general population samples [1]. Findings have indicated that students who enter college with significant distress due to a history of traumatic events may be at high risk for academic difficulties and college dropout, which is especially important to consider for patients with a history of childhood sexual trauma [2, 3]. Additional studies revealed significant variability in PTSD symptom course over the first year of college. Exposure to trauma during this period contributed to this variability, exerting an influence on the maintenance and worsening of PTSD symptoms (usually observed in the second semester). Alcohol involvement also showed a deleterious influence on PTSD symptom status over time [4]. Students with PTSD were found to be at an increased risk of developing problematic use of drugs and alcohol, which may be related to negative coping patterns [5]. Alcohol use may also predispose students with PTSD to victimization and sexual assault. Additionally, drinking alcohol for college men has been shown to increase the likelihood of perpetrating sexual assault [6, 7].

A complicating factor for transitioning students with PTSD to college is the prevalence of sexual violence on college campuses and thus risk of further exposure to trauma and revictimization. Approximately 20% of college women and 6% of college men have been victims of an attempted or committed sexual assault [7, 8]. Federal legislation such as the Clery Act of 1990 and its amendment, the Campus Sexual Violence Act of 2013, are geared to preventing sexual violence and promoting safety on campus. These laws address guidelines for reporting of sexual crimes, implementation of primary prevention and awareness programs, and disciplinary proceedings that are prompt and fair for both accuser and the accused (Clery Center) [9]. Additionally, Title IX of the Higher Education Act (1972) prohibits discrimination based on gender within all institutions that receive federal aid and includes sexual violence as a form of discrimination. This law requires colleges to respond promptly and effectively to sexual harassment and sexual violence. In 2014, The White House established the Task Force to Protect Students from Sexual Assault in order to address sexual violence on college campuses by strengthening federal enforcement efforts and providing schools with additional tools to develop primary prevention strategies (Center for Changing Our Campus Culture) [9]. Bystander intervention training are community-/campus-based programs that teach individuals to recognize situations or behaviors that may become violent or that reinforce social norms supportive of violence and safely and effectively intervene by becoming potential witnesses to violence rather than as possible victims or perpetrators. Green Dot and Bringing in the Bystander are two examples of evidence-based bystander intervention programs [9, 10]; Center for Changing Our Campus Culture).

Access to appropriate treatment on college campuses for students with PTSD can also be challenging. Evidence-based psychological treatments for PTSD include Cognitive Processing Therapy (CPT), Trauma Focused CBT (TF-CBT), Prolonged Exposure Therapy (PE), and Eye Movement Desensitization and Reprocessing (EMDR) [11]. Although some of these treatments are short term and could potentially be carried out in college-counseling settings, they are very specialized and require staff training, which may not be readily available. There is limited data on treatment of PTSD in college student-counseling centers. Additionally, due to the severity, intermittent acuity, and often chronic nature of post-traumatic symptoms, counseling centers tend to refer students to community providers for ongoing, long-term work. Students who exhibit self-harm behaviors may be referred to psychiatric inpatient or partial-hospitalization programs in order to ensure safety and most colleges are not able to provide this level of care on campus.

Helpful Resources

Resources for Clinicians and Families

- Moving Into Adulthood Resource Center http://www.aacap.org/AACAP/Families_and_Youth/Resource_Centers/Moving_Into_Adulthood_Resource_Center/Moving_Into_Adulthood_Resource_Center.aspx
- Casey Life Skills http://www.casey.org/casey-life-skills-resources/
- http://healthymindsnetwork.org/
- National Center for PTSD https://www.ptsd.va.gov—resources related to assessment, treatment
- https://www.justice.gov/ovw/protecting-students-sexual-assault

Resources for Families

- AACAP Facts for Families on PTSD and Sexual Abuse www.aacap.org
- www.ulifeline.org/ Mental Health Resources for College Students
- http://www.doe.virginia.gov/special_ed/transition_svcs/outcomes_project/college_guide.pdf
- Endrapeoncampus.org—describes Title IX legislation
- KnowyourIX.org
- Changingourcampus.org
- National Sexual Violence Resource Center—www.nsvrc.org

Office-Based Tools

- College readiness assessment: https://www.iidc.indiana.edu/styles/iidc/defiles/instrc/webinars/college-readiness_assessment.pdf
- The Posttraumatic Stress Disorder Checklist for DSM-5 (PCL-5) https://www.ptsd.va.gov/professional/assessment/adult-sr/ptsd-checklist.asp

References

1. Read JP, Ouimette P, White J, Colder CR, Farrow S. Rates of DSM-IV-TR trauma exposure and posttraumatic stress disorder among newly matriculated college students. Psychol Trauma. 2011;3:148–56.
2. Duncan RD. Childhood maltreatment and college dropout rates. J Interpers Violence. 2000;15:987–95.
3. Jordan CE, Combs JL, Smith GT. An exploration of sexual victimization and academic performance among college women. Trauma Violence Abuse. 2014;15(3):191–200.
4. Read JP, Bachrach RL, Wright AG, Colder CR. PTSD symptom course during the first year of college. Psychol Trauma. 2016;8(3):393–403.
5. Read JP, Griffin MJ, Wardell JD, Ouimette P. Coping, PTSD symptoms, and alcohol involvement in trauma-exposed college students in the first three years of college. Psychol Addict Behav. 2014;28(4):1052–64.
6. Gilmore AK, Lewis MA, George WH. A randomized controlled trial targeting alcohol use and sexual assault risk among college women at high risk for victimization. Behav Res Ther. 2015;74:38–49.
7. Krebs CP, Lindquist C, Warner T, Fisher B, Martin S. The campus sexual assault (CSA) study: final report. 2007. Retrieved from the National Criminal Justice Reference Service: http://www.ncjrs.gov/pdffiles1/nij/grants/221153.pdf
8. Krebs CP, Lindquist CH, Berzofsky M, Shook-SA B, Peterson K, Planty M, Langon L, Stroop J. Campus climate survey validation study: final technical report. Washington, DC: U.S. Department of Justice, Bureau of Justice Statistics; 2016.
9. Clerycenter.org   http://www.changingourcampus.org/resources/not-alone/WH_Task_Force_First_Report.pdf
10. Banyard VL, Plante EG, Moynihan MM. Bystander education: bringing a broader community perspective to sexual violence prevention. J Community Psychol. 2004;32(1):61–79.
11. Department of Veterans Affairs and Department of Defense. VA/DoD clinical practice guideline for the management of post-traumatic stress. Washington, DC: Department of Veterans Affairs and Department of Defense; 2010.

"Too Much on My Plate": Transitioning to College with an Eating Disorder

Jennifer Derenne

Case History

Sally is an 18-year-old Caucasian female, eldest of three girls, who presented for an initial consultation the June following her high school graduation from a small, rural, Midwestern public high school. She was active in theater, sports, took multiple advanced placement classes and was the valedictorian of her graduating class of 200 students. She was diagnosed with Anorexia Nervosa, Binge-Purge Type at age 16, and underwent a 2-week medical hospitalization for low weight (BMI of 15.1) and vital sign dysregulation. She was successfully treated with family-based therapy (FBT). Sally was fully weight restored to a BMI of 20 for the 6 months prior to the consultation and was completely abstinent from purging behaviors for that time as well. She did not require psychotropic medication and transitioned to individual psychotherapy shortly after completing FBT to work on "perfectionism" issues.

Sally was accepted to an Ivy League school located in an urban center across the country from her parents' home. She planned to major in biology, in preparation for medical school in the future. Sally asked her parents to schedule the evaluation so that she could request an exception from the college to live off campus in her first year. She felt that this was necessary so that she could have her own kitchen and would be able to feel comfortable that she was eating healthfully and could prepare her own meals. She was looking forward to getting back into running; she was required to stop cross-country when she was restoring weight in the course of FBT and had not gone back to it after being medically stabilized because she was so busy with other obligations. The family wanted to establish care with

J. Derenne, M.D.
Division of Child and Adolescent Psychiatry, Department of Psychiatry and Behavioral Sciences, Stanford University School of Medicine, Lucile Packard Children's Hospital, Stanford, CA, USA
e-mail: jderenne@stanford.edu

© Springer International Publishing AG, part of Springer Nature 2018
A. Martel et al. (eds.), *Promoting Safe and Effective Transitions to College for Youth with Mental Health Conditions*, https://doi.org/10.1007/978-3-319-68894-7_17

someone near home and requested documentation to support Sally living alone and being exempted from the university meal plan. They did not want the administration to know about her eating disorder as it was "all in the past" and feared that it would affect her academic future.

Sally did not want to establish psychiatric care on campus, stating "I don't want it to affect me becoming a doctor." She also believed it unnecessary, given that she was doing so well and thought that it would be too difficult to connect to new providers. She preferred to "check in" with the home provider on an as-needed basis via Skype.

The family was given feedback that, while she had put a lot of work into recovery and seemed to be doing well, there were a number of potential challenges in the upcoming transition. They were encouraged to return for several visits over the course of the summer so that they could work together on crafting a transition care plan that would provide a safety net for her in her first year and make it more likely that she would be able to remain in school. While they understood the clinician's concern that living off campus might make Sally vulnerable to relapse (given that there would be very limited oversight), the family was disappointed that they would not be given a letter to support their request. Nonetheless, they agreed to return in 2 weeks' time.

At the end of August, they presented again 2 weeks prior to traveling for move-in weekend. Sally was apologetic, but stated that she had gotten caught up with her summer job and could not take time away for doctor's visits. However, she did take the concerns to heart and reported wanting to do whatever she could to be successful with the transition. She had started running about three miles three times per week, continued to eat what her parents prepared, and said that she felt well, both physically and mentally. She had her pre-college physical a couple of weeks earlier and was told that her vital signs and weight remained stable. Sally was able to meet her roommates online and was happy about her living situation; she was looking forward to registering for classes and her parents were feeling very confident as well.

They knew that the university had a student health center and had seen something on the website about mental health services. Given that the college was in an urban center and was associated with a major medical school, they felt comfortable that there would be options available if she thought that she needed more support. They decided against telling the university about the eating disorder.

The family was encouraged to talk about ways that they might notice that Sally was slipping or in need of more support. Sally noted that she would video chat with her parents regularly, and they would notice if she looked thinner. She also felt that she would be able to let them know if she was having urges to lose weight. She was strongly encouraged to set up an appointment with the student health center to monitor her weight and vital signs throughout the transition.

Sally's mother called in early November after receiving a concerning call from the Vice President of Student Affairs. They were Skyping regularly, but did not notice that Sally had lost weight because she wore baggy sweatshirts and assured them that she was doing well. She had been a little homesick in the beginning of the year, but had been able to get through that fairly quickly. According to university administration, Sally was identified as a student at risk after she passed out while running on the treadmill at the recreation (rec) center. She refused medical assessment at the time. The rec center noted that she was spending hours each day exercising. Residence Life had also raised concerns that her toilet was clogged multiple times and her roommates noted that she ate very little, drank multiple cups of coffee each day, and stuck to a very rigid routine. She continued to earn *As* in all of her classes, was active in campus organizations, and was friendly with her classmates and neighbors. They wanted her to complete a mandated assessment to make sure that she was medically healthy enough to remain enrolled in school. Sally said that she was fine and did not see any need for evaluation. However, she did agree to have parents visit, after it was clear that her access to the recreation center was restricted.

While there, Sally's parents accompanied her to visits at the Student Health Center and Counseling Center, where she signed releases of information for the administration. Her vital signs were unstable, her BMI was 14.3, her potassium was low, and the physician recommended a medical admission. She did not want to miss school, but agreed to be hospitalized so that she would not be forced to take a medical leave of absence. While in the hospital, she admitted that her eating disorder had resurfaced as she felt anxious about the increased academic workload and felt intimidated by her peers, whom, she believed, were much more talented. She also acknowledged that, without her parents around to hold her accountable, it was far easier to skip meals and restrict her portions.

While in the hospital, Sally kept up with homework assignments and listened to online recordings of lectures. The inpatient team encouraged her and her parents to consider taking a voluntary leave so that she could focus more completely on recovery. However, Sally and her parents were resistant to doing so, as she did not want to waste money and time on the work she had already completed. Parents did not feel empowered to enforce any limits as she was over 18, and they wanted her to learn to be more independent and learn how to manage her illness.

Sally agreed to drop a lab class and enrolled in a local eating disorder intensive outpatient program near the college for added support. This 3 hour per day program allowed her to have meal support at dinner and a snack and provided individual and group psychotherapy as well. She signed a contract with her parents and team, in which she agreed to a higher level of care if she was unable to meet specific standards for vital sign stability and weight restoration. She also agreed to a leave of absence if she was unable to maintain her health with this plan in place.

Sally's motivation to stay in school proved to be strong. She felt uncomfortable about having to drop a class, but attended the program as recommended and was able to restore her health. There were a number of other college students in the program she chose (it was very close to campus), and they were able to support each other with meals at other times as well. Her team communicated with the case manager on the student of concern team to confirm that she was adhering to the contract, and she transitioned to an outpatient eating disorders team once she finished the intensive outpatient program. She was able to see a medical provider and dietitian in the student health center and found an eating disorders therapist in the community who was accessible via public transportation.

Analysis of Transition

There were a number of factors in Sally's case that are predictive of a negative transition outcome. She presented for consultation very shortly before she was scheduled to depart for college, she had only a few months of medical stability before the planned transition, and the family had done very little to establish a relapse prevention plan. They had not allowed Sally to practice being more independent with her meals and snacks with some parent oversight in place, and both Sally and her parents had strong feelings about not sharing her history with the university. It was also concerning that they did not follow through on recommendations to work with a provider over the summer to put a more solid transition care plan into place. Perhaps this was partly related to their disappointment in not being given the letter they requested to support off-campus housing.

Positive predictors of a healthy transition to college include: Sally's excellent academic history and her ability to meet deadlines; Sally's ability to work over the summer, while also exercising regularly and maintaining her weight; she attended a school with a strong student of concern team that identified worrisome behaviors early; and, the student of concern team had a clear plan about how to address Sally's mental and medical health issues. In addition, the location of the university was ideal in that there were subspecialty care services readily available very close to campus.

While this is officially considered a "failed" transition in the sense that Sally experienced a significant relapse of eating disorder symptoms and required additional care, it is also a good example of how the university can work effectively with students to identify concerning behaviors and develop a reasonable treatment plan with clearly defined contingencies in place.

In an ideal world, this family would have been talking about future plans when they were still in treatment for Sally's initial presentation of anorexia nervosa. It is important to let families know that eating disorders often reappear in times of life stress and transition, and to remind them that the transition to college is particularly difficult, even in individuals who do not have a history of medical or mental health problems. In addition, it would have been helpful for Sally and her parents to keep her mental health needs in mind as Sally visited schools, completed applications, and made her final college choice. Students and parents need to understand that health and counseling records are kept separate from the academic record; therefore, if the student seeks help the counseling and medical records will not appear on the transcript and will not affect graduate school plans. While the decision about whether to inform the school of her diagnosis ultimately rests with Sally as she is over 18, it is helpful for the family to understand that the vast majority of universities are invested in keeping students healthy and supported so that they are able to earn their degrees. Luckily for Sally, she decided on a university that was affiliated with a major medical center and had the full array of eating disorder treatment options nearby. This would not have been nearly as likely if she had gone to school in a more rural area.

From the provider perspective, it was unfortunate that Sally presented for a new consultation so soon before leaving for school and was not able to return for the suggested preparatory visits. Unfortunately, this is not uncommon. To be fair, she was medically stable and doing well. However, she and her family underestimated how much her stability depended on the structure of regular meals and snacks and oversight that her parents provided. It was important that the clinician attempted to engage them in some relapse prevention planning. It can be very helpful for the student to identify signs that they are slipping and to have input from parents about ways that they have noticed when things were not going well. If the student had returned for planning sessions, it would have been important to investigate the eating disorder services on campus, to consider making an appointment to establish providers to develop a safety net, and for the student to sign releases of information so that the university care team could contact the parents and/or home providers in the event that there was a significant clinical deterioration.

From the university perspective, Student of Concern teams can identify at risk students who may present in all sorts of ways. Faculty, residence life, the recreation center, cafeteria staff, and environmental services may have concerns about students and can make these concerns known to the Student of Concern team. Students may also present via the student health and/or counseling centers although providers there are limited by confidentiality (unless there is significant risk to self or others). If the committee feels there is significant risk, they can reach out to the student to express concern and to determine whether further investigation or intervention is needed. Because eating disorders are common in the teenage and young adult years, most colleges recognize the need for medical and mental health providers to have training in eating disorders and to be well versed in local treatment options. Many universities have multidisciplinary eating disorder care teams (consisting of a medical provider, psychotherapist, and dietitian) on campus that meet regularly to coordinate care.

Clinical Pearls

- Eating disorders have the highest mortality rate of any mental illness due to medical complications of malnutrition. Regular medical follow-up of weight, vital signs, and laboratory data while attending university is essential, and it is important that the student is medically stable and eating independently prior to making the transition.
- Multidisciplinary eating disorder care teams function optimally when roles are clearly defined, and there is close communication to prevent splitting and ensure that consistent messages are being given.
- Treatment contracts that spell out the frequency of visits to treatment team providers and clear relapse prevention plans can hold students accountable to consequences if they are deteriorating. It is important that family and providers are willing to follow through on the plan (i.e., the student will withdraw and seek a higher level of care if they drop below a certain weight).
- It is more likely that subspecialty providers and programs (like intensive outpatient and partial hospital programs, residential treatment programs) will be available in urban areas that are served by major medical centers.

- Having the student sign releases of information for the university team to communicate with parents and the home team is very important. There should be a clear plan as to who is directing treatment during the school year and whether the student will see the home team during school breaks. It is helpful for information (including a clinical summary) to be exchanged prior to matriculation.
- Parents have more influence than they think over whether their child seeks medical care after turning 18. Most college students continue to depend on their parents for financial and emotional support. Parents cannot legally force an adult child into treatment, but they can insist on medical stability and ongoing care as a requirement for staying enrolled in school if they are paying tuition.
- Many counseling centers have limits on the number of sessions available and will refer to community therapists when it is clear that long-term specialty treatment is necessary. It is important to know this from the start so that appropriate clinicians can be identified and insurance coverage for the community providers can be confirmed.

Brief Literature Review

According to the Spring 2016 American College Health Association's National College Health Assessment survey, in the prior 12 months, 1.3% of students report having been diagnosed with or treated for Anorexia Nervosa by a professional; another 1.1% report having been diagnosed or treated for Bulimia Nervosa. 1.4% reported that an eating disorder had significantly interfered with academic functioning [1]. In addition to having a profound effect on overall function in academic and social realms, the eating disorders can put medical health at significant risk due to concerns about malnutrition. Electrolyte abnormalities and atrophy of the cardiac muscle can lead to arrhythmia and sudden death. In addition, approximately half of deaths in anorexia nervosa are due to completed suicide [2].

Students with a history of disordered eating are at risk of relapse in times of stress and transition. New onset eating disorders are also common in the college years, especially with the focus on developing romantic relationships and being attractive to peers. The transition to college introduces a fairly abrupt change in structure and autonomy, while also dramatically increasing academic expectations. Students who previously participated in gym class or organized sports may no longer make time for regular exercise [3]. Others are so worried about gaining the "freshman fifteen" that they pre-emptively begin restricting intake and may engage in compulsive exercise [4]. Binge drinking may lead to overeating and weight gain. Misuse of stimulant medications and caffeine to increase academic productivity can have deleterious effects on appetite and lead to weight loss as well.

There are a number of outreach and prevention efforts that look promising but need further study. The Body Project is a cognitive-dissonance-based approach that encourages students to consider the harmful effects of the thin ideal and promotes advocacy and body positivity efforts in a small group setting [5]. Many campuses observe "Love your Body" Week during February's eating disorder awareness month, and may offer clinical screenings, advocacy projects, and panel discussions to promote awareness and encourage those with symptoms to consider treatment.

Helpful Resources

- AACAP Facts for Families—Eating Disorders in Teens https://www.aacap.org/AACAP/Families_and_Youth/Facts_for_Families/FFF-Guide/Teenagers-With-Eating-Disorders-002.aspx
- Academy for Eating Disorders Medical Guidelines http://www.aedweb.org/images/updatedmedicalcareguidelines/AED-Medical-Care-Guidelines_English_02.28.17_NEW.pdf
- Medical Management of Restrictive Eating Disorders in Adolescents & Young Adults http://www.jahonline.org/article/S1054-139X%2814%2900686-7/fulltext

References

1. Association, A. C. National College Health Assessment II: Spring 2016. 2016. http://www.acha-ncha.org/docs/ACHA-NCHA-II_ReferenceGroup_ExecutiveSummary_Spring2016.pdf
2. Birmingham CS. The mortality rate from anorexia nervosa. Int J Eat Disord. 2005;38:143–6.
3. Derenne J. Successsfully launching adolescents with eating disorders to college: the child and adolescent psychiatrist's perspective. J Am Acad Child Adolesc Psychiatry. 2013;52(6):559–61.
4. Schaumberg K, Anderson LM. Patterns of compensatory behaviors and disordered eating in college students. J Am Coll Health. 2014;62(8):526–33.
5. Rohde P, Shaw H. Assessing program sustainability in an eating disorder prevention effectiveness trial delivered by college clinicians. Behav Res Ther. 2015;72:1–8.

Transition in the Weeds: Heading to College with a Cannabis Use Disorder

18

Timothy VanDeusen

Case History

Joe is an 18-year-old Caucasian male, only child, recent public high school graduate who had educational supports through a 504 Plan, and a 5 year history of outpatient mental health treatment. He also had a very recent, lengthy, psychiatric inpatient stay and was about to attend a small university near a major metropolitan area. He was referred by his biological parents 1 month prior to the beginning of freshman year in college for combination therapy and medication management with a psychiatrist located near his new school.

Joe easily engaged in his initial evaluation, which took place over two sessions just 1 week after the referral. His parents were also seen at this time. He clearly described the symptoms which resulted in his hospitalization and presented other past treatment history, his educational history, and some social history in an organized fashion. Two weeks after his high school graduation Joe was hospitalized for a first episode of "psychosis and mania" when he smoked ½ ounce of marijuana in a period of 3 days by himself playing video games when his parents took a long weekend trip out of state. His usual use of marijuana had been 2–3 times per week sharing about 1/8 of an ounce with two or three friends. He experienced insomnia, paranoia, and racing thoughts. He thought people were trying to kill him which he described as "the most terrifying thing I've ever been through." He spent 1 month on a locked inpatient unit followed by 1 month in an intensive outpatient program (IOP) for comorbid mental health and substance use disorder diagnoses. His medications in the hospital included ziprasidone and clonazepam, which he reported in

T. VanDeusen, M.D.
Department of Psychiatry, Connecticut Mental Health Center, Yale School of Medicine, West Haven, CT, USA
e-mail: timothy.vandeusen@yale.edu

© Springer International Publishing AG, part of Springer Nature 2018
A. Martel et al. (eds.), *Promoting Safe and Effective Transitions to College for Youth with Mental Health Conditions*, https://doi.org/10.1007/978-3-319-68894-7_18

combination helped his anxiety. However, his mother insisted he not continue clonazepam after discharge for fear of its "addictive" potential. An amphetamine salt combination (ASC) he had been taking was temporarily stopped given the concern that it may have contributed to the psychotic symptoms. His "psychosis and mania" resolved in the hospital and he reported abstinence from marijuana and other illicit substances. He was discharged from the IOP on ziprasidone 40 mg at bedtime.

Joe was treated intermittently for depression, anxiety, and ADHD by a community outpatient psychiatrist and two therapists since the eighth grade. He said his parents forced him to go to therapy and talking about his feelings made him feel worse. One therapist did CBT but he was not motivated to do the homework. There was no report of family therapy, but when his parents were brought into a session, Joe felt uncomfortable and refused to talk. He was diagnosed with generalized anxiety disorder and ADHD in eighth grade and was prescribed an ASC which both he and parents report helped him. The dose of that medication was adjusted multiple times during high school with no untoward effects or dependency.

In ninth grade, he was treated for a depressive episode precipitated by family conflict which resulted in a 6 month separation of his parents. This also coincided with the death of his maternal grandfather, who had a close relationship with Joe. He struggled with mood and anxiety symptoms throughout high school, but treatment remained sporadic. In 12th grade, he was fatigued much of the time, had a noticeable drop in grades and an increased frequency of anxiety symptoms. He was prescribed lurasidone for "mood swings" which he did not take regularly because it made him more depressed, tired, and suicidal (his first and only experience of suicidal ideation). Joe denied any history of suicide attempts. It was unclear if other med trials were suggested by his outpatient psychiatrist. There was no report of separation anxiety or panic attacks. His mother is currently in treatment for anxiety.

Joe began smoking marijuana in ninth grade as a way to fit in at the new high school. At times, he smoked daily, which led to two high school suspensions, both unknown to his parents. He denied using substances to his providers, thinking they would tell his parents. No urine toxicology screens were ordered by his providers including his primary care physician. He drank alcohol once or twice per month and had never been intoxicated. He denied using any opiates or hallucinogens. He used a high dosage of an ASC, up to 70 mg daily, stating "it was prescribed that way." There was no report of legal charges or any referral to a substance abuse rehabilitation program. Maternal uncle had a history of substance dependence.

Joe grew up as an only child in a small town 90 min away from a major city. His mother and father worked full-time with his mother commuting to the city. His dad had a sales job requiring international travel with many weeks away from home. Joe was cared for by a full-time nanny from infancy until eighth grade when his mother quit her job to stay at home and spend more time with him. This resulted in an abrupt dismissal of the nanny, with Joe having no opportunity to say goodbye. Joe reported that this led to feelings of sadness and anger towards his mother, which he attributes to the beginning of his anxiety and depression. He rarely saw his father, yet always felt he was a disappointment to him. His father told him "if you played sports you would feel better." Joe was surprised that his recent hospitalization resulted in his father taking a major supportive role in his recovery and in planning for his care as he transitioned to college.

Joe stated he always felt "stupid," and struggled through elementary, middle, and secondary school. He attended a public school for grades K-4 and was bullied by other boys because "of my small size." He recalls periods of stomach aches and headaches which caused him to miss school. He entered a small, private school for grades 5–8. His attendance and mood improved, he was calmer and had fewer physical symptoms. He still had few friends and lacked confidence in most subjects except art and music. Per his request, he left private school and entered Grade 9 at the local public midsize high school. He initially had anxiety when switching schools, but it did not prevent him from attending school. He made some new male friendships leading to use of marijuana and alcohol. Joe's academic struggles resurfaced so his psychiatrist recommended neuropsychological testing. Testing revealed an above average IQ and confirmed the diagnosis of ADHD. Joe received accommodations for ADHD including extended time for tests, a quiet area to take exams to decrease distractions, and twice weekly support to help him track assignments under a 504 plan, all of which were helpful. Testing reports and 504 plans were not available for review.

The differential diagnosis at his pre-college psychiatric evaluation included cannabis use disorder, moderate, cannabis induced psychotic disorder, with onset during intoxication, generalized anxiety disorder, ADHD, persistent depressive disorder (formerly dysthymia), R/O major depressive disorder and R/O bipolar disorder. Certainly it was going to be important to track any psychotic symptoms, especially while abstinent from cannabis, to rule out a primary psychotic disorder. Joe signed releases of information authorizing information transfer from his former providers and allowing communication with parents about treatment compliance. No prior records were ever received and calls were not returned. Once college started, he would attend weekly psychotherapy/medication management sessions. Specific crisis management plans were not established although the new provider felt comfortable about accessing more intensive services, if needed, given that Joe had health insurance and was near a large medical center.

When applying to college, Joe took into consideration the location and size of the school and the availability of a pre-med curriculum (he wanted to be a physician like his grandfather). His mental health providers did not suggest that he consider the availability of academic supports or mental health services on various campuses. It is unclear if the high school attempted to develop Joe's self-advocacy skills regarding his ADHD. Joe applied very late and was admitted to only his current institution, a small private university which was a 3 h drive from home. He was excited to move into the dorm and experience college life. He registered for a full course load of five classes, two of these being biology and chemistry. The IOP treatment team attempted to discharge Joe to his long-term outpatient psychiatrist but that practice did not see young people over the age of 18 or once they graduated from high school. The IOP urged Joe and his parents to find treatment provider(s) on or near the college and to register for accommodations through the campus' disability office, all of which were set up in the weeks prior to the start of school.

In the next few sessions, Joe revealed that his roommate was caught by campus police with possession of marijuana found in his backpack which led to a 1 week suspension and was told the next time would be expulsion. This incident appeared to upset Joe, and he affirmed that he would not consider smoking marijuana for fear of similar consequences.

Despite attending all classes, including his 9 a.m. English class, Joe gradually began to have doubts about his ability to keep up with his coursework, and was very discouraged when he failed his first chemistry exam. He also had trouble keeping organized in biology lab. He complained of difficulty focusing in class and distractibility when doing homework. He was encouraged to follow-up at Disabilities Services which he had avoided due to stigma, denial of illness, and wanting to "make it on my own like most other kids." He was prescribed ASC which seemed to work. However, 2 weeks later, he began having panic attacks at night so ziprasidone was increased to 80 mg at bedtime. Joe was also given clonazepam 1 mg prn for insomnia. Both the ASC and the clonazepam were dispensed in carefully meted out amounts. Joe was cautioned to store these medications in a safe place and to not share any of his medication with peers. Both these pharmacological interventions were necessary to help prevent Joe from relapsing into using cannabis. He continued to firmly deny cannabis use given it might also explain his "panic attacks." He also denied paranoia and other perceptual disturbances.

As Joe started feeling more depressed, he shared the sense of loneliness he felt as an only child, amplified by his mother and father working full-time and traveling. He failed both midterms in biology and chemistry, had doubts about the pre-med major, and thought about switching to English, which he enjoyed. Treatment focus shifted to understanding and accepting his mental health issues and advocating for him to decrease his course load which he resisted as tuition was not prorated or reimbursable. A session with Joe and his father proved helpful when Dad reassured him that his health took priority. Joe's dad contacted the Dean who requested a letter from the psychiatrist recommending withdrawal from the science classes. Joe ended the term with 2 B's in humanities classes.

Joe's mother phoned the office during January break stating that Joe had decided to stay home winter semester and take classes at the local community college. His parents helped him connect to outpatient psychiatric services near his home. A random urine toxicology screen done by the new physician was positive for cannabinoids.

Analysis of Transition

There were a few factors predictive of a positive transition to college. Joe and his parents had secured a treatment provider who was near his new school and easily accessible via a campus shuttle. The region offered a full range of mental health services, at various levels of care, which accepted Joe's insurance. Accommodations had been established with the Office of Disabilities. He was taking ziprasidone regularly and on his own. Joe seemed committed to refrain from further cannabis use.

In contrast, there were many factors predictive of a poor transition outcome. Joe had a recent hospitalization and IOP stay with questionable mental health stability in the context of an upcoming major developmental transition. Despite this, he registered for a full load of classes. Although Joe had a treatment provider in place, a detailed relapse prevention plan, regarding cannabis use, was not specified. There was diagnostic uncertainty at the time of transition, given such a short time from the "psychotic" episode. Treatment throughout high school was inconsistent, there were gaps in the treatment history regarding clinical decision-making and medication choices, and his use of cannabis (partly from his nondisclosure) had gone undetected/unaddressed until after high school graduation. These factors made it difficult for Joe and his parents to begin to grasp the impact of his mental health issues in the college environment and to help him plan how to avoid cannabis use at college. He had a long history of impaired peer relationships and used substances to fit in. He had an unclear attachment to his parents and there was little attempt to address his mixed feelings towards them during high school and in preparation for transition. Joe had not fully processed the losses of his nanny and grandfather. Lastly, Joe seemed to have some ambivalence about attending college.

Joe had a suboptimal transition. Symptoms of anxiety, depression, and ADHD interfered with his academic functioning to the point that he needed to withdraw from some classes. He was unable to remain abstinent from cannabis, despite his scary experience a few months earlier, which likely exacerbated his symptoms. He qualified and had registered for academic supports but did not follow through and use them. On a positive note, he engaged with his new provider near campus, captured some credits for the semester, voluntarily established a new plan for second semester, and may have the opportunity to do some family work since he will be living at home.

There appeared to be many deficiencies in preparing Joe and his family for the transition to college. Given the recent hospital stay, the mental health providers at the IOP, along with those who had worked with Joe throughout high school, should have had frank discussions with Joe and his family about other postsecondary options besides going to a residential college and taking a full load. Joe could have asked to delay matriculation for one semester and taken one or two classes locally or worked part-time to maintain a low level of stress and to work on extending his abstinence and devising a relapse prevention plan. Alternatively, he could have requested a reduced course load at his college of choice and participated in more extensive substance use treatment near campus. Although Joe and his parents could provide a cogent history, treatment planning would be improved with better information transfer among former and new providers. The only information that was received came from the IOP and consisted of a list of his current medications and a few written progress notes. More nuanced information from Joe's former, longitudinal care providers, would have been helpful.

It is important for home providers to educate college-bound patients and their parents on ways the young person can manage their psychiatric issues in college. In Joe's case, education about (1) the prevalence of substances on college campuses, (2) situations to avoid in order to decrease access to substances and irresponsible use of substances, and (3) the availability of substance-free housing on some campuses would be important topics to cover. In addition, education about ADHD and the use of academic support services to promote success in the college academic environment may have been useful. Providers should remind patients that the stress of college might not be experienced initially but may occur about 4–6 weeks into the semester, the time of their first exams and deadlines for research projects or papers.

Joe was resistant to individual therapy and family therapy throughout high school. Perhaps a group therapy approach would have been more appealing to Joe to address his anxiety, social skills, and self-esteem. More sustained efforts to address family issues/relationships may have promoted autonomous functioning and separation from parents.

Joe's mental health providers should have taken a more active role in guiding both Joe and his parents in their decisions about college. The young person should be encouraged over time to explore his interests, strengths, and vulnerabilities. For this case, Joe may have pursued a humanities curriculum earlier and avoided academic failure. Ideally, the academic supports and mental health services at the chosen college should match the patient's needs. Other considerations that might ease the transition to college include the size of the college, the culture of the school regarding substance use, academic rigor, availability of flexible scheduling, proximity to home, and the availability of loans for part-time students.

Clinical Pearls

- Pre-college providers should provide psychoeducation to the prospective college student about the availability of cannabis on campus, high risk situations and how to manage them (relapse prevention), consequences of use/abuse, the possible cognitive and motivational effects of long-term cannabis use, and possible "no drugs" policy on most college campuses.
- When patients and parents begin visiting college campuses, they should inquire about treatment options on and off campus for substance abuse and mental health disorders, and if the family's insurance covers these services. Marijuana Anonymous or other 12-step groups, IOP programs for young adults with comorbid disorders, and providers with experience in MI/MET and MET/CBT therapies focused on marijuana dependence can all be useful.
- When working with TAY who are potentially abusing cannabis, consider collecting random urine toxicology screens. Normalize this by saying, "I request random urine specimens from all my patients that have a history of substance use." Some patients with substance use issues can benefit from urine collection to maintain sobriety.
- To improve a college student's motivation for decreasing cannabis use, providers may want to perform a quick screening test which can be a valuable way to show patients if they indeed meet criteria for cannabis use disorder. The most widely used screen, the CUDIT-R (Cannabis Use Disorder Identification Test-revised),

is an eight-item questionnaire, validated for DSM-5 cannabis use disorder and when used regularly can track effectiveness of treatment.

- Providers need to be aware that patients with co-occurring psychiatric illness and cannabis use disorder or other substance use disorders are at risk for relapse when psychiatric symptoms worsen. Also, symptoms of substance misuse may mimic those of comorbid psychiatric disorders or make it difficult to diagnose comorbid conditions, particularly if limited history is available.
- Pre-college providers can help TAY improve their self-advocacy skills by discussing their diagnoses, current and future treatments, overall functioning, and their rights and responsibilities under the Americans with Disabilities Act to access academic accommodations on campus.
- When psychiatrists on or near campus accept a new patient enrolling in college, it is very important to receive written/verbal records from former providers to design the most effective treatment for the student and to devise successful relapse prevention strategies.
- With the patient's permission, involving parents in the campus mental health intake process, to review the patient's past psychiatric history, identify triggers to relapse, and devise emergency plans can prove essential to a successful transition to college. Alternatively, providers may solicit the help of the family (with the patient's permission) in securing prior medical records.
- Students coming to campus with a diagnosed mental illness should ideally be seen by their new providers weekly for the first few weeks of school for a quality transfer of care. Determining what ongoing support will be needed for the patient after the initial transition should consider the patient's current adjustment to college, his/her past history of compliance with treatment, and ability to seek help when distressed or relapsing.
- For all students taking psychotropic medications, but especially those taking controlled substances, the provider should advise the student to store medications carefully (such as in a locked box) and caution that prescription refills will not be given out early.

Brief Literature Review

Cannabis is the most commonly used illicit drug by adults and adolescents in the United States [1]. It is also the most frequently reported substance misused on campus [2] and the rate of cannabis use by college students is rising. Among full-time college students surveyed in 2015 by the National Institute of Drug Abuse, as part of the Monitoring the Future Study [1], the annual prevalence of marijuana use was 38%, with prevalence rates in males higher than in females, 40% and 37%, respectively. Annual prevalence rates have been climbing over the past several years with the 2015 rate similar to those of the mid-1980s. Prevalence of daily marijuana use among college students in 2015 was 4.6%.

Various factors may have contributed to the increased use in cannabis: an increase in perceived safety and acceptability of cannabis [1]; increased potency of cannabis, from about 4% in 1995 to about 12% in 2014 [3]; a possible potentiation effect between cannabis and other substances of abuse [4]; and an increase in states with medical marijuana laws which appears to be associated with an increase in cannabis use and cannabis use disorders in those states [5].

The rising rate of marijuana use in adolescents and college students is also of concern as long-term marijuana use can have adverse impacts on brain development, particularly in adolescents [6]. Animal and human studies have documented cognitive effects such as decreased memory, compromised concentration, difficulties in information processing, and changes in motivation [6]. In a retrospective study, marijuana use during the first year of college was associated with poorer attendance in class, lower grade point averages, and longer time to graduation [7].

In a general population study [4], there was an increased risk of other substance use disorders with cannabis use. Cannabis may also represent a significant risk factor for the development of a psychotic illness in at-risk individuals [8]. Longitudinal studies have found that early onset of cannabis use was associated with a greater risk of developing psychotic symptoms compared to cannabis use begun at an older age [9]. Furthermore, "in adolescents and young adults with a first episode of psychosis, co-occurring substance use has been reported in as many as 74%, and this comorbidity has been associated with less effective treatment responses, decreased medication adherence, and a worsened course of illness" [8].

Because of increased marijuana use on campus, practitioners treating college students should routinely screen for alcohol and drug use, monitoring those at risk of abuse, and referring those with abuse disorders for treatment. Currently the most effective treatment and best evaluated intervention for cannabis abuse is CBT which is often used with MI or MET, with significant decreases in cannabis use and an increase in negative toxicology screens [10]. These interventions work best when the individual wants to decrease cannabis use frequency and amount. Pharmacologic interventions have shown no to modest effects in decreasing cannabis use [10]. A brief, in-person MET intervention in college students reduced marijuana use over a short-term period of 3 months [2]. Given current trends for use of marijuana by adolescents and young adults, cannabis use disorders require increased attention from medical and mental health practitioners, researchers, educators, as well as policy and law makers.

Helpful Resources

- National Institute on Drug Abuse https://www.drugabuse.gov/drugs-abuse/marijuana
- Chart of Evidence-Based Screening Tools for Adults and Adolescents https://www.drugabuse.gov/nidamed-medical-health-professionals/tool-resources-your-practice/screening-assessment-drug-testing-resources/chart-evidence-based-screening-tools-adults

- Screening and Assessment of Cannabis Use Disorders (CUDIT-R)
  Adamson SJ, Kay-Lambkin FJ, Baker AL, Lewin TJ, Thornton L, Kelly BJ, and Sellman JD. (2010). An Improved Brief Measure of Cannabis Misuse: The Cannabis Use Disorders Identification Test—Revised (CUDIT-R). Drug and Alcohol Depend. 110:137–143.
  http://www.warecoveryhelpline.org/wp-content/uploads/2016/11/CUDIT-R-revised-with-scoring.pdf
- Pew Research Center, "6 Facts About Marijuana" http://www.pewresearch.org/fact-tank/2015/04/14/6-facts-about-marijuana/
- https://findtreatment.samhsa.gov
- http://www.integration.samhsa.gov/clinical-practice/sbirt/brief_counseling_for_marijuana_dependence.pdf

References

1. Johnston LD, O'Malley PM, Bachman JG, Schulenberg JE, Miech RA. Monitoring the Future national survey results on drug use, 1975–2015: Volume College students and adults ages 19–55. Ann Arbor: Institute for Social Research, The University of Michigan; 2016. http://www.monitoringthefuture.org/pubs/monographs/mtf-vol2_2015.pdf
2. Lee CM, Kilmer JR, Neighbors C, Atkins DC, Zheng C, Walker DD, Larimer ME. Indicated prevention for college student marijuana use: a randomized controlled trial. J Consult Clin Psychol. 2013;81(4):702–9.
3. El Sohly MA, Mehmedic Z, Foster S, Gon C, Chandra S, Church JC. Changes in cannabis potency over last two decades (1995–2014) analysis of current data in United States. Biol Psychiatry. 2016;79(7):613–9.
4. Blanco C, Hasin DS, Wall MM, Florez-Salamanca L, Hoertel N, Wang S, Kerridge BT, Olfson M. Cannabis use and risk of psychiatric disorders: prospective evidence from a US National Longitudinal study. JAMA Psychiatry. 2016;73(4):388–95.
5. Hasin DS, Wall M, Keyes KM, Cerdá M, Schulenberg J, O'Malley PM, Galea S, Pacula R, Feng T. Medical marijuana laws and adolescent marijuana use in the USA from 1991 to 2014: results from annual, repeated cross-sectional surveys. Lancet Psychiatry. 2015;2(7):601–8.
6. Lisdahl KM, Wright NE, Medina-Kirchner C, Maple KE, Shollenbarger S. Considering cannabis: the effects of regular cannabis use on neurocognition in adolescents and young adults. Curr Addict Rep. 2014;1:144–56.
7. Aura AM, Caldeira KM, Bugbee BA, Vincent KB, O'Grady KE. The academic consequences of marijuana use during college. Psychol Addict Behav. 2015;29(3):564–75.
8. Goerke D, Kumra S. Substance abuse and psychosis. Child Adolesc Psychiatr Clin N Am. 2013;22(4):643–54.
9. Parakh P, Basu D. Cannabis and psychosis: have we found the missing links? Asian J Psychiatr. 2013;6:281–7.
10. Walther L, Gantner A, Heinz A, Majic T. Evidence-based treatment options in cannabis dependency. Dtsch Arztebl Int. 2016;113(39):653–9. https://doi.org/10.3238/arztebl.2016.0653.

Stealing Youth: Personality Disorder Goes to College

19

Vivien Chan

Case History

Jimmy was a slender, 19-year-old Filipino-American cisgender single heterosexual male, third of four children, born to middle-class, married-but-estranged parents. He enrolled in a large suburban in-state public research university, the most reputable IHE to which he got accepted (per his account), located 400 miles from his hometown after graduating in the top 20% of his elite private high school which was highly ranked and considered academically rigorous. He entered initially with a major in physics, with the intent to study "pre-med" but later changed his major to psychology due to a declining grade point average (GPA). At the time of college entry, he carried diagnoses of Oppositional Defiant Disorder; Other Specified Depressive Disorder; Social Anxiety Disorder; Parent–Child Relational Problem; r/o Cluster B (Borderline) Traits; r/o Cluster C (Avoidant) traits. Jimmy was first seen by the campus counseling service during the first semester of his freshman year of college. Later, he transferred to the campus insurance-based service for longer term care, and this service sought records of past treatment.

Jimmy saw a high school counselor sporadically (~5 visits) during his first 2 years of high school for complaints of rebellious behavior (e.g., not talking to parents, walking out of the home when angry, yelling at parents, being "mouthy" to teachers, and refusing to complete assignments). Despite these behaviors, he maintained his A/A- grades, even in his Advanced Placement classes, by achieving high scores on tests. His externalizing behaviors were thought to be in reaction to overly strict parenting, so he and his family were referred to a concierge-type licensed

V. Chan, M.D.
Student Health Center, University of California Irvine, Irvine, CA, USA

Department of Psychiatry and Human Behavior, UCI Health, Orange, CA, USA
e-mail: Vchan1@uci.edu

© Springer International Publishing AG, part of Springer Nature 2018
A. Martel et al. (eds.), *Promoting Safe and Effective Transitions to College for Youth with Mental Health Conditions*, https://doi.org/10.1007/978-3-319-68894-7_19

professional counselor (LPC) therapist in the community. In response to a request for records by the campus insurance-based comprehensive service, the LPC initially wanted to give a verbal summary in lieu of a written one. While a phone call was arranged, the service also repeated its request for records. Eventually, the LPC sent a brief handwritten summary which indicated that subsequent to the first session, an attempted family session was unproductive due to each family member's stonewalling of verbal engagement as well as reticence to talking about emotional and family issues. In the following two sessions, Jimmy shared with the LPC that in the context of feeling high levels of distress, frustration, and loneliness, he had engaged in intermittent self-asphyxiation and superficial cutting in the recent past. He denied current urges to harm himself and denied suicidal intent. The LPC informed the parents and referred Jimmy and his family to a psychologist for family work and a child and adolescent psychiatrist in the community. The working diagnosis appeared to be Parent–Child Relational Problem and Personal History of Self-Harm. Despite Jimmy's parents' perceived stigma about mental health treatment, given that the high school was made aware of their son's self-harming behaviors by the LPC, they felt obliged to follow through with the referrals.

The psychologist and psychiatrist, after their independent evaluations and consent-authorized consultations with each other, diagnosed Jimmy with Oppositional Defiant Disorder; Other Specified Depressive Disorder; Social Anxiety Disorder; Parent–Child Relational Problem; r/o Cluster B (Borderline) Traits; r/o Cluster C (Avoidant) traits. Medical and substance use history were noncontributory. Jimmy denied having any current legal problems or past trouble with the law. He denied a history of physical or sexual abuse, and his parents denied a family history of mental illness. Individual and family psychotherapy were recommended as well as pharmacotherapy. Jimmy and his parents were adamantly opposed to medication, and they discontinued psychiatry visits after the initial consultation. Jimmy and his parents presented intermittently to the psychologist for family work, which was characterized by talking over one another. The family eventually dropped out of psychological treatment.

However, Jimmy met with his LPC, on average, one to two times a month through junior and senior years of high school. Therapy was primarily supportive, focusing on self-esteem. Jimmy discussed his feelings of inadequacy as compared with his peers. He did not have any sustained friendships. He lamented not having a girlfriend. He externalized blame, stating that his siblings belittled him for his slender size. He felt distant from his older siblings, who were almost a decade older than he, and he did not relate to his youngest sister, whom he described as "annoyingly perfect." He expressed discontent that his parents did not acknowledge his efforts and accomplishments as praiseworthy and that they did not chastise his siblings for their (perceived) derogatory comments. When revealing a family secret that his father conducted extramarital affairs, he seemed apathetic about it. Jimmy reported intermittent episodes of self-asphyxiation and cutting, denying these were suicide attempts, stating he engaged in them when he examined his lonely existence. He would report these events post-fact and without physical evidence of harm and was not hospitalized psychiatrically. His LPC encouraged him to attend an outpatient adolescent dialectical behavioral therapy (DBT) group; Jimmy attended about half of the sessions and reported that he stopped self-harm behaviors. He and his parents did not feel that he needed to continue extra treatment and stopped DBT groups prematurely.

At first glance, Jimmy appeared prepared to go to college from high school. He had independent, albeit haphazard academic functioning, and he managed his own schedule, grooming and transportation. He had not required any academic accommodations throughout high school. His trouble with authority figures had diminished. However, Jimmy was underdeveloped in his own identity and in social relationships. The LPC attempted to advance Jimmy's psychosocial development by encouraging him to get a part-time job, to volunteer at a local animal shelter, or to join a gaming club at school. Jimmy joined a video game interest club at school, under heavy therapeutic pressure.

In therapy, some time was spent on looking at aspects of the college environment which were different from high school and which might pose problems for Jimmy, like having a roommate. The LPC also remarked that Jimmy might benefit from continuing therapy on campus and that he should look into the availability, accessibility, and cost of mental health services on or near campus, but Jimmy felt this was not necessary. He applied to several schools, all of which were a full-day car ride from home. Parents declined to get involved with college transition activities, with Jimmy's father revealing on the phone that he expected Jimmy's family relationships to improve once he was away at college, predicting a similar experience to what the Father had with his own parents.

At the penultimate planned session, Jimmy revealed a long-standing history of theft. Since starting high school, he had regularly stolen small electronics in the form of cell phones, tablets, gaming equipment, and other mobile electronics, and he either fenced them whole or dismantled them, selling off parts. This activity was one source where he derived positive self-esteem. He believed that other students who were "stupid enough" to leave their items unsecured deserved to lose them. Since he had turned 18 years old, the therapist could not now share this information with Jimmy's parents. Jimmy also revoked all consents and did not present to his termination visit. He did not respond to further phone calls, nor to a letter from the LPC.

Jimmy presented to the campus counseling service sporadically throughout freshman year with complaints of dysphoria related to low self-esteem, comparing his academic, social, and dating abilities to peers and feeling inadequate. Given the infrequency of his appointments, he was seen by serial supervised trainees but was not referred to the in-house psychiatrist. Jimmy complained that going home on holidays was "boring" and a waste of time; however, he never made alternative plans. When home, he isolated himself and passed the time playing video games. His parents had little input in his day-to-day campus life other than to pay the tuition and fees. At the counseling service, Jimmy's diagnosis was Adjustment Disorder with Depressed Mood, ruling out Major Depressive Disorder. His counseling service providers did not raise any diagnostic questions, did not describe any personality disordered features, and did not request any prior treatment records. Early in his sophomore year, he presented again to the counseling service and due to the recurrent nature of his complaints he was quickly referred for "long term" care services, to the insurance-based mental health program on campus. There, he established care with a psychiatrist and psychologist, and he also was assisted by a licensed clinical social worker for complex case management needs. Counseling services did not have a shared treatment record with the insurance-based mental health program on campus, so Jimmy signed an authorization for information to be exchanged with the counseling service as well as with his past treatment providers.

The counseling service records documented an unusual event. Jimmy had requested help from his mental health counselor regarding his first C grade (in a physics class). Despite receiving a signed consent to speak with the counselor about Jimmy's grades, the senior academic advisor refused to exchange information. The advisor became fixated on the medical terminology on the authorization form, which primarily followed health privacy rules to meet state professional privacy regulations. However, as a university facility providing services exclusively to students, the counseling records were governed by FERPA as were the student's academic records. It also was evident that the student was presenting different stories to different people. In session, Jimmy agreed to the psychological counselor's plans to assist and support him about his C grade. To the academic advisor, Jimmy portrayed that he had been coerced to share his academic information, about which he was very ashamed, going so far as to claim that his counselor raised his voice at him and pressured him into consent. The academic advising team aligned with Jimmy's portrayal that the helping services were unhelpful, and even, aggressive.

A similar scenario was reenacted when his insurance-based psychiatrist and psychologist later sought an authorization for release of information from the same academic advisor. Instead of seeing the larger perspective that collaboration and information assisted clinical providers in treatment planning, the advisor made various allegations based on Jimmy's hearsay about unprofessional behavior by the clinicians. This layperson did not have any insight into the pathological defense mechanisms that appeared to be occurring. Due to the hostile, unfounded, escalating claims of the senior academic advisor, the clinical team sought administrative and legal consultation. Jimmy himself denied any provocative speech that would have given the academic advisor such a misleading perception of treatment and portrayed himself as innocently misunderstood to the clinical team. Ultimately, the advisor was counseled by administrative and legal personnel to facilitate communication. The advisor saw his own role as the lone supportive individual who was keeping Jimmy successfully engaged in college and remained hostile toward clinical staff, rebuffing psychoeducation from the clinical team about the student's communication patterns.

Concerned about his dropping grades, Jimmy elected to change his major to psychology (and to a different academic advising team). After doing so, he attended class more regularly and remained in good academic standing. His change in major buoyed his GPA. He did not register for nor receive any disability accommodations at university. He lived with a male roommate in campus-adjacent apartment housing. He yearned to date and socialize, but other than his friendship with his roommate, he was quite socially isolated. Although he reported feeling fine speaking up in class when called upon, he was unwilling to explore campus groups, attend intramural sports, or engage in leadership development. He was fearful of making any social overtures at the risk of embarrassing himself. He refused to sign consent for the clinical team to speak with his family. After the home-based treatment records arrived, Jimmy was able to talk with the psychologist, psychiatrist, and social worker about his long-standing depression, self-injury, and thefts. Although he could describe long-standing depression, he had a difficult time seeing major depressive disorder and anxiety as legitimate medical conditions. He admitted that he and his roommate had bonded more because they had started stealing items together. Despite his pride in stealing, he continued to experience neurovegetative symptoms of depression and was started on antidepressant medication which was also hoped to address his anxiety. Jimmy reported compliance with oral medications and came to every scheduled psychiatric, psychological, and social worker appointment.

Within 4 months of his transition of care to the insurance-based clinic, Jimmy and his roommate were arrested for shoplifting. Jimmy was terrified that the police would examine his mobile phone where he kept a "trophy list" of all of his crimes. Subsequent to that time and through to the resolution of his court case, he was intermittently suicidal, with sudden attacks of dysphoria and hopelessness. He believed that death by suicide was preferable to incarceration, reporting that he would complete suicide if he were sentenced to jail. He continually refused consents to speak with his family and with his roommate, and he kept his legal problems and treatment hidden from his parents. His roommate started to distance himself from Jimmy due to their legal issues. Jimmy questioned the value of interpersonal relationships and expressed hopelessness about his ability to maintain them.

Occasionally through the next academic year, he continued deliberate self-harm, again in the form of self-asphyxiation and, once, used a razor to cut superficial vertical lines on the flexor aspect of his forearms, stating that "it would make the veins and arteries bleed out faster." He would report these events grudgingly, often evading and falling silent when asked. He denied that these were suicide attempts and stated he engaged in them to relieve psychic pain when he examined his lonely existence. Jimmy did not initially agree to voluntary hospitalization, citing a need to maintain his schoolwork. He later was involuntarily hospitalized psychiatrically twice for self-asphyxiation when discovered by his roommate. He claimed these as rehearsal for hanging in jail. He was discharged both times within 72 h. The hospital attributed his repeated suicidality to the prolonged, uncertain outcome of his legal case.

As his court date drew nearer, Jimmy wondered aloud if a psychiatric hospitalization would help a judge be more sympathetic to his plight. The psychiatric bed shortage limited voluntary hospitalization when he was ready to consider it. However, he was not open to higher levels of care, such as partial hospitalization (PHP) or intensive outpatient treatment (IOP). The two local DBT centers were cash-only. Despite exploring options with the social worker, Jimmy prioritized his attorney fees over DBT. Jimmy eventually reported that his attorney did not recommend using mental health problems as a legal strategy, but this did not change his fears about possible incarceration. As his court date became imminent, Jimmy's providers alerted the campus Student of Concern team of his chronic suicidality and his risk of suicide pending legal outcome of the case. The Student of Concern team did not take any active action but remained alerted to Jimmy's risk. Jimmy's academic progress remained steady, holding between a 3.2 and 3.4 GPA.

By the end of his junior year, Jimmy's attorney was able to plead the case to a misdemeanor with probation. His cell phone trophy list was never discovered in police investigation. Recklessly, Jimmy continued to steal items while his court case was pending and afterward. His depression lingered past the resolution of his court case and diminished over the course of his senior year but still impaired his socialization activities. Although he was less contemplative of suicidal plans, he continued to doubt his romantic and social abilities. Jimmy remained quite isolated socially. He required adjunctive antipsychotic medication to improve depressive symptoms. After addition of antipsychotic medication, he stopped self-injurious behaviors. He never permitted consent to obtain collateral information from his family.

Jimmy continued to be selective in reporting his history. One day, he came to treatment and announced to his psychologist that he was fearful he would not get a good reference check from his internship. He had been employed for some time and had independently gotten hired as a scribe in a medical office. He stated he needed the job in order to pay for his legal bills. When asked why he did not reveal this earlier, or to the social worker when exploring DBT referral, he claimed it was the fault of the treatment team for not asking explicitly enough. After graduation, he managed to interview for and secure a job, and he continued community-based psychiatric and psychological services, having finally acknowledged the benefit and need for ongoing mental health care. In fact, he asked to remain with his current treatment team, which could not occur due to college policies of treating students only.

Analysis of Transition

Jimmy had a number of strengths that may be viewed as predictive of a positive transition outcome. He was a strong student, who had undergone previous treatment, and he had a companionable, yet concerning, relationship with his roommate. He demonstrated a history of reaching out for assistance with mental health and academic concerns on his own once in college. Despite this, there were also numerous challenges that can be seen as predictive of a negative transition. He had adolescent-onset problematic behaviors and no transition care plan. His family was not involved in treatment, and Jimmy characterized his family as unsupportive and overly harsh. There appeared to be stigma against mental health disorders within the family. In addition, he was engaged in active illegal behavior and active deliberate self-harm with suicidal ideation, and his depression had been suboptimally treated. Finally, there was inadequate sharing of records across treatment settings and limited options to validate Jimmy's history given his refusal to grant consent for the treatment team to speak with his parents.

This case represents a failed transition to college because Jimmy's education was significantly affected by his mental health difficulties and legal challenges. Although he sought treatment throughout high school and college, inadequate sharing of records, suboptimal history taking, selective reporting, and marginal adherence to the high school treatment plan by the patient made it challenging to properly diagnose and fully treat his symptoms. Unfortunately, this can be quite common.

It is possible that if the LPC who worked with Jimmy in his high school years had framed transition tasks as being important for future academic success, he and his family may have been more willing to develop a transition care plan that would have improved continuity of care. A safe and predictable transfer of care plan, which included crisis management and an overlap of treatment teams, may have provided a holding environment across settings and been helpful to Jimmy. Given that Jimmy attended individual sessions regularly in high school, a therapeutic approach beyond supportive therapy, such as CBT or DBT, done in a planned and progressive fashion, may have helped identify precedents to episodes of self-harm, diminish the frequency of such episodes, and build self-regulation skills in preparation for the transition to college.

Some providers are reluctant to acknowledge and discuss maladaptive personality traits with patients and families. Sometimes, provider bias lends itself to overlooking personality problems or treating them as lesser forms of brain pathology. Transient maladaptive personality characteristics may arise in the developmental period of late adolescence and early adulthood. Clinicians can highlight at-risk personality traits, interpersonal styles and behaviors in hopes of engaging emerging adults into necessary therapeutic treatments before traits blossom into full-blown personality disorders. Providers should help patients and families with personality problems look for IHE that have experienced providers of specific evidence-based, manualized treatments on campus or nearby. Although it may be very challenging to replicate all the components of intensive evidence-based treatments, like DBT, CBT, or Multisystemic Therapy (MST) on an outpatient service, a firm understanding of development and family dynamics can often modify outcomes. In particular, family coaching and psychoeducation is key to successful management of personality disorders.

When transitioning patients with maladaptive personality traits or personality disorders, providers may need to broach a conversation about the different levels of care available. Depending on the level of insight, motivation, and overall functioning, patients may require regular or intensive outpatient treatment, or partial hospitalization. In more severe cases, patients may need inpatient hospitalization and may even benefit from postponing matriculation or taking a medical leave of absence to devote time to residential treatment. Relapse prevention discussions aimed at helping patients identify the signs and symptoms that would require a higher level of care should be routinely incorporated into treatment discussions as anticipatory guidance. Such conversations can helpfully realign patients' concept of the severity of their own illness.

Clinical Pearls

- Clinicians should help patients with personality disorders develop a Wellness Recovery Action Plan (WRAP) (http://mentalhealthrecovery.com/) and a Wellness Toolbox early on, so that more adaptive coping strategies may be learned and refined well in advance of transition to college. The free app, Virtual Hope Box (http://t2health.dcoe.mil/apps/virtual-hope-box) offers a modern way to do this.
- When considering and applying to college, patients with personality disorders and their families should consider the proximity, availability, and feasibility of outpatient services, as well as IOP, PHP, residential treatment programs, and psychiatric hospitals in the area. It is important that there are accessible practitioners of evidence-based treatments such as DBT, CBT, and MST nearby.
- When there is a strong treatment relationship already in place, families and clinicians may want to consider encouraging the youth to apply to competitive colleges close to home. This may allow the student to remain in a consistent therapeutic relationship throughout the college years.
- Maladaptive personality traits may surface in late adolescence and young adulthood and resolve over time with ongoing brain maturation, new developmental experiences in new environments, removal from a negative or toxic environment, and/or treatment.
- Patients with personality disorders may be disruptive on campus. Due to sharing inconsistent information with different staff members, splitting and other pathological defense mechanisms may occur. It is important that team members communicate freely and frequently to present a unified, cohesive plan. Extra consultation or team meetings may be required, especially if the multidisciplinary providers are not colocated.
- Safety concerns such as self-injury and suicidality must be addressed early and often, and the Student of Concern team may need to be involved to communicate and enforce firm and consistent limits around how to handle at-risk and unsafe behavior.
- Administrative and legal consultation may be necessary to clarify FERPA and HIPAA when dealing with counseling centers, health care clinics, and academic offices that are bound by different privacy laws. Releases of information can have language that is specific to only one privacy law and may be needed between two mental health services on the same campus.
- In observing confidentiality and ethical rules, mental health providers cannot report committed crimes revealed in the course of psychotherapy except as required by law (e.g., duty to warn/harm to a specific target, or instances of preventing child or elder abuse). Providers working on campuses may be subject to the federal Clery Act which requires aggregate crime statistic reporting.
- Continuity of information from one provider to the next can be inadequate and difficult to access. Even within campus entities, records may be in "information silos," behind firewalls. Providers may need to prepare consents for each individual within a system, and case managers may more easily contact key stakeholders across disciplines.

- Prompt responses to requests for information from other mental health providers can facilitate timely development of a differential diagnosis and appropriate treatment plan. For clinicians, there is value even in brief off-service summary notes with a future treatment provider in mind. Sample off-service notes are shown under office-based tools.
- It is important for clinicians with the appropriate training and experience to be involved in complicated cases. There is a balance between providing sound care within effective boundaries and in determining when failures in treatment engagement have occurred. Inadequate history taking about self-injury and legal issues may lead to a delay in optimal treatment.
- While child and adolescent psychiatrists typically advocate for involving parents in care, there are certain situations (e.g., abuse, neglect, overly harsh, or demeaning interactions) where parental involvement may not be in the young person's best interests. It is necessary to follow the young person's lead and "roll with resistance" unless there are critical safety and ethical factors.

Brief Literature Review

Personality disorders, where effective treatments are primarily psychosocial [1–3], are often comorbid with other psychiatric conditions, where effective treatments may include medications. Although personality disorders are often considered chronic and immutable, up to 45% of BPD patients remitted in 2 years and 85% remitted in a 10-year longitudinal study [4]. Even though BPD is not often diagnosed until adulthood, it often begins in adolescence [5]. According to Gunderson, the age of onset of BPD is 15% in adolescence (13–17 years), 50% in early adulthood (18–25 years), 25% in young adulthood (26–30 years), and 10% in adulthood (31–48 years) [6]. The temporal stability of borderline personality disorder diagnosis is lower than that of other personality disorders, and BPD carries significant heritability (up to 68%) [5]. This may lead to provider bias in choosing to refer to time-intensive psychotherapies, like DBT, mentalization-based therapies, MST, or family psychoeducation. One randomized controlled trial unsurprisingly found DBT efficacious in college students [7]. Even though manualized therapies, like STEPPS (http://www.steppsforbpd.com/), are more studied for personality disorders, psychodynamic therapies and transference-based therapies are also effective [6]. Mentalization-based therapies are also showing promise for antisocial personality disorder [8]. Despite the optimistic prognostic data, personality traits and disorders nonetheless are associated with higher interpersonal and partner conflict compared with age-matched peers [9]. The repository of high quality literature on personality disorders, college transition, and this population is scanty. However, there is a strong body of literature on the treatment of personality disorders in general, and BPD in specific. In this case, the patient engaged in a less well-studied but high-risk-for fatality behavior, self-asphyxiation [10].

The principles of self-care are important for both patients and practitioners and are embodied in WRAP. Comprised of an inventory of wellness tools, daily maintenance plan, and identification of triggers, regular implementation of WRAP should be considered. When working with personality disorders, clinicians should also regularly seek professional consultation to manage boundaries, as well as the conscious and unconscious demands of therapeutic work.

Helpful Resources

Resources for Clinicians

- Casey Life Skills helpfully outline domains that are important to living independently: https://www.casey.org/casey-life-skills-resources/
- WRAP: http://mentalhealthrecovery.com/
- National Education Alliance for Borderline Personality Disorder: http://www.borderlinepersonalitydisorder.com

Resources for Families

- "Transition Resources A-Z" https://www.ahead.org/students-parents/transitions
- College and Career Readiness Standards http://www.parentcenterhub.org/priority-cc-readiness/
- Borderline Personality http://www.ulifeline.org/topics/149-borderline-personality
- How Borderline Personality Disorder Can Impact College https://www.verywell.com/how-borderline-personality-disorder-can-impact-college-425150

Office-Based Tools: Sample Off-Service Notes

Documentation in progress notes and an "off service" summary are important for future providers to understand the transition plan of care. For providers too rushed to compose an entire treatment summary, communication can be quickly facilitated by planning ahead. Regularly in the progress note, an abbreviated summary, such as "Jimmy, who entered this service in 201x and who received brief counseling in 200x and 201x was started on [medication] in [month/year] and reached a stable dose of [milligram] by [month/year]," can be tremendously helpful, even to cross-covering providers and consultants. When transitioning patients off service, another plan, such as "Discussed with Jimmy maintaining dosages of current medications for at least an additional 6-month period or until psychosocial events, such as the start and maintenance of a new job, are going well. In addition, he was given a [xx day] supply of medications and was advised that all services will cease based on his eligibility as a nonstudent pending [date]. He was referred to [resources] on how to [find/use] his next insurance service and encouraged to have all records transferred to his new provider directly prior to his first appointment."

References

1. Linehan M. DBT® skills training manual. 2nd ed. New York: The Guildford Press; 2014.
2. Henggeler S, Schoenwald S, Borduin C, et al. Multisystemic therapy for antisocial behavior in children and adolescents. 2nd ed. New York: The Guildford Press; 2009.
3. Bleiberg E. Treating personality disorders in children and adolescents: a relational approach. New York: The Guildford Press; 2001.
4. Gunderson J, Stout R, McGlashan T, et al. Ten-year course of borderline personality disorder. Arch Gen Psychiatry. 2011;68(8):827–37.
5. Biskin R. The lifetime course of borderline personality disorder. Can J Psychiatry. 2015; 60(7):303–8.
6. Gunderson JG, Links P. Borderline personality disorder: a clinical guide. 2nd ed. Washington, DC: American Psychiatric Publishing; 2008.
7. Pistorello J, Fruzetti A, MacLane C, et al. Dialectical Beahvior Therapy (DBT) applied to college students: a randomized clinical trial. J Consult Clin Psychol. 2012;80(6):982–94.
8. Bateman A, O'Connell J, Lorenzini N, et al. A randomized controlled trial of mentalization-based treatment versus structured clinical management for patients with comorbid borderline personality disorder and antisocial personality disorder. BMC Psychiatry. 2016;16:304. https://doi.org/10.1186/s12888-061-1000-9.
9. Chen H, Cohen P, Johnson J, et al. Adolescent personality disorders and conflict with romantic partners during the transition to adulthood. J Pers Disord. 2004;18(6):507–25.
10. Busse H, Harrop T, Gunnel D, et al. Prevalence and associated harm of engagement in self-asphyxial behaviors ('choking game') in young people: a systematic review. Arch Dis Child. 2015;100:1106–14.

Part III

Clinical Cases Focusing on Special Populations and Situations

"Baby, Please Don't Change": Transitioning Squared, Transgender in College

20

Ludmila De Faria

Case History

Jay is a 19 y/o Caucasian transgender male (born female), only child, born and raised in urban NY state. His parents report an uneventful childhood and normal development. He reported no problems growing up and graduated in the top 10% of his high school class. He had never seen a psychiatrist before coming to college, despite ongoing anxiety and history of self-injurious behavior, and a diagnosis of Attention Deficit Hyperactivity Disorder (ADHD) given by his pediatrician.

Jay reported that he had struggled with gender and body issues most of his life. When he was around 7 or 8 y/o he used to pray to wake up as a boy. In addition to that, he had a degenerative muscular illness (Charcot-Marie-Tooth) that caused significant physical impairment. These issues significantly interfered with social life, school, and self-esteem. Jay reported being "weird at making friends" and having no social interaction with peers outside school. He developed symptoms of what he now realizes was depression around age nine or ten, but was never formally diagnosed or treated.

He also admitted to increased anxiety since middle school, and had difficulties with making friends, especially outside of the school day. He worried too much, especially in social situations, where he felt "too self-conscious" and "judged" to connect with others. He had difficulty sustaining attention in school and based on parental report of behavioral issues, was eventually diagnosed with ADHD by his pediatrician. The school did not feel that he needed testing or accommodations given that his grades were so good. He was started on Strattera, but according to his

L. De Faria, M.D.
University Health Services, Florida State University College of Medicine,
Tallahassee, FL, USA
e-mail: Ldefaria@fsu.edu

© Springer International Publishing AG, part of Springer Nature 2018
A. Martel et al. (eds.), *Promoting Safe and Effective Transitions to College for Youth
with Mental Health Conditions*, https://doi.org/10.1007/978-3-319-68894-7_20

parents, experienced severe and intolerable side effects and parents decided to stop medication after a very short time and work on structuring his schedule instead. They reportedly did not want him to see a psychiatrist. According to Jay, home life was not "the best" and added to his feelings of anxiety. He was born into an upper middle-class family that reinforced traditional gender roles. His father was a professional with a graduate degree and the main bread winner and his mother was a stay at home parent, who made sure Jay stayed on track in school. According to Jay, his mother had "a lot of emotional issues, but refused to get help." She would often display irritable mood and was hypercritical of Jay. He had a better relationship with Father, whom he described as supportive. Mother made all decisions concerning home life and the children. During the middle and high school years, he achieved academic success thanks to Mother's strict managing of his schedule and assignments. They often clashed about Jay's appearance (he insisted on wearing shorts and pants and avoided dresses) and the friction between Jay and his mother contributed to his anxiety. He reported frequent arguments that ended in meltdowns and self-injurious behaviors (cutting). During those arguments, Mother also became agitated and Father later told the psychiatrist that he feared they would "kill each other."

Although he began to inform himself about transgender issues and "contemplate" the idea of being a male throughout high school, he never discussed it with his parents. The summer between junior and senior year in high school he attended a camp where he met and fell in love with his first girlfriend. They maintained a long-distance relationship for half a year. During that time, as he still lived as a woman, he decided to come out as transgender to his friends and as a lesbian to his family. According to Jay, his parents thought it was "a phase" and chalked it up to the fact that Jay did not have boyfriends and did not feel pretty as a girl. Being openly lesbian caused more social difficulties. He was ostracized by peers and had a very small circle of friends. After he broke up with his girlfriend, he did not date again. He blamed his lack of dating experience on his social awkwardness. Despite being forced to participate in several extra-curricular activities, he reported feeling uncomfortable in most settings. He now thinks that people were not sure if he was "boy" or "girl" and did not approach him. Although he was resentful of their attitude, he also internalized some of their transphobia. He often remarked that he could not find a date because "girls don't like feminine-looking trans men." He denied explicit bullying, though. Once he came to college, he decided to live openly as a transgender male.

Jay saw college as an escape from home life and was invested in staying in school. Unfortunately, most of his academic success in high school had been achieved under the close supervision of his mother. She supervised him while he worked, selected the classes for him to take, communicated with teachers, and reviewed all his assignments. She insisted that he participate in extracurricular activities to build up his resume and college application. At the end of high school, he had the grades to attend an academically rigorous state university with over 40,000 students. He chose this school for the undergraduate music program and intended to eventually apply to law school. Both Jay and his family focused mainly on academic success to the detriment of addressing his mental health issues. Jay never utilized accommodations during high school, and both he and his parents assumed that he would do well without them in college as well. Despite the previous issues identified by his pediatrician, including ADHD and anxiety, they did not see the need to explore mental health or academic support resources available at his college of choice. Nor did they consider having a backup care plan in case these issues resurfaced during the transition to college. Jay's parents had a "wishful thinking" approach: once Jay was enrolled in his dream college and doing what he liked best, all would fall into place and he would grow and mature. Jay, on his side, felt that once he was away from parents and able to "live his own life," everything would improve.

Unfortunately, as soon as he entered college, symptoms started to get out of control. He had difficulty managing day-to-day life and organizing his schedule. As anxiety increased and he started to struggle with "passing" (being perceived as preferred gender), he began to avoid going to classes and social activities, and his grades began to suffer. Even though substance abuse had not been an issue at home, once in college, where he had easy access to it, he began to use alcohol and cannabis to manage anxiety. Alcohol worsened motor impairment caused by CMT. When his parents realized the severity of Jay's condition, they again turned to the pediatrician at home. Jay was instructed to seek help at school, where he first went to the counseling center and eventually to the psychiatric clinic for treatment.

During the first encounter, he was still struggling to define his gender identity. He dressed in male clothes but did not insist on using masculine pronouns. He reported that he was still living as a woman to most people, including faculty and peers, because he had not disclosed to his parents that he was transgender. The school roster and medical records still used his female given name and biological gender. He reported symptoms of depression, including feeling tired all the time, decreased motivation and energy, irritability, and mood fluctuations. He expressed feelings of worthlessness and often needed external validation to feel good about himself. He also ruminated excessively about academic failure. He reported frequent meltdowns, especially when he felt rejected by friends ("I hate when they cancel plans") and ongoing self-injurious behaviors. He was unable to regulate emotional reactions and had very little resiliency. He often acted out his emotions in a dramatic manner. Whenever he became angry, he threatened to kill himself. When upset, he punched the walls of the dorm or used a pocket-knife to cut himself.

He was diagnosed with Gender Dysphoria, Major Depressive Disorder, recurrent, moderate, history of ADHD, and Anxiety Disorder, unspecified. His inability to sustain a stable self-image, his extreme reaction to perceived abandonment, and frequent episodes of self-injurious behavior suggested a diagnosis of Borderline Personality Disorder as well.

At the end of the session, the resources available were reviewed, including counseling, life coaching, and accommodations. Treatment with an antidepressant was also recommended. He said that he had to discuss all this information with parents and would only take an antidepressant "if my parents agree." Jay had significant issues adequately separating and individuating from his parents. He was unable to make decisions about school and his own medical care without explicit parental guidance and approval. Eventually, after allowing the psychiatrist to speak with his parents, he began medication, with only a modest response. During treatment Jay displayed a pattern of frequent drop in visits between scheduled ones and accessed multiple resources simultaneously. At one point, he was going to the counseling center every 2 weeks, and to a local therapist weekly.

Once in treatment, Jay insisted on focusing on gender dysphoria and transitioning. He believed that most of the anxiety and depression was related to that and that once he started hormone therapy, it would all resolve. He decided to come out to his parents and it did not go well. They made him shut down his social media accounts and forbade him to tell extended family and faculty at his school. Mother was particularly troubled and threatened to take him out of school. Father was concerned about Jay's future career as a lawyer, and how it would be impacted. They came in person to the counseling center and the clinic, accusing providers of "putting ideas in his head through therapy." They assumed Jay would be referred to gender reassignment surgery right away and forbade Jay to proceed with transitioning until they were satisfied that this was not the case. They continued to insist that this was a phase, and his mother stopped speaking to him. Jay became difficult to engage in treatment due to family interference. He was devastated by their lack of support.

Jay made a few friends through Pride Union events but isolated himself from most people in his academic program. As the parents interfered with the transitioning process by forbidding him to come out to faculty and students, they created a situation of isolation. Jay could dress and behave like a man for a handful of Pride Union friends, but had to use his female name in class and to the rest of the school body. This situation created a significant stressor for Jay, ultimately increasing symptoms of depression and anxiety that he treated with alcohol and cannabis.

Several different medications were tried but were either not effective or caused significant side effects. It is possible that Jay was not compliant with medications, and that he was also using more alcohol and cannabis than he was reporting. There was significant academic decline and Jay considered a leave of absence from school. However, the idea of returning home was devastating to him. During a particularly difficult week of conversation with parents regarding his ability to stay in school given his poor academic performance, Jay expressed suicidal ideation to the RA in his dorm and was hospitalized. Following discharge from the hospital, he was referred to intensive outpatient treatment.

A positive outcome of the hospitalization was that it prompted parents to engage in treatment, although Mother remained against the transitioning. Jay signed a release of information allowing providers to talk to both parents openly. This allowed for family education. They knew very little about gender dysphoria and Father welcomed the opportunity to ask questions and share his concerns. Over time, his father became the spokesperson for the family and was very protective of Jay. He began to use male pronouns and Jay's preferred name. He reflected that he just wanted "for his kid to be happy." They received information about local and national resources, including support groups for them. As the gender dysphoria was addressed, Jay was more accepting of treatment for his other diagnoses. He was referred to the Student with Disabilities Resource Center for accommodations and could remain enrolled, on a reduced class scheduled while he attended the intensive outpatient program.

Analysis of Transition

Jay's transition into college was clearly unsuccessful and tumultuous, as evidenced by academic decline and worsening mood and anxiety symptoms leading to psychiatric hospitalization. Many factors were predictive of a negative transition. Although he had clear mental health needs that manifested in different ways since childhood, they had not been fully addressed. He had shown significant social anxiety from an early age and was also unable to manage academic demands without the assistance of a supervising adult. In addition to that, Jay was enmeshed with his mother and never explored being more independent. He did not acquire the skills necessary to individuate and transition into adulthood. Even though he expressed weariness of being controlled by parents, he tried to replicate the home dynamic at school, seeking advice and reassurance from those that appeared to be in position of authority (resident assistant, advisors, counselor, and even psychiatrist). He was unable to organize his schedule, manage his health, or even articulate his needs. In addition to that, his social anxiety made it hard for him to engage with others outside the confines of treatment. Jay lacked complete understanding of his diagnoses, thinking instead that his mood and anxiety symptoms would improve with the resolution of his gender dysphoria.

Positive predictors included Jay's intelligence and participation in extracurricular activities. He excelled when given direction and adequate structure. Despite the difficult dynamics, his family was intact and supportive, and, while they did not wish for him to see a psychiatrist, they did seek out care with the pediatrician when necessary. When it was clear that Jay was struggling at college, his pediatrician directed him to the appropriate supports on campus.

In retrospect, it would have been helpful for the family to prepare Jay to live independently. He should have developed skills to manage his finances, household tasks, personal care, and academic functioning. It would also have been helpful for the family to gradually withdraw the amount of structure they were providing so that Jay could see how much he relied on their help to earn good grades. This may also have prompted the school to complete educational testing and potentially provide accommodations. Having this support in place during high school may have allowed the family to explore the resources available at the university. However, given the nature of Jay's chronic medical illness, it is easy to understand how protective his parents were, and that it may have been difficult for them to "let go." Working with a psychotherapist and a child psychiatrist may also have helped Jay identify and begin to discuss his gender concerns earlier on, and the clinicians could have helped the family formulate a transfer care plan prior to matriculation. Referring Jay to the counseling center and ODS from the beginning may have helped to avert symptom exacerbation and academic decline.

Thankfully, Jay ultimately followed his pediatrician's recommendation to seek mental health services and once he was at college and that he agreed to seek academic supports for his ADHD. This allowed him to work through family issues preventing adequate separation and individuation, as well as homing in on gender issues and seeking appropriate care for his anxiety and depression. The hospitalization seemed to serve as a wake-up call for his parents, and helped engage them effectively in the treatment process.

Clinical Pearls

- Despite most colleges offering safe zones for LGBTQ patients and access to peer support groups, this population remains at higher risk to be victims of violence, to be diagnosed with a mental health issue, and to attempt or complete suicide. They are more likely to experiment with drugs and alcohol and engage in promiscuous behavior.
- Addressing gender dysphoria in college can be daunting for both patients and families, even in the best-case scenario, when families are supportive.
- Helping transgender patients and their parents become informed about their rights and available resources is extremely important. It can help them successfully transition into college and adulthood on their own terms.
- Helping the patient develop the ability to advocate for themselves is crucial. For anyone suffering with a mental health illness, articulating needs, navigating the care system, and securing access to treatment will be a lifelong necessity. For patients who belong to sexual minorities, this is often difficult as there are structural barriers preventing access. Supporting their endeavors and connecting them with appropriate resources may be pivotal in allowing them to graduate.
- Treating a patient with complex clinical issues who received little to no prior psychiatric care prior to coming to college can be quite challenging. It is much like putting a puzzle together. At times, parents are unwilling or unable to corroborate history and provide information. In those situations, it is important to collaborate with other resources at the university/college to amplify the pool of clinical information available.
- Involving parents in treatment remains a challenge in the college age population, as the patients are often attempting to individuate and may resent parental involvement. However, in moments of crisis, emerging adults will sometimes demand parental involvement, only to reject it when parents' goals turn out to be different than patient's goals. For the treating psychiatrist, navigating this fine line can be difficult.
- Parental involvement increases positive outcome, but it should always be balanced against the patient's need for independence. Encouraging emerging adult patients to think about when parents (or who, if not parents) should be involved and what can be discussed early on, before a crisis ensues, becomes central to the treatment plan. It allows the provider to act according to the patient's desires, if the need arises.
- A college with a culture which supports mental health and wellness may allow some young people to seek treatment that had been stigmatized in their families.

Brief Literature Review

Despite increased visibility and more clinical practice interest due to higher demand, the transgender population, especially transgender youth, remain at-risk for poor physical and mental health outcomes [1]. This presents an interesting paradox, where lesbian, gay, bisexual, transgender (LGBT) youth feel more comfortable to "come out" at an earlier age because of societal acceptance, and yet face increased risk of mental health issues. This may be in part because adolescence is a developmental period characterized by strong peer influence and opinion that makes them, especially younger adolescents, more susceptible to social exclusion behavior. It is possible to find stronger prejudice, including homophobia [2]. Today sexual minority youth is more likely to face peer victimization when they come out, with long-lasting developmental consequences.

As early as 1995, the Institute of Medicine recognized the need to increase data regarding specific health risks associated to being a sexual minority [3]. Research studies completed since then have consistently shown that sexual minority groups experience "lower levels of self-esteem, higher levels of psychological stress, and a lower level of general well-being" [4]. This is particularly true to emerging adults and adolescents, who may experience lack of support at home in addition to more stigmatization from society in general. This population, sexual minority transitional age youth, is at higher risk for health, mental health, and social problems, including STDs, school difficulties, addiction, depression, and suicide [5, 6, 7]. Gender nonconformity not only increases stigmatization and induces more health risk behaviors, but it worsens psychosocial adjustment due to adding further stressors during a particularly difficult developmental stage. The prevalence of mental health, substance dependence, and comorbid psychiatric disorders in a community sample of sexual minority youth can be as high as two to four times that of the general US population [4, 5, 8], with nearly half reporting suicidal ideation and one-third reporting suicide attempt within the preceding 12 months.

According to the American College Health Association (ACHA) report, 17.5% of college students describe themselves as non-gender conforming. Transgender youth may perceive college as a more accepting and less judging environment. Unfortunately, there are still structural stigma that increases victimization. Access to college itself can be denied or made more difficult, from scrutinizing applications to being refused campus housing. The transitioning process itself can be traumatizing, from the burdensome process for name changes to lack of access to trained and knowledgeable health care providers. Mental health care, and managing suicidality in particular, can pose some challenges in managing college students. According to the American Foundation for Suicide Prevention report on suicide rates in transgender population (2014), 41% of the respondents said they had attempted suicide (compared to just 4.6% of the general population). Prevalence of suicide attempts was highest among those who are younger (18–24: 45%), and multiracial (54%) or American Indian or Alaska Native (56%). On the other hand, family connectedness and support, as well as school safety can be significantly protective of reported suicide attempts in youth with same-sex sexual experience [9].

Finally, one important aspect of improving health outcomes in transgender youth (including mental health outcomes) is facilitating access to care. Transgender youth, much like their adult counterparts, have decreased access to care, due to both personal and structural barriers, including internalized stigma, lack of access to health insurance or knowledgeable providers [7]. Although colleges are trying to close the gap and promote awareness, much remains to be changed.

Helpful Resources

Resources for Clinicians

- The Health of Lesbian, Gay, Bisexual, and Transgender People: Building a Foundation for Better Understanding
  http://www.nap.edu/catalog/13128/the-health-of-lesbian-gay-bisexual-and-transgender-people-building
- Violence Against the Transgender Community
  https://origins.asu.edu/origins-portal/violence/violence-gender/transgender-violence
- Injustice at Every Turn—A Report of the National Transgender Discrimination Survey
  http://thetaskforce.org/static_html/downloads/reports/reports/ntds_full.pdf

Resources for Families and Students

- FAQ About Transgender Students at Colleges and Universities
  http://www.lambdalegal.org/know-your-rights/article/trans-in-college-faq

References

1. Olson-Kennedy J. Mental health disparities among transgender youth: rethinking the role of professionals. JAMA Pediatr. 2016;170(5):423–4.
2. Russell ST, Fish JN. Mental health in lesbian, gay, bisexual, and transgender (LGBT) youth. Annu Rev Clin Psychol. 2016;12:465–89.
3. National Academies of Sciences Report: the health of lesbian, gay, bisexual and transgender people. www.nap.edu/catalog/13128/the-health-of-lesbian-gay-bisexual-and-transgender-people-building
4. Rodgers SM. Transitional age lesbian, gay, bisexual, transgender and questioning youth. Issues of diversity, integrated identity and mental health. Child Adolesc Psychiatr Clin N Am. 2017;26:297–309.
5. Centers for Disease Control and Prevention. Health risks among sexual minority youth. 2016. http://www.cdc.gov/healthyyouth/disparities/smy.htm. Accessed May 2017.
6. Talley AE, et al. Addressing gaps on risk and resilience factors for alcohol use outcomes in sexual and gender minority populations. Drug Alcohol Rev. 2016;35:484–93.
7. Higa D, Hoppe MJ, Lindhorst T, Mincer S, Beadnell B, Morrison DM, Wells EA, Todd A, Mountz S. Negative and Positive Factors Associated With the Well-Being of Lesbian, Gay, Bisexual, Transgender, Queer, and Questioning (LGBTQ) Youth. Youth & Society 2012; 46(5):663–687.
8. Reisner SL, Biello KB, Hughto JMW, Kuhns L, Mayer KH, Garofalo R, Mimiaga MJ. Psychiatric diagnoses and comorbidities in a diverse, multicity cohort of young transgender women baseline findings from project lifeskills. JAMA Pediatr. 2016;170(5):481–6.
9. Zaza S, Kann L, Barrios LC. Lesbian, Gay, and Bisexual adolescents: population estimate and prevalence of health behaviors. JAMA. 2016;316(22):2355–6.

Juggling Priorities: Staying Sober in College as a Nontraditional Student

21

Jennifer Derenne

Case History

Sam, a 25-year-old Caucasian male with a history of Alcohol Use Disorder, presented to the university counseling center on recommendation of the Office of Disability Services (ODS). A professor encouraged him to approach ODS two months after the start of his freshman year of college when he began to experience significant difficulty managing his course load. This led to anxiety that was starting to impair his relationships, and he was beginning to question whether college was right for him.

Sam grew up in the surrounding area near the university. He was the youngest of four children, who were primarily raised by their mother after his parents divorced. They split soon after his birth, so Sam was comfortable with the custody plan, which entailed spending every other weekend with his father and stepmother. He got along with his family and found them to be supportive. He recalled having some difficulty sitting still in classes but earned good grades in elementary and middle school and teachers praised his curiosity and enthusiasm for learning. As high school approached, his mother moved to a more affluent neighborhood, which made it necessary for Sam to change schools. His siblings had already graduated and were working and living independently. They moved from a large metropolitan school district to a small town with social cliques. While he had never before had trouble fitting in, he felt that his new classmates were materialistic and he did not feel accepted by them. As a result, he felt dysphoric and lost interest in school work. His

J. Derenne, M.D.
Division of Child and Adolescent Psychiatry, Department of Psychiatry and Behavioral Sciences, Stanford University School of Medicine, Lucile Packard Children's Hospital, Stanford, CA, USA
e-mail: jderenne@stanford.edu

© Springer International Publishing AG, part of Springer Nature 2018
A. Martel et al. (eds.), *Promoting Safe and Effective Transitions to College for Youth with Mental Health Conditions*, https://doi.org/10.1007/978-3-319-68894-7_21

mother was busy working and was not particularly distressed by the drop in his grades. When he was able to obtain a work permit, Sam decided to devote his free time to working and earning money. A strong work ethic was valued by both parents, and they liked that he was being productive. He started working in the kitchen of a local restaurant and began to hang out with his older coworkers after hours. They were happy to buy alcohol for him and he began to drink heavily after his shifts. Because he came home late from work, his mother did not realize the extent of his drinking. He experimented with cocaine and marijuana, but did not like how they made him feel.

Sam was able to finish high school with a barely adequate GPA. While he did not find the work particularly difficult, he devoted the bare minimum to his education. He was able to save a lot of money, but was not sure what he wanted to do with his life. He elected to attend the local community college and continued to work at the restaurant. His work friends were dismissive of higher education, and he struggled to balance work and school. He decided to leave community college after a few weeks, and continued to work full time. His sister became worried after he shared his own concerns about the amount he was drinking, and helped connect him to an outpatient addictions therapist. Despite his efforts to cut down on his alcohol use, Sam continued to be tempted by his coworkers. After getting a DUI one night after a long shift, he and his therapist decided that a residential program would be helpful. His family was supportive and he found an out of state rehabilitation program that appealed to him.

His mother's insurance covered 60 days, and he was invested in the recovery process. Sam connected to Alcoholics Anonymous and attended meetings religiously. He slipped a few times, but ultimately learned that he was much more functional when he did not drink, and was able to remain sober with the help of the structure and support offered by AA. He quit his job at the restaurant, started a local lawn and gardening business, and continued to live with his mother for the next few years. He was independent with life skills, did not require any outpatient mental health treatment, and began seriously dating his future wife. With sustained sobriety (5 years), he was interested in returning to school. His dismal high school GPA made it impossible to attend the local 4-year university, so he returned to the community college to gradually complete the general studies curriculum with the intent to transfer his credits. This time, he earned mostly As and was invested in completing his work. He was connected to his classmates, as he felt that they had shared life experience, and felt motivated to transfer to a 4-year college to study finance.

Sam was accepted to the local university, and got married the summer before classes started. His wife was a college graduate who was working at a public relations firm, and agreed to support them financially while he finished school. His father agreed to help him with loans, and Sam had saved a substantial amount of money in the time that he was working. While supportive of his educational goals, his wife was also insistent that they spend time together, and that he contribute equally to household chores. He attended an orientation for transfer students and remained friendly with a few of the other students he met there, but they were younger and he felt that they had little in common.

Sam was thrilled to take advantage of classes that he felt were intellectually stimulating, but also felt pressure to be practical and to finish his degree as quickly as possible. He was irritated by the 18- and 19-year-old first year students in his classes who seemed entitled, did not appear to appreciate their educational opportunities, and seemed more focused on frat parties than on studying. He also found it challenging to balance the increased academic load with his relationships and hours spent maintaining sobriety (AA meetings, activities with sober friends). His wife expected him to plan regular date nights with her, and he needed to help out around the house. He yearned to make friends in his classes, but felt that the campus culture was largely focused on partying, and he felt like an outsider. When he did join events, people encouraged him to "just have one," and he did not feel that they were understanding or supportive of his situation. Sam was not aware of any alcohol-free activities on campus.

Given his history, ODS recommended neuropsychological testing to rule out learning disorders and ADHD. His wife's insurance covered the services, and he was relieved to learn that he did not meet criteria for any learning or attention disorders. He was referred to the study skills center for help with organization and time management after determining that he had never developed the necessary study skills when he was in high school. Sam decided to take classes over the summer so that he could do fewer courses each semester, and could have more time with his family. He attended sessions with a psychologist in the counseling center focused on navigating his relationship with his wife, and improving his communication skills.

Sam continued to attend AA meetings both on and off campus and maintained his sobriety. With the help of his therapist, he was able to connect to student organizations focused on activities that he was passionate about, such as volunteering and hiking. He invited his wife to join in these activities, and she was welcomed by the other students. He met other students who did not drink through meet up activities and the on-campus AA meeting, which met most weeks classes were in session. He spent 5 years at the university, graduated, and went on to get a job in finance for a local company. He and his wife had their first baby at the end of his senior year.

Analysis of Transition

There were a number of predictors in Sam's history that suggested that he was at risk of a negative transition outcome. These include the fact that he had a suboptimal transition from high school to his initial attempt at community college, as well as poorly developed organizational and study skills. In addition, at age 25, he was a nontraditional student, who would likely have difficulty connecting to classmates who were much younger and had different life experiences. While he was not in formal mental health treatment, he was spending hours each week attending AA meetings, talking with his sponsor, and participating in sober activities with other members of his AA community. This provided substantial support, but also decreased the time Sam had available to study and socialize with classmates. Many college students experiment with alcohol and other substances; this environment could potentially trigger a relapse of drinking which could jeopardize his ability to remain enrolled.

From a more positive standpoint, Sam was independent, mature, and motivated to work hard. He had a strong sober community to rely on, as well as the structure and support of his marriage. While his study skills were initially inadequate for the demands of a 4-year college, he was receptive to refining and building them. He did not have a learning disorder or ADHD. His sobriety was early, yet solid enough to withstand the stresses of the transition and the temptations of campus party culture. He was self-aware enough to recognize that he was struggling academically and sought help appropriately. Sam was willing to follow through on the referral to the counseling center, and used his sessions effectively.

Sam's story highlights the unanticipated difficulties that can arise when nontraditional students without current mental health treatment transition to college. His transition was suboptimal, in that he lacked preparation. He really had no idea how challenging it might be to try to balance school and relationships, while also trying to maintain his sobriety. While his history of addiction was significant, he was engaged in a peer support community rather than working with more traditional mental health providers that could have helped engage him in transition care planning.

Given his difficulty with the transition from high school to community college, Sam might have anticipated having some trouble transitioning to 4-year college. He could have proactively sought out an individual tutoring consultation or attended a study skills session prior to beginning classes. Working with an upper class mentor could have alerted him to the potential difficulties faced by other nontraditional students and could have given him another avenue for support and consultation. Similarly, an orientation specifically geared for nontraditional students (or a break-out session at the transfer student orientation) could have connected Sam to other students who might face similar challenges.

In addition to providing programming to optimize support for nontraditional students, the university can also work to make the campus environment feel safe and welcoming to those students who are managing addictions issues. This can be accomplished by facilitating student groups and activities that do not focus on alcohol or other substances, as well as supporting sober residence halls and an active 12-step community on campus. Of note, it can be difficult to have consistent campus AA meetings, given that students typically lead meetings and can have difficulty adhering to schedules during busy times like midterms and finals. They also often do not meet during holidays and vacations.

Clinical Pearls

- Nontraditional students may have difficulty feeling part of the campus community, especially when they are married, have children, or are much older than their classmates.
- Mentoring programs and targeted orientation sessions may help nontraditional students anticipate challenges and develop skills to manage them. They can also connect students who may have similar life experiences.

- Nontraditional students should be aware of campus tutoring and study skills centers, especially if they struggled with classes in high school or at community college. Students who do not finish their degrees the first time around *may* have underdeveloped study skills or undiagnosed attention or learning disorders.
- Attentive faculty and administrative staff can be instrumental in connecting students to the appropriate resources and services on campus. Older students are often very invested in their education, and, as a result, may be more self-aware and willing to follow through on referrals.
- Underage drinking and substance use can be rampant on college campuses and may be a significant trigger for students trying to manage substance use disorders. Students need to anticipate this and develop strategies to maintain sobriety in the face of peer pressure and high stress.
- Universities may offer sober living environments and on-campus 12-step meetings, but these may be inconsistent and dependent on the academic calendar. Students may need to investigate community 12-step meetings and activities near campus to ensure that they have access to support at all times, even during exams and breaks.

Brief Literature Review

At 4-year degree granting postsecondary institutions in 2015, 11% of students at public universities and 14% of students at private nonprofit universities were nontraditional aged. At private for-profit 4-year universities, 69% of undergraduate students were older than 25 years [1]. According to Horn and Carroll [2], nontraditional students are those who have one or more of the following characteristics: (1) >24 years old, (2) financially independent from their parents, (3) working full time, (4) attending classes part time, (5) having dependents, (6) being single parents, and (7) possessing GED or high school equivalent. Students are further classified as mildly [one trait], moderately [2–3 traits], or highly [4 or more traits] nontraditional based on the number of characteristics they possess. The more nontraditional the student, the less likely he or she is to earn a degree. They are more likely to be female, ethnic/racial minorities, and first-generation college students. Nontraditional students are also more likely to leave school before completing their degrees [3]. A recent study [4] comparing traditional and nontraditional undergraduate students found that the nontraditional students scored significantly higher on measures of life stress, anxiety, and depression, and therefore may have a higher need for counseling services. The authors go on to clarify that the increased stress may also be related to lower socioeconomic status, which does tend to be more common in nontraditional students. The two groups did not appear to differ on alcohol use as measured by the AUDIT-C (Alcohol Use and Disorders Identification Test-Consumption).

Given that nontraditional students are making up an increasingly large percentage of the university population, and are also more likely to experience stresses that may lead to attrition, campuses need to devote more resources to optimizing their transition and graduation rates. Dropping out without a degree has serious economic ramifications for those who choose for-profit institutions—both in terms of ability to get a job and in terms of debt burden [5] Daycare on campus, financial planning seminars, and "mentorship" programs may help decrease life stress and improve retention in this population. This is especially important, because higher educational attainment is associated with better health outcomes. Life expectancy is increased by approximately 10 years in those who earn a college degree as compared to those who do not finish high school [6].

Problematic alcohol use continues to be a significant issue on college campuses, but not much has been written about sober students and how best to support them [7]. The literature tends to focus rates of abuse and dependence, as well as some studies looking at outreach, prevention, detection, intervention, and outcomes. The Fall 2016 American College Health Association National Health Assessment [8] reported that 3.3% of students reported that alcohol had a negative effect on their academics in the preceding 12 months, and 50.3% experienced other untoward outcomes (such as getting in trouble with police, doing something they regretted, or forgetting where they were or what they did). While 49.6% of students reported having used alcohol within the last 1–9 days, 21.4% reported that they had never used alcohol.

Helpful Resources

Support Groups

- Alcoholics Anonymous http://www.aa.org/ includes search for local meetings

Sobriety Apps

- Sober Grid https://itunes.apple.com/us/app/sober-grid/id912632260?mt=8
- Sobriety Support. https://play.google.com/store/apps/details?id=com.capstone 2015.sobrietysupport&hl=en
- Quit That https://itunes.apple.com/us/app/quit-that!-track-how-long/id909400800? mt=8
- Recovery Box. https://itunes.apple.com/us/app/recoveryBox/id538010611
- Sober Tool. https://itunes.apple.com/us/app/sober-tool-alcoholism-addiction/ id863872931?mt=8

Frequently Asked Questions

- Frequently Asked Questions for Child, Adolescent, and Adult Psychiatrists and Other Professionals Working with Transitional Age Youth with Substance Use Disorders. http://www.aacap.org/App_Themes/AACAP/Docs/clinical_practice_ center/systems_of_care/sud-tay.pdf

Web-based Articles

- "Best Practices in Advising Non-traditional students". http://www.nacada.ksu. edu/Resources/Academic-Advising-Today/View-Articles/Best-Practices-in-Advising-Non-traditional-Students.aspx
- "Five Essential Mechanisms Supporting Non-traditional Student Success". https://evolllution.com/opinions/essential-mechanisms-supporting-non-traditional-student-success/
- "Staying Sober on Campus: College Students in Recovery". https://www.pyra-midhealthcarepa.com/recovery-college/

References

1. McFarland J, Hussa B. The condition of education. Washington, DC: National Center for Education Statistics; 2017.
2. Horn LJ, Carroll DC. Nontraditional undergraduates: trends in enrollment from 1986–1992 and persistence and attainment among 1989–90 beginning postsecondary students. Washington, DC: US Department of Education Office of Educational Research and Improvement; 1996.
3. Choy S. National Center for Education Statistics. 2002. Retrieved from https://nces.ed.gov/pubsearch/pubsinfo.asp?pubid=2002012.
4. Trenz RC, Ecklund-Flores L, Rapoza K. A comparison of mental health and alcohol use between traditional and nontraditional students. J Am Coll Health. 2015;63:584–6.
5. Dwyer R. Gender, debt, and dropping out of college. Gend Soc. 2013;27:30–55.
6. Bravemen P, Laura G. The social determinants of health: it's time to consider the causes of the causes. Public Health Rep. 2014;129:19–31.
7. Misch D. On-campus programs to support college students in recovery. J Am Coll Health. 2010;58:279–80.
8. American College Health Association. American College Health Association-National College Health Assessment II: Reference Group Executive Summary Fall 2016. Hanover: American College Health Association; 2017.

Moving Forward by Taking Medical Leave: A Paradoxical Path to Success

D. Catherine Fuchs

Case History

Joe is a 21-year-old Caucasian male, college junior, from a large Northern city in the U.S. middle of three siblings, who was required to take a Medical Leave of Absence (MLOA) twice during his time in college. He came to college with a history of Bipolar I Disorder (BP I Disorder) and Obsessive Compulsive Disorder (OCD) first diagnosed in 6th grade.

Joe was a term baby with normal developmental milestones, described as bright and engaging. In 6th grade parents noticed irritability both at school and at home, progressing to episodes of rage, dysregulated sleep, and a decline in academic performance. Parents also began to notice excessive focus on cleanliness with fear of germs, long showers, and avoidance of social settings. He was diagnosed with BP I Disorder and OCD. Treatment included both psychotherapy for the patient and his family as well as pharmacologic intervention with fluoxetine and valproic acid. He had a good response to treatment and both academic performance and social interactions improved.

As his co-occurring illnesses progressed, he struggled with school attendance and academic work. He increasingly misread social cues leading to progressive social isolation and loneliness. He lacked motivation, had depressed mood, and increased rituals regarding cleanliness including multiple showers per day lasting up to an hour each time.

At age 15, he developed symptoms of severe depression with refusal to eat or drink, refusal to get out of bed, and extreme social withdrawal, leading to inpatient psychiatric hospitalization. Joe initially lacked insight but gradually became more

D.C. Fuchs, M.D.
Department of Psychiatry and Behavioral Sciences, Vanderbilt University Medical Center, Nashville, TN, USA
e-mail: Catherine.fuchs@vanderbilt.edu

© Springer International Publishing AG, part of Springer Nature 2018
A. Martel et al. (eds.), *Promoting Safe and Effective Transitions to College for Youth with Mental Health Conditions*, https://doi.org/10.1007/978-3-319-68894-7_22

insightful and engaged in treatment. He was discharged on fluvoxamine, lamotrigine, and risperidone with an outpatient treatment plan.

Joe returned to high school with implementation of an IEP and classification as ED. He received accommodations targeting his difficulty dealing with transitions, challenges with getting out of bed in the morning resulting in tardiness, inefficiency in completion of academic work due to obsessional focus on details, and social difficulties resulting from rigidity in relationships.

He functioned adequately for approximately 1 year then began to struggle significantly with loneliness as he experienced social rejections. Compliance became sporadic leading to a second hospitalization at age 17 and at the start of his senior year of high school. He again was stabilized with therapy and the same medication regimen.

Medical history was unremarkable. Family history was notable for OCD, anxiety, and BP I disorder. Joe has an intact family with good social supports.

The CAP recommended that Joe delay going to college for a year to develop skills to manage stress and to demonstrate ability to effectively manage a schedule. Joe did not want to delay and went directly from high school to college, attending a mid-sized academically rigorous school that emphasizes academics, leadership, and social involvement on campus. Prior to heading to college Joe and his family worked with the home psychiatrist to identify a psychiatrist and therapist in the community within walking distance from his college. The CAP worked with Joe and his family to develop goals, focusing on transition and independent management of illness. Joe also created goals for his work with a treatment team at college, and tried to identify resources on campus, specifically identifying disability services. With Joe's written permission, the CAP agreed to share clinical information with the new providers and to remain available for consultation. The CAP arranged to continue working with Joe on school breaks.

Joe moved into a dorm room with a roommate who was socially active. The roommate had peers over to the room frequently, complicating Joe's need for order and cleanliness. Joe was not prepared for the lack of control over his physical environment and began to experience distress expressed through increasing rigidity. He began to miss doses of his medicines and to sleep through classes. In high school, he had initial insomnia with late morning awakening; in the dorm, he did not have the parental supervision to help him maintain a healthy pattern of sleep which contributed to the poor class attendance. Joe did not seek help with accommodations due to his desire to be "normal." It was reported to the Director of Housing that Joe lacked social connections and, in turn, he expressed this concern at the university Student of Concern Committee (SOC). By mid-semester of his freshman year, he was reviewed by the university SOC given additional concerns with academic deficiency. The SOC tasked the Director of Housing with following up on social and behavioral concerns through communication with the Area Coordinators (AC) for the residential housing system. The ACs receive "gatekeeper training" annually to develop skills needed to guide students at risk. The Academic Dean reported that he had requested Joe schedule a meeting to review his academic status. The Director of the Counseling Services is often a member of the SOC providing consultation regarding general patterns of concern (while safeguarding HIPAA protected information thereby not revealing any contact the student may have had with the counseling center). The Director of Counseling Services suggested to the SOC that they consider mental health issues when a student presents with an academic and behavioral pattern similar to that reported about Joe.

Joe had met with the psychiatrist when he and his parents moved him to campus and Joe followed up with both the psychiatrist as well as the therapist for the first few weeks. His compliance then became sporadic. Despite having a release to talk with Joe's parents, the providers did not inform them of his lack of attendance with the expectation that Joe function as an independent young adult. The parents assumed that he was attending his appointments since they did not receive any communication.

In early November, Joe was struggling to get out of bed and expressed hopelessness. Parents were contacted by the university housing team; they came to campus and accompanied Joe to the university counseling center (UCC) for assessment. The UCC recommended to the Dean that Joe take a voluntary MLOA. The Dean granted the request with specific expectations for a treatment plan to address his mental health issues and a requirement that Joe demonstrate ability to function effectively in a structured and productive activity while on leave.

Joe met with his home psychiatrist and expressed anger at his parents for agreeing to the medical leave. He initially minimized his non-compliance with medication. Gradually, Joe began to engage in problem solving rather than blaming of others. He was able to express his frustration and sadness at needing to be "different," citing the need to have a regular sleep schedule when his peers were staying up late at night. He used the next 9 months to explore his decision-making and his understanding of his psychiatric needs as he prepared to return to school. He participated in a volunteer job to provide structure to his day.

In preparation for return, Joe was required to provide a personal statement conveying his progress and demonstrating his plan for behavioral changes to help him manage his illness on campus. The home CAP was asked to submit a progress report using a structured university form addressing specific clinical and behavioral questions. Joe and the CAP re-evaluated his support system on campus as well as the need for a treatment contract that would include communication with the parents. It was determined that he should have a therapist in the community with knowledge of OCD as well as a case manager at the UCC to help coordinate communication and care. They developed a plan for the CAP to consult with the primary care provider at the Student Health Center, creating a consultation model for medication management. This allowed Joe to consolidate his care in a setting that would also address his general health care needs and he could continue to interact with his home-based psychiatrist. The parents arranged with Joe and the Academic Dean to ensure that the Dean and the professors were aware of academic accommodations through the Office of Disability Services. Joe signed a FERPA waiver and parents requested that the Academic Dean inform them if there was concern about his academic performance.

Upon his return, Joe initially did well academically but avoided social interactions because he did not want to answer questions about his absence. As the semester progressed, he again began to miss classes, initially because he had not completed the assignments and did not want to submit less than perfect work. Parents were informed of these concerns. As this pattern continued, he became self-critical and discouraged and became increasingly irritable. Sleep became a concern as he began to stay up late at night and to sleep during the day. Gradually, his sleep pattern worsened and he became expansive and grandiose. He missed appointments with the various members of his support team who attempted unsuccessfully to reach out to Joe, emphasizing the goal of independence. Joe did not respond to these efforts but did seek help at the Student Health Center where he focused on physical symptoms compounded by his lack of self-care. The primary care provider recognized Joe's deterioration in mental status and contacted his home CAP. As agreed upon in the student success plan, parents were informed and again MLOA was recommended. The need for this MLOA was identified in early October, earlier in the process of symptom presentation, enabling a decision focused on proactive care rather than in response to academic failure.

Once home again Joe, his parents, and the CAP collaborated with the university treatment team to identify key challenges impacting Joe's success at college. They identified the impact of his mental health needs on his approach to academics. It was clear that Joe needed an external support system to provide academic guidance. The university team recommended an academic "coach," paid for by the family, who could meet with Joe 2–3 times per week to focus on study skills and management of anxiety and avoidance. Joe spent another 10 months at home working on his psychosocial challenges and potential for growth. When he returned to school, he began meeting with a private academic "coach" three times per week. This provided a structured safety net for him regarding his academic work contributing to a growth in self-confidence as he began to experience success. This also created an environment for academic accountability without parents needing to be directly involved. Joe consistently worked with the Wellness program to develop strategies for managing stress.

After two MLOAs, he completed college and continued his education, successfully attending graduate school.

Analysis of Transition

There were several aspects of this case that were predictive of an ultimately successful transition to college. A key factor was his engagement in treatment throughout high school; though he often rejected expectations placed upon him, he had a positive relationship with the CAP. Joe's family was supportive and open to guidance during his multi-step transition to college. Another positive predictor was the establishment of channels of communication, including coordinated follow-up care, with releases signed proactively. It was also fortunate, although Joe did not make his college choice based on this, that the IHE and nearby community, offered an array of supportive services and mental health treatment options. Finally, often students with BP I Disorder struggle with thoughts of suicide; this was not an issue with Joe, contributing to the potential for successful transition.

Joe also had negative predictors for success, most strikingly his lack of acceptance of his illness as a risk factor during his transition. This was compounded by parental denial of the level of risk. Intermittently his illness destabilized, increasingly his risk for problematic transition.

Joe wanted to individuate from parents, a normal developmental drive, which to him meant not being sick and not being at home. Parents wanted him to be able to go to college and at some level hoped that the actual step of going to college would symbolize success and control over the illness. Joe needed to consider how his study skills in high school would translate to the study skills necessary for success in college. This was difficult for Joe while in high school due to his sense of failure and vulnerability when talking about his academic struggles. Denial of these challenges interfered with preparation for obtaining disability support services and prevented adequate development of a safety net. Colleges are not required to identify the need for accommodations [1] so it is necessary to educate students and families about the need for self-advocacy. The problem was exacerbated significantly by his desire to believe that going to college demonstrated that he had conquered his illness; with that belief, he convinced himself that he no longer needed to take medication, utilize academic supports, or engage in the treatment process.

In the case of Joe, the home psychiatrist served as a consultant who was familiar with the longitudinal pattern of illness, Joe's strengths, and the risk factors entering college. The initial transition care plan included a community therapist and psychiatrist. This receiving team did not have adequate understanding of the university system to implement a safety net for the student. Upon return to school after the first medical leave, the home psychiatrist provided consultation to arrange a broader system of care, including case management and utilization of campus partners. By providing consultation to the primary care student health system, the CAP addressed Joe's resistance to engaging with a new psychiatrist while ensuring that Joe had face-to-face assessments as part of the prescribing of medications. The return to school was difficult for Joe, and he soon began to struggle academically leading to destabilization of his illness. However, unlike the first MLOA, which occurred at a time of marked social and academic failure, the structure in place served as a safety net and his need for additional stabilization was more quickly identified. He took a second MLOA to continue to focus on skill development and identified an additional team member for his success plan, an academic coach. With this plan, Joe was successful in his college experience. The transition outcome was a process of failed attempts balanced by continued work to increase Joe's insight and level of accountability for his mental health, resulting in successful graduation from college.

Clinical Pearls

- Lack of insight into the impact of mental illness in the context of the college environment frequently compounds academic and social engagement, often resulting in a need for medical leave from school, but often only once failure occurs.

- MLOAs can become more complicated when the student and parents struggle with denial regarding the severity of the illness and its impact on college success
- MLOAs should be structured, addressing both positive and negative predictors for success. MLOA guidelines should include: (a) exit instructions, (b) return policies, and (c) a plan for student success [2].
- It is not uncommon for multiple MLOAs to be necessary to cement the student's and family's learning about the severity of illness and need for a structured and supportive safety net.
- Interdisciplinary teams of professionals, often referred to as Student of Concern Teams, meet on a regular basis to identify students who are struggling, establish a system of supports for those students, and monitor their progress [3]. The mental health professional on the team provides consultation regarding clinical scenarios while maintaining confidentiality of any specific student.
- Campus "gatekeepers," including faculty, residential life staff, campus security and others, interface with students on a regular basis, are typically trained to engage, support, and refer students at risk.
- The drive toward autonomy is normal and can override logical and practical decision-making; missteps should be reframed as learning experiences, particularly for this age group.
- The student with mental illness needs to develop independence but may need additional "bridges" (such as an academic coach) to accomplish their independence.
- Despite age of majority, involvement of parents can be very useful, and providers need to flexibly look at cases on an individual basis about parent involvement in treatment planning and ongoing monitoring.
- The consultation model of medication management may be useful for treating patients at a distance.
- Releases of information to allow communication among treatment providers, including reports on compliance with treatment, may prove helpful for students with mental illness as they transition to college.
- It is critical for the mental health system to assess transitional needs through a lens of prevention, management, and collaboration to develop a safety net in which the student can continue to progress developmentally while exploring academic opportunities.

Brief Literature Review

Medical leaves should be requested when the student has mental health concerns contributing to inability to function safely or effectively as a student. The mental health condition may negatively impact student welfare and academic engagement even if grades are acceptable. Georgetown University recently reviewed MLOAs based on disability law [2]. The model, consistent with many schools, is a partnership between the clinical or wellness system and the Dean with the leave granted by the Dean who typically writes a letter defining expectations while the student is on leave. The school must individualize the expectations with clear rationale for each one. The exit letter often defines a recommended length of time away, expectation for engagement in a "productive activity," and participation in treatment. Grades are typically not recorded during the semester in which the leave occurs. Financial aid offices work with students to avoid penalties for MLOA. International student offices work with students to inform them of protections regarding visa status. Many schools have a structure for MLOA returns which includes a personal statement by the student and recommendations by the home provider, ideally using a structured form. The CAP should identify factors in the college environment that contributed to destabilization of the student in order to avoid the bias of assuming the rapid stabilization once home means the student is ready for return. At Georgetown, even with careful review of exit and return, 30–40% of returning students need a second MLOA, consistent with reports from other schools. However, studies suggest that medical leaves often contribute to ultimate academic success [2]. Communication between the home-based provider(s) and the university clinical system is useful to ensure understanding of the university stressors and resources.

The vast majority of MLOAs are voluntary with federal disability law [4] no longer supporting direct threat to self as a reason for mandatory leave. A school must demonstrate "A significant risk to the health or safety of others that cannot be eliminated by a modification of policies, practices or procedures, or by the provision of auxiliary aids or services." As a result, involuntary MLOAs are difficult to implement. University policies differ but must follow the Office of Civil Rights Section 504 of Rehabilitation Act of 1973 and the Department of Justice new direct threat regulation under Title II of the American with Disabilities Act [4].

Many schools require review of activities while on leave and recommendations by home providers before the student can register for classes. Often students are required to meet with a clinician or wellness representative to develop a student success plan (for example, see Resource section at end of chapter) designed to identify support services facilitating a successful "return to school" transition. The information from the home provider helps to inform the planning, emphasizing the importance of communication by the CAP. Students returning from MLOA are often monitored by the campus SOC team typically for the initial return semester with reassessment of level of need based on observed level of success.

Child and Adolescent psychiatrists working with TAY must understand the complexities facing institutions of higher education when dealing with students diagnosed with mental illness and are encouraged to participate in a collaborative approach to include prevention and consultation.

Helpful Resources

- Medical Leave of Absence Process
  https://www.vanderbilt.edu/healthydores/taking-time-off/

References

1. Thomas SB. College students and disability law. J Special Educ. 2000;33(4):248–57.
2. Meilman PW. Conforming a voluntary medical leave of absence policy to recent disability law. J College Stud Psychother. 2016;30(1):54–63.
3. http://hemha.org/campus_teams_guide.pdf
4. http://counsel.cua.edu/nacuanotes/titleIIregulations.cfm

Half a World Away: The Mental Health Journey of an International Student

23

Doris Iarovici

Case History

Meihui, an 18-year-old freshman of Chinese heritage whose family currently resided in Hong Kong, was referred to the counseling center by the student health service in October of her freshman year, after a work-up for persistent fatigue found no clear etiology. A professor, concerned about the student missing class and not responding to emails, had contacted the office of case management. (This office, housed within Student Affairs, serves as a centralized place for reporting worrisome student behaviors; it helps link students to services and provides follow-up.) In advance of Meihui's first psychiatry appointment, but after the work-up for fatigue, there was a message from case management. The case manager had broached the option of dropping a class, or considering a medical leave. The latter suggestion precipitated an episode of chest pain and shortness of breath for which Meihui's roommates took her to the emergency department located on campus.

Meihui came to her first psychiatric appointment and tearfully complained of increased difficulty concentrating, oversleeping, missing class, and dropping grades. She was planning to major in engineering and was taking all science and math classes.

She did not have any formal past psychiatric diagnosis, but in the fall of her senior year of high school she had a similar bout of oversleeping and problems with concentration. Frantic about not being "competitive for college," she cut herself, but her mother did not share that information with the pediatrician to whom she was taken for fatigue and the inability to concentrate. Without rendering a formal

D. Iarovici, M.D.
Counseling and Mental Health Services, Harvard University Health Services,
Cambridge, MA, USA
e-mail: doris@dorisiarovici.com

© Springer International Publishing AG, part of Springer Nature 2018
A. Martel et al. (eds.), *Promoting Safe and Effective Transitions to College for Youth with Mental Health Conditions*, https://doi.org/10.1007/978-3-319-68894-7_23

diagnosis, the pediatrician prescribed a stimulant for a few months. Once college acceptances rolled in, Meihui felt better, and discontinued medicine. She then had a rough summer with episodes of dizziness, trembling, shortness of breath, and fear of dying. The pediatrician gave her a medicine whose name she did not recall, and referred her to a therapist at that time, but there was a long waitlist and her father was skeptical of the recommendation. She left for college before being seen.

Meihui was the older of two girls in a family that had moved several times due to her father's career in international banking. Her mother did not work outside the home. Meihui had been in the top 10% of her class. In college, however, she felt her class-mates were smarter, and that it took her much longer to do her work, especially reading. Although fluent in English, she had never previously lived in the U.S. and she still struggled to understand nuances. She did not find classes interesting, was finding less and less enjoyment in anything, and was beginning to feel hopeless about her future.

She was not aware of any family psychiatric history, but noted her family did not discuss such matters. Her mother occasionally took to bed for stretches of days, and there was talk of a maternal aunt who had a "nervous breakdown" in China. Meihui denied any trauma history, but tearfully recounted how in the past year, she discov-ered her father was having an affair and confronted him. He assured her it was over and made her promise not to tell her mother, as "she couldn't take it." Although she kept her promise, Meihui found it increasingly difficult to be around her father and was relieved to come to college. She felt better the first few weeks. She was sur-prised at the openness of her peers in discussing emotional challenges and divulging details of personal and family matters. Her peers also questioned her early commit-ment to a career and field of study. Her family, and many peers at home, had always implied that the best careers were in science and math fields.   Increasingly   tired, she began to keep to herself. She avoided phone conversations with her parents until the recent ER visit; now her mother was planning to come to the U.S. to spend a few weeks taking care of her. The student did not want to sign a consent for release of information to her mother, fearing that it would disclose her father's secret. At the same time, having heard from her sister that her parents were fighting more, she was afraid that perhaps her mother already knew.

Meihui met criteria for a diagnosis of Major Depressive Disorder, single episode, moderate, and the psychiatrist recommended a selective serotonin reuptake inhibi-tor (SSRI) antidepressant and cognitive behavioral therapy. She was very reluctant to take a daily medication, instead hoping to get a stimulant again, to take as needed so she could "just focus on my work." She was not sure she had time for psycho-therapy. She definitely did not want to take a medical leave, and in fact did not want to go back to Hong Kong for winter break. With psychoeducation, she eventually agreed to start an SSRI, but continued to voice concerns about concentration and felt significant time pressure to salvage the semester.

Diagnostic questions included the possibility that Meihui may have had undiag-nosed ADHD, inattentive presentation. Although she performed well in school as a child and adolescent, she had enormous help structuring her time from both her mother and various tutors hired by the family over the years. Her mother frequently brought to school papers or lunches that Meihui forgot at home. She described impulsivity, but it was difficult to sort out whether that was the result of a mood disorder, or Attention-Deficit/Hyperactivity Disorder (ADHD), or both. She had done well in the second half of her senior year of high school without continuing stimulant medication although she did still take it occasionally before an exam. Generalized Anxiety Disorder was also in the differential diagnosis, with the recognition that the long-standing academic anxiety and pressure to perform that Meihui described might have been a normal back-drop in the high-pressure school she attended in Hong Kong. Neuropsychological testing was considered, but the student balked at the cost, and it was not covered by the student insurance plan.

Because Meihui had received minimal mental health care only through her pediatrician, no formal transition readiness evaluation, transition planning, or transfer of care plan had been done. Her pediatrician had filled out the required health form for college, but identified "mild situational anxiety" as the only mental health concern.

Meihui had been drawn to American colleges because of their excellent reputation, but had not visited colleges during the application process or after admission. It's not uncommon for international students to first set foot on the campus where they will spend the next 4 years when they arrive to start school. Because the family moved often and Meihui seemed to weather these transitions, neither she nor her family considered the potential impact of moving alone, a great distance from home.

She ultimately was able to remain in school without taking a medical leave, but like many international students, relied on others to notice her struggles, help identify her issues and direct her to appropriate resources for help. She required case management, student health and student counseling services, and had the ER visit. Had peers and faculty members not become directly involved in her care, she might have failed out or had a more serious health consequence.

Analysis of Transition

There are a number of predictors that bode well for Meihui's transition. She is an intelligent, hard-working student, with good mastery of the English language. Her family is supportive in that they made efforts to get her some help in China and her mother is coming to the U.S. in response to her crisis. And fortunately, Meihui is at a school with a range of on-site services and with faculty, peers, and administrators who noticed her distress and reached out to her.

Many aspects of this case were predictive of a negative transition outcome. Meihui did not have a clear understanding of her mental health issues, which impacted her ability to advocate for herself. She seemed ambivalent about her major. She experienced the added stress of keeping "family secrets." By withholding clinically pertinent information from her pediatrician, her family highlighted stigma regarding mental illness. She faced increased academic demands and a significant increase in responsibility to meet those demands in the absence of previous supports (tutors, Mother). Meihui had limited knowledge of how to negotiate college resources. Finally, once on campus, she experienced acculturation issues and social isolation.

As with many international students who become a focus of clinical attention, no one identified Meihui's existing mental health vulnerabilities as such in order to communicate about them with the student herself, her family, or with providers at her college. Many international students who struggle in transitioning have experienced some hint of potential difficulties during the years before college, but have no formal mental health diagnosis. Not only do the students themselves lack an understanding of the link between emotional health and academic functioning, but often so do their families, communities, and even health care providers. Family problems, such as infidelity or addiction or withdrawal from daily activities in a parent, are seen as sources of shame to be concealed, rather than potential indicators of mental illness, which may be biologically (and behaviorally) passed down to offspring.

This young woman had a rocky transition, with academic difficulties that led to dropping a class, social isolation, and emotional distress. In the absence of a formal past diagnosis of ADHD, it was harder to tease out the degree to which her mood disorder was the primary factor in her disrupted concentration.

Meihui showed signs of new-onset difficulties in the year preceding college, both at school and at home, with new-onset cutting. Families respond to such difficulties according to the cultural norms of their countries, and an extensive literature suggests that mental health concerns and psychiatric treatment continues to be stigmatized in many parts of the world. Especially in Asian countries which place high emphasis on academic achievement, (but not exclusive to those countries), families may attend to academic obstacles—in Meihui's case, her fatigue and difficulty concentrating—without pursuing a more holistic evaluation of the potentially complex diagnostic picture (developmental maturity, emotional health, individual goals, or family stressors and dynamics.) Health care providers, both domestically and abroad, have a wide range of attitudes and biases themselves toward mental health services. Meihui's pediatrician could have referred her to more specialized mental health care earlier in her senior year or could have given a more detailed account of the student's difficulties on the health forms to the host college. Had a full evaluation for ADHD been performed and a diagnosis of ADHD confirmed, plans for any needed accommodations might have been addressed ahead of the student's transition to college. Cultural norms around what is appropriate disclosure vary significantly, so colleges may have less information about international students than they do about domestic ones.

There are many things that universities can do—and often are already doing—to improve transition outcomes for international students, especially those with difficulties. Problems might be diminished if colleges communicated with families, once students were accepted, about what increases the risk of acculturation stress, and about how to access resources for students with any pre-existing difficulties or when problems arise. Such communications might be especially helpful if provided in the family's language of origin. Many schools are also increasing opportunities for international students to interact with students and others from their host culture.

Clinical Pearls

- Clear communication of any health issues with campus health services before the student arrives on campus facilitates connection to appropriate resources before crisis strikes. This rarely happens in general and seems even less common for international students.
- Although generalizations about particular international student cohorts are often made, remember that within-group differences can be as important as between-group differences (students bring their own family traumas, socioeconomic factors, complex multi-national histories.)
- There is growing diversity in the specific cultural factors which affect students' attitudes regarding mental health and help-seeking, making it impossible for clinicians to be culturally well versed in all the potential obstacles or issues. However, an attitude of humility and allowing the student to educate the clinician about relevant cultural norms can facilitate culturally competent care.
- International students who come from collectivistic, rather than individualistic, cultures may experience more stress as they acculturate to an environment where they are encouraged to pursue their own goals.
- International students may be more reluctant to seek health care in general, and counseling services in particular, than domestic students. Still, they may be more comfortable accessing help through health services rather than counseling centers.
- They do often benefit similarly from the same services as domestic students, even if they are initially more fearful or reluctant to engage in treatment.
- International students may not view prior care they received as mental health care, making it important for clinicians to ask very specific questions.
- They may be taking non-Western treatments (such as medicinal teas) and not even consider them medications.
- They may have used prn medications, such as stimulants for focus or sedative-hypnotics for sleep, without necessarily understanding the need to meet certain diagnostic criteria, or the risks of taking such medicines, because of a strong cultural emphasis on academic achievement at any cost.
- International students are often much more reluctant to consider medical leave because it often jeopardizes their visa status, and may make it difficult for them to return.
- Collaboration among multiple campus services is important for all students who are having difficulties and is critical in successful work with international students.
- Most schools now have additional orientation events for international students, which include an introduction to the concept of acculturation stress, familiarize students with existing resources, and try to link students with shared identity groups on campus.

Brief Literature Review

International students comprise an increasingly large percentage of the student body at American, Canadian, British, and Australian universities [1, 2]. The literature on international student adjustment is somewhat limited with regard to empirical data, though there is clear recognition that acculturation, a transition that all international students must make, provides an additional stressor. Language difficulties and loss of social support systems have been consistently recognized as particular risk factors for acculturative stress; isolation from students of the host culture seems to particularly exacerbate problems [3]. Counseling centers might use an acculturative stress rating scale to help guide treatment efforts [3]. Acculturation appears to be less difficult when the culture of the host country and the student's home country are more similar, as when Western European students study in the U.S. But some studies suggest that within person characteristics weigh more heavily in determining who will struggle than do within-group differences. Clearly, the enormous heterogeneity among students from different countries, and even within-country variability, makes the very notion of "international" difficult to study, and makes generalizations risky. Yet certain notions do emerge from existing studies.

Stressors unique to this population include language barriers, wide cultural differences with regard to social norms—including how to form friendships—differing beliefs about health and health care, and significant financial pressures [4]. They must contend with loneliness, racism, discrimination, and the microaggressions that exist in society in general, and on campus more specifically [5]. Some studies suggest that international students constitute a high-risk group with regard to mental health issues, having more depressive, anxiety, and irritability symptoms along with sleep and appetite disturbances and low energy, while other studies have questioned those claims [2]. One study of 218 international students at a large public university in New York found that compared to US born students, the international students used crisis hours more, were more likely to have been hospitalized for psychiatric reasons or express suicidal ideation, were more likely to be referred by a professor or other professional, and more frequently presented problems such as grief, loneliness, or academic worries. They less frequently had substance abuse diagnoses [1].

One explanation for the higher severity of mental health concerns in this population is that they underutilize health services in general, and counseling services in particular, leading to worsening of problems by the time they rise to clinical attention. One large Australian study found that of the international students who felt they had a health issue, only 62% actually accessed health services, but of those who felt they needed counseling services, less than 20% ever sought that treatment [2]. Students who took action in response to their own sense of needing help tended to be older, suggesting that young adults transitioning to college may be at particular risk of not seeking help. The rate of counseling center utilization appears to be somewhat lower than rates found among domestic students: comparing pooled self-report data from the Healthy Minds survey, for example, one study found that only 36% of students who screened positive for a mental health problem ever received any kind of treatment in the past year [6].

Trends toward expressing more somatic symptoms, rather than emotional symptoms, described in previous literature, also may be reflected in the international student's tendency to seek "medical" rather than "counseling" help. Students accustomed to hierarchical societal structures may be more comfortable with more directive treatment styles, more common to traditional medical models than to counseling models; they may even view nondirective clinicians as incompetent [7]. Yet it's a balancing act: intelligent young adults from all over the world respond poorly to overly rushed, authoritarian communication styles and are interested in data that can help them make decisions about what they may consider a new framework for health [8]. Thus, the same relationship-building skills that can be helpful with other groups also apply to work with international students.

Helpful Resources

- To help in outreach efforts on campus, NAFSA's guide:
  https://www.nafsa.org/findresources/Default.aspx?id=27117
- To help international students whose financial worries affect mental health:
  http://www.nafsa.org/About_Us/About_International_Education/For_Students/
  Financial_Aid_for_Undergraduate_International_Students/

References

1. Mitchell SL, Greenwood AK, Guglielmi MC. Utilization of counseling services: comparing international and US college students. J College Couns. 2007;10:117–29.
2. Russell J, Thomson G, Rosenthal D. International student use of university health and counseling services. Higher Educ. 2008;56:59–75. https://doi.org/10.1007/s10734-007-9089-x.
3. Poyrazli S, Kavanaugh PR, Baker A, Al-Timimi N. Social support and demographic correlates of acculturative stress in international students. J College Couns. 2004;7(1):73–82. Retrieved from http://search.proquest.com.ezp-prod1.hul.harvard.edu/docview/213731973?accountid=11311
4. Mori SC. Addressing the mental health concerns of international students. J Couns Dev. 2000;78:137–44.
5. Prieto-Welch SL. International student mental health. Stud Services. 2016;2016:53–63. https://doi.org/10.1002/ss.20191.
6. Eisenberg D, Hunt J, Speer N. Help seeking for mental health on college campuses: review of evidence and next steps for research and practice. Harv Rev Psychiatry. 2012;20(4):222–32.
7. Essanoh P. Counseling issues with African college students in US colleges and universities. Couns Psychol. 1995;23:348.
8. Iarovici D. Clash of cultures: international students. In: Mental health issues and the university student. Baltimore, MD: Johns Hopkins University Press; 2014.

"If I Am Not an Athlete, Then Who Am I?" Portrait of a Depressed Student-Athlete

24

Ryan C. Mast

Case History

Laura is an 18-year-old Caucasian female who is a college freshman and a student-athlete on scholarship. She is the youngest of three children to go to college, from a suburban, middle-class upbringing in the Midwest; and she hates her sport. She graduated from high school in the top 25% of her class. In her junior year of high school, she was diagnosed with Major Depressive Disorder, and she also was noted at that time to have significant anxiety symptoms including excessive worry that disrupted normal sleep patterns.

Laura described that she had always had a natural talent for most sports, and with significant effort in her junior year of high school, she became the best female basketball player in the city. While her family, friends, classmates, and others were congratulating and praising her, she internally felt hollow and fake. Reflecting upon her childhood now, she stated that she received a lot of positive attention for her abilities as an athlete even as a very young child. She found that the harder she worked, the better the results, and the more attention she received. Her grandmother notably was extremely proud of her athletic accomplishments, and Laura described not wanting to disappoint her. Dedication to her sport soon evolved into a drive toward perfectionism, and Laura became very hard on herself for mistakes. One coach fueled that fire and blamed her for losses since "the whole team is counting on you."

The childhood joy of games and sports soon became a nightmare that was all-encompassing and seemingly inescapable. Laura identified that her love for basketball died in the sixth grade, but she continued to play while suffering silently.

R.C. Mast, D.O., M.B.A.
Department of Psychiatry, Wright State University, Boonshoft School of Medicine,
Dayton, OH, USA
e-mail: ryan.mast@wright.edu

© Springer International Publishing AG, part of Springer Nature 2018
A. Martel et al. (eds.), *Promoting Safe and Effective Transitions to College for Youth with Mental Health Conditions*, https://doi.org/10.1007/978-3-319-68894-7_24

243

As the years passed, she publicly wore a mask in the spotlight, but privately, she cried most nights during her junior year of high school. She eventually confided in a teammate and a friend, and they encouraged her to tell her parents and the coach, and Laura agreed to do so. While her parents and coach seemed supportive of her, Laura felt as though they really did not listen to her or try to understand. As a result, she did not share all of the details of her struggles with them. Consequently, her parents and coach were unaware that she was struggling with her identity as an athlete, and they did not know that basketball had completely crossed over from enjoyable play to tedious work for her. While they might not have understood completely, Laura's parents did subsequently arrange for her to see a psychologist (specializing in sports psychology) for weekly therapy, and this was helpful, but many symptoms of anxiety and depression persisted. The combination of poor concentration, sadness, apathy, and a lack of time left over for academics led to a significant and rapid decline in her grades to the point that she was at risk for not meeting the minimum GPA to play on the team. Noticing that she was still symptomatic, her parents consulted her pediatrician and then took Laura to see a psychiatrist.

The CAP who Laura saw in her junior year of high school diagnosed Major Depressive Disorder (moderate) noting her significant anxiety symptoms before games and excessive guilt after games. Laura told the CAP more about her symptoms than anyone else, but she also withheld some symptoms and concerns because she worried about her parents' potential reaction if they found out. She denied a history of bullying and of physical or sexual abuse. She denied ever having suicidal thoughts, but admitted to morbid ideation that "maybe it would be easier if I were not here." Laura denied plan and intent. She denied alcohol, tobacco, and illicit drug use stating that substances would likely impair her athletic abilities and jeopardize her chances at an athletic scholarship. This was important to her since she worried constantly about her parents' finances. While she knew that her parents would be supportive and take out personal loans to help (like they had for her two older siblings), she did not want to burden her parents in that way.

At the end of the intake session with the CAP during high school, he recommended: continued weekly therapy (CBT), melatonin to help with sleep, a 504 Plan limiting make up school work to essential assignments only with extended due dates, and baseline blood work. Laura's parents appreciated the recommendation of melatonin since they were hesitant about starting any medications except for natural supplements, and they had read that "Athletes should take helpful, safe, legal supplements." So, they reportedly reasoned that melatonin would improve sleep, which should enhance concentration and mood; therefore, leading to better performance in both sports and academics. Certainly, this could have been the result if Laura's depressive symptoms had not been so prominent. At the time, Laura's only other medication was a multivitamin. She was not taking birth control since she erroneously believed that they all caused weight gain. She identified as cis-gender and heterosexual but was not sexually active and had no plans for that since she had no time to pursue a relationship. She also had amenorrhea at the time presumably from playing sports (but she had not told anyone of her amenorrhea).

Baseline labs came back normal, and by the next appointment Laura reported some improvement in sleep with melatonin and a reduction in her depressive symptoms, but not a significant improvement. Because of her continued symptomatology, her psychiatrist subsequently recommended an SSRI, but Laura reported that her parents declined to start it because "they said that I need some healthy anxiety to be a good athlete, they did not want my personality to change, that an SSRI would do that, and that the National Collegiate Athletic Association (NCAA) probably will not allow me to take an SSRI" (which is inaccurate). Laura stated that it certainly did not feel like healthy anxiety at all, and she expressed frustration again that her parents neither understood her struggles nor the actual risks and benefits of the medication. Her coach was supportive in general, but once during his half-time locker-room speech to the team, he reportedly stated, "You saw what happened when Laura blocked those shots. They are too anxious, weak-minded, and timid to even shoot now." She stated that when he delivered that last line, he looked at her and immediately flushed red with the weight and impact of his own words suddenly realized.

By the end of junior year in high school, Laura had a good understanding of her own mental health needs, but lacked both the ability and desire to share those needs with her parents, providers, coaches, or friends. She spent time reading about sports psychology, and she tried to use coping tools (breathing techniques and guided imagery) that she learned from books and in therapy. She developed a short-memory for her "failures" stating that like a kicker in football, all athletes need to learn from the past, but not dwell on the past because they cannot afford to be "in their own heads all of the time." She also realized that perfectionism was unattainable, and that idea was freeing.

In senior year of high school, she was no longer the best player in the city, and she was okay with that. She spent less time practicing and tried to have some fun and enjoy her final year of high school. Though her parents discouraged her, she took a part-time summer job at a local amusement park in the games department between her junior and senior years. The job seemed to lift her spirits and she made friends outside of school and basketball. The job also helped her learn about paychecks and taxes, and start thinking about her transition from dependent high school student to somewhat independent college freshman. Outside of basketball and school, she spent time in the public library doing practice SAT and ACT questions hoping to earn an academic scholarship; ultimately, the most she was offered was a $2000 academic scholarship. At the same time, she was also looking at college websites and materials, and paying attention to the counseling services available at the schools in which she had the most interest.

Laura was heavily recruited by colleges for basketball in her senior year, and she was offered many sizeable athletic scholarships. Though her parents did not fully understand her difficulties, they valued her mental health. They hoped she would choose the local college and live at home freshman year so they could help ease her transition to college (and possibly also their own transition to empty nest). They asked her therapist, CAP, and pediatrician for input on Laura's college options and transition plan. Laura appreciated that her parents were involved and talking with the right people. However, she wanted some distance from family, and asked her

CAP and therapist to help her develop a plan that would allow her to thrive away from home and would ease her parents' minds about her ability to be far from them. The CAP and therapist met with Laura and her parents and offered general psycho-education on depression. They encouraged her parents to attend college visits with Laura paying special attention to mental health services available on campus. The importance of Laura being honest with her parents was emphasized so that parents could help monitor for the need of an SSRI. Her parents gained a better appreciation of Laura's struggles through these discussions though Laura carefully managed what was disclosed during the sessions. During college visits, both Laura and her parents made special note of the value that each coach and athletic department placed on mental health and wellness.

Ultimately, Laura chose a Division I university that was a 3 hour drive from home. She later revealed to her new psychiatrist at the college that she chose that school both by feel and with four guiding principles in mind: (1) Mental health services available, (2) Academics (she wanted to study psychology), (3) Distance (she wanted a school that was far enough away that her parents would not constantly visit, but that she could still drive home on a weekend), and (4) Athletics (did the athletics department seem supportive). Overall goodness of fit with all four domains was more important than a university that was exceptional in three domains, but suboptimal in the fourth domain.

It was the university's policy that incoming students could not schedule appointments at the UCC until they matriculated and were on campus. The wait time for an appointment was unpredictable. So, the initial plan for ongoing care was for Laura to see her home providers 2 weeks into the semester and then monthly. Once she established care on campus, home providers would be available during school breaks and the summer if needed. Laura would also Skype with her parents weekly. Her providers requested that she sign release of information forms so they could communicate with the UCC. Laura chose not to sign any forms at that time, noting she would prefer such releases to be for specific campus providers and not a global release for the UCC.

Her first week on campus, Laura went to the UCC and scheduled an appointment with a psychologist for the following week. She was soon also scheduled with a psychiatrist. At her first psychiatric appointment she stated, "I am 18 now, and as an adult I would like to start an SSRI for depression. My parents never let me take one." She went on to state, "I am listed as a student-athlete, but my parents think that athlete is the first word: 'athlete-student'. I basically play for the scholarship and to make others happy." She identified the dilemma as: "If I continue to play, I will feel like a phony. If I quit, a lot of people would be disappointed, and they would see me as a failure who threw away a golden ticket. Some people might call this an existential crisis, and they would probably be right because I wonder what my identity is if I am not an athlete. Perhaps I am destined to be depressed in college because these questions will always be on my mind." She asked for an inexpensive SSRI because she planned to pay out-of-pocket so that her parents would not find out. She stated that she loved her parents and already knew their opinion on the matter but would inform them over the winter break or sooner if symptoms worsened. Also at the intake, Laura declined to sign consents for her previous providers or for her family. She felt that her home therapist was more aligned with her parents than with her, and did not want any word of the SSRI to get back to Mom. Laura also worried about the limits of confidentiality and whether the athletic department would have access to her records. She was assured that they would not have access unless she chose to allow it.

Feeling listened to turned out to be perhaps the most essential part of the treatment because she now felt free to say anything without worrying that it might get back to her parents. Laura continued melatonin and started an SSRI. She was switched to a second SSRI because of side effects. This medication was titrated over a few weeks and by mid semester she reported moderate improvement in her depressive symptoms. Laura was passing her classes and she was playing well.

In the fourth game of the basketball season, Laura had a scary fall and suffered both a concussion and back injury. Concussion protocol was followed, and she sat out significant time while recovering. She exercised very little because it exacerbated symptoms (including headaches). She presented to a psychiatric appointment during that time and was not doing well with her symptoms of depression and anxiety. "I have always been a pretty healthy athlete until now. I feel depressed, and cannot go for a run to take my mind off it. I have unlimited time to be in my own head, and that is not really a good thing right now." Medication was titrated, and she returned feeling much better. She had also started yoga to get low-impact exercise and to work on mindfulness. Her first yoga session made her very sad and worried. She stated, "The instructor guided us through a body inventory exercise telling us to concentrate first on our toes and how they felt, then our feet, etc. I realized for the first time that most of my joints genuinely hurt. I always played through pain and tried to ignore it." She began to wonder aloud, "Will I need new knees when I am 40? Why am I putting my body on the line if I am not good enough to play in the WNBA?"

While her symptoms from the concussion resolved, her back injury did not improve and she required minor surgery. The surgery was successful, but the surgeon suggested she would likely have some residual limitations that would prevent her from ever fully returning to her original level of performance, and there was real concern about the risk of reinjury. So, Laura (the leading scorer in the history of her high school) finished her college career with a total of 10 points, 4 rebounds, and 1 block.

She returned to the next psychiatry appointment stating that, "My identity as an athlete is over. While I am happy that the decision is made, I am not happy it ended with an injury. An injury made the decision for me, and as someone who likes control, I did not like that." She added that people might feel bad for her, but looking on the bright side, no one would be mad or disappointed in her "for just quitting and throwing my talent away."

That semester, given her physical and mental health symptoms, she had to drop two classes and passed the others without any accommodations. The next semester, her physical symptoms were better, but she continued to struggle with mental health concerns and again had to drop a class. Laura lost her scholarship after leaving the team so she took out loans and worked part-time. The following year, she returned and was doing much better after adjusting to her new identity and dreams. In the end, it turned out that everyone was supportive. Laura said, "Grandma is just happy that I am happy." Grades for that year were a 4.0 (and were the best that she had ever had in high school or college).

Laura graduated in 4 years with a major in psychology. She worked in the summers at a shelter for homeless and runaway youth. She had felt pressure as an athlete to be a good role model since she represented her school and city; now she was content being a good role model for kids. She joined a co-ed rec basketball team, and she enjoyed basketball for the first time in more than 6 years. Since quitting the team, she had what seemed like limitless free time to do homework, find a job, volunteer, attend parties, briefly experiment with alcohol, and find a boyfriend. At her request, during senior year the SSRI was tapered off with good success. In therapy, she pondered what would have been different if she had really opened up to her mental health providers and parents in high school. "Was there a way for me to enjoy basketball? Would I have tried to make a comeback after my injury?"

Analysis of Transition

Reflecting back on Laura's case, there were many factors predictive of a successful transition to college. Laura engaged in mental health treatment prior to college and demonstrated initiative for self-help. She was adherent with taking melatonin. She showed desire for and efforts toward independence and autonomy. During the college application and selection process, she investigated mental health services on different campuses and developed a transition care plan. She tended toward healthy coping strategies such as physical exercise. She had solid abilities in organizing and structuring her time.

There were also some negative predictive factors operating in this case. Laura's depression was not fully treated at the time of transition. She had poor communication with her parents. Even after revealing her struggles in junior year of high school, she continued to hide some symptoms from her parents, coach, and providers. She was unable to confide in her parents about her feelings toward basketball. Laura took on some responsibilities under the guise of not wanting to worry or bother her parents without discussing matters with them. She was overly focused on the opinion of others and had concerns about stigma. With her transition to college, she continued to hide some symptoms and treatment details from her parents.

Laura's transition to college could be considered suboptimal. She arrived on campus with an inadequately treated depression and functioned below her abilities academically. However, away from home, Laura advocated for herself and was started on antidepressant medication for her depression which can be considered a positive outcome of her transition to college.

In retrospect, there were a few things that could have been done differently to improve Laura's transition outcome. Laura's parents would have benefitted from earlier and more advanced psychoeducation on depression, its treatment (including the risks, benefits, and potential side effects of medications), and its impact on Laura's function. Earlier intervention with psychotropic medication would have improved Laura's outcome. Also, not challenging the parents' rationale for using or not using a medication, which was based on how it would impact her immediate performance on the court or her eligibility 18 months into the future, probably contributed to Laura's impression that her provider was more aligned with her parents. Even the fact that parents had Laura see a sports psychologist in high school may have inadvertently reinforced Laura's opinion that they considered her an "athlete-student." Highlighting these issues for the parents may have encouraged them to be better listeners.

If Laura had been more forthcoming about her symptoms and feelings, a better understanding of her identity development, depression, and anxiety would have allowed for improved planning and a better outcome. One possible strategy for getting Laura to open up would have been to address her worry about burdening her parents. Subsequently, family therapy might have proven beneficial in uncovering her misconceptions and improving communication.

Clinical Pearls

- Psychoeducation for the student-athlete and their parents is important. This should include education about common developmental and phase of life challenges that a student-athlete faces. Many athletes struggle with identity development and managing internal and external motivations and pressures. Transition *to* a college athletic program and life *after* college athletics includes processing identity changes and maintaining a healthy lifestyle.
- At some point, for most athletes play becomes work. Injuries are ubiquitous, and most have experience playing with and through injuries. Learning to balance athletics, academics, and social life is key.
- Many athletes struggle with depression, anxiety, eating disorders, substance use disorders, insomnia, and body image issues. Some avoid seeking help for reasons such as stigma and fear of being perceived as "weak." It is important to also recognize that team dynamics can have an effect on mental health.
- Many LGBT athletes worry that coming out about their sexual orientation will negatively impact about how teammates and opponents will treat them.
- Mental health screening is recommended for all athletes. In addition to screening for depression, anxiety, alcohol and other substance use, experiences around hazing, sexual abuse, physical aggression, and gambling should be addressed.
- Since there is often a close connection between team physicians, sports medicine, sports psychologists, and coaches, the college-athlete often has questions about the limits of confidentiality, and boundaries must be adeptly managed by clinicians.
- College-athletes often have questions about acceptable and banned substances and medications. Most psychotropic medications, including SSRIs, are *not* on the banned substances list. Patients should be counseled to check with the

designated official on campus before taking any substance. Exceptions can be made if certain medications are clinically indicated, and this includes stimulants, for which there is a *medical exception documentation* form on the NCAA website.

- For students headed to college with an already diagnosed mental illness, creation of a clear and comprehensive transfer of care plan is essential. Engaging with the campus mental health clinic early in the first semester often leads to better outcomes.

- Impaired communication between parents and children can impact the adjustment to college life. Remind parents to be available to talk or just listen and to focus their attention when approached by their teen/young adult. When greater barriers to communication exist, family therapy is indicated. Expectations for communication while away at college should be discussed before the student heads to campus. Parents may pick up nuanced changes in their child that signal a mental health concern.

- All patients headed to college should be educated about navigating normal phase of life tasks and challenges (increased independence from parents, developing and maintaining relationships, managing schedules, struggling with deciding who they will be and how they will get there).

Brief Literature Review

The NCAA notes that there are approximately 460,000 college student-athletes in the United States participating in 24 sports at more than 1000 member institutions, and the need for providers trained in the care of the student-athlete is therefore paramount and on the mind of all IHE. Both the NCAA and many college-athletes have identified mental health and wellness as areas of serious concern. Anxiety, depression, substance use issues, and eating disorders are not uncommon in this population [1–3]. The NCAA has created numerous programs and documents with the goals of improving student-athlete mental health and promoting wellness across campuses.

Suicide accounted for 7.3% of all college-athlete deaths between 2003 and 2012 (35 total identified suicides) [4]. Male college football players had the highest suicide rate of all college-athletes. Male college-athletes were significantly more likely to commit suicide than female college-athletes, both in terms of total number (29 of the 35 suicides were males) and in terms of relative risk. African American college-athletes have a higher incidence than Caucasian college-athletes with regard to suicide.

It should be noted that the incidence of suicide for college-athletes is less than that of college non-athletes and also less than that of non-college same age peers. It is thought that the lower incidence in college-athletes is due at least in part to better social connectivity and the antidepressant effects of exercise. While the incidence is lower, it is still extremely concerning and the fourth leading cause of death of college-athletes [4].

The NCAA has published additional documents for the treatment of injuries (including concussion protocols) especially in light of the risk of post-concussion depression and suicidality. Special attention is also being paid to the time required to heal from injuries (including the very variable amount of time required to heal from a concussion before returning to competition). Physical injuries can certainly have psychological consequences, and the opposite is also true; psychiatric conditions (including depression, anxiety, eating disorders) can affect physical health and therefore athletic performance [5–7].

College-athletes are at a high risk for aggression/violence [8], hazing, and substance use. Twelve percent of all college males reported being in a physical fight in the preceding 12 months compared to 24% of male college-athletes [9]. Also, 74% of college student-athletes experienced at least one form of hazing during their time in college. Participating in drinking games was the leading form of hazing (47%) with 23% reporting having to drink alcohol to the point of becoming sick or passing out [10]. The NCAA is also focused on sexual violence awareness and prevention [11].

In addition to common mental health and physical concerns of all athletes, the "female athlete triad" has also been emphasized and addressed with documents created by the NCAA. This triad consists of the following three interrelated conditions: (1) energy deficiency with or without disordered eating, (2) menstrual disturbances/amenorrhea, and (3) bone loss/osteoporosis.

Helpful Resources

- The NCAA has created many helpful documents related to student-athlete mental health and wellness. The documents listed below can be accessed at: http://www.ncaa.org/health-and-safety/medical-conditions/mental-health
  Mental Health Best Practices, Mind Body and Sport—Understanding and Supporting Student-Athlete Mental Wellness, Sports Medicine Handbook, Managing Student-Athlete Mental Health Issues, Addressing Sexual Assault and Interpersonal Violence, Helping Support Student-Athlete Mental Health: A Primer for Campus Stakeholders Outside of Athletics
- NCAA drug testing program, banned substances, and ADHD Medical Exception Reporting Form http://www.ncaa.org/sport-science-institute/ncaa-drug-testing-program
- Concussion Safety Protocol Management. http://www.ncaa.org/sport-science-institute/concussion-diagnosis-and-management-best-practices
- NCAA Coaches Handbook: Managing the Female Athlete Triad. http://www.femaleathletetriad.org/wp-content/uploads/2008/10/NCAA-Managing-the-Female-Athlete-Triad.pdf
- International Society for Sport Psychiatry (ISSP): https://sportspsychiatry.org/
- The NCAA Sports Science Institute has both a newsletter and is active on twitter @NCAA_SSI

Office-Based Tools

- The NCAA website includes screening tools for: General Index, ADHD, Alcohol Use, Anxiety, Sleep Apnea, Cannabis Use, Depression, Disordered Eating, Insomnia, and NATA Recommendations for Pre-Participation Exams. https://www.ncaa.org/sites/default/files/HS_Mental-Health-Best-Practices_20160317.pdf

References

1. Greenleaf C, Petrie T, Carter J, Reel J. Female collegiate athletes: prevalence of eating disorders and disordered eating behaviors. J Am Coll Health. 2009;57:489–95.
2. Weigand S, Cohen J, Merenstein D. Susceptibility for depression in current and retired student athletes. Sports Health. 2013;5:263–66.
3. Barry AE, Howell SM, Riplinger A, Piazza-Gardner AK. Alcohol use among college athletes: do intercollegiate, club, or intramural student athletes drink differently? Subst Use Misuse. 2015;50(3):302–07.
4. Rao A, Asif I, Drezner J, Toresdahl B, Harmon K. Suicide in National Collegiate Athletic Association (NCAA) Athletes: a 9-year analysis of the NCAA Resolutions Database. Sports Health. 2015;7(5):452–57.
5. Fauman B, Hopkinson M. Special populations. In: Kay J, Schwartz V, editors. Mental health care in the college community. West Sussex: Wiley; 2010. p. 247–65.
6. NCAA Multidisciplinary Taskforce. Mental health best practices: inter-association consensus document: best practices for understanding and supporting student-athlete mental wellness. NCAA Handbook. 2016. https://www.ncaa.org/sites/default/files/HS_Mental-Health-Best-Practices_20160317.pdf.
7. Yang J, Cheng G, Zhang Y, et al. Influence of symptoms of depression and anxiety on injury hazard among collegiate American football players. Res Sports Med. 2014;22:147–60.
8. Murnen S, Kohlman M. Athletic participation, fraternity membership, and sexual aggression among college men: a meta-analytic review. Sex Roles. 2007;57(1):145–57.
9. The mental health landscape in sport. https://www.nata.org/sites/default/files/mentalhealth-landscape.pdf.
10. Addressing student athlete hazing. http://www.ncaa.org/sport-science-institute/addressing-student-athlete-hazing.
11. Sexual violence prevention: an athletics tool kit for a healthy and safe culture. http://www.ncaa.org/sport-science-institute/sexual-violence-prevention-tool-kit.

The Challenge of Coming in First: Helping First-Generation College Students Win Beyond Getting In

25

Jessica Moore

Case History

Noel is a 17-year-old African-American female from a low income, urban area in the Midwest. She is the second oldest child of five with three much younger siblings. Noel lived with her maternal aunt during high school, which was 300 miles from her family; she played on the school's volleyball team. In high school, she participated in regular education classes without accommodations and graduated in the bottom one third of her class. She is a first-generation college student (FGCS) and is enrolled in an Historically Black College and University (HBCU). At the time of her transition to college, Noel's Diagnosis was Major Depressive Disorder single episode, in partial remission.

Her mother and father work minimum wage jobs. Hoping to escape the gun violence in their community, for several years Noel's parents moved the entire family around to several different cities. Despite this, Noel did well academically in elementary and middle school. Though her parents had little involvement or interest in her school work, she was motivated by teachers' praise. With their encouragement, she excelled on state testing allowing her to participate in the Gifted and Talented program. She spent most of her time with her older brother or babysitting her younger siblings. She had few friends in middle school as she often felt too embarrassed by her poor living conditions and tattered clothes to invite others to her home. By the end of middle school, amidst increasing financial burdens including near homelessness, her parents sent Noel and her old brother to live with a maternal aunt to complete high school, hoping for a safer and more stable environment.

J. Moore, M.D.
PGY5 Child and Adolescent Psychiatry, UT-Southwestern Medical Center, Dallas, TX, USA
e-mail: jessica.moore@utsouthwestern.edu

© Springer International Publishing AG, part of Springer Nature 2018
A. Martel et al. (eds.), *Promoting Safe and Effective Transitions to College for Youth with Mental Health Conditions*, https://doi.org/10.1007/978-3-319-68894-7_25

Noel was referred to psychiatric care at the start of her junior year of high school by her guidance counselor after a physical fight with another student. At that time, she had symptoms of depression: a depressed and irritable mood, insomnia, hopelessness, and thoughts about death. She had begun to put less effort into school, maintaining only the minimum 2.0 grade point average (GPA) required to play on the volleyball team, the one activity she maintained interest in. Noel was diagnosed with major depressive disorder, without psychotic features. She declined medications, but attended weekly psychotherapy with a psychiatrist, focusing on reframing negative thoughts from a CBT approach. As therapy continued, she noticed that as her depression improved her grades and the ability to get along with her teammates improved, motivating her to attend weekly visits. Her biggest success was being named captain of the volleyball team by her peers.

Despite poor grades in general, Noel's coach recognized her math talent and leadership skills, so encouraged her to apply to college. Her math teacher noticed that she was self-motivated in mathematics and self-sufficient in daily activities such as getting to school on time, tending to hygiene, using public transportation, keeping to a budget, and preparing light meals. Given this, she felt that she might excel in a college environment, away from her familial demands. Although not convinced that college was the right place for her, she reluctantly agreed to apply, not wanting to disappoint her coach and teacher. She only applied to one college, a mid-size HBCU with low cost tuition and rolling admissions, which her cousin attended in a nearby city. She hoped that by attending a small college with other students of color she might feel more at home and supported. Though she hoped they would assist her in filling out the college application and taking her for a campus visit, her aunt and parents were not involved in the application or transition process, except to provide the necessary fees.

Noel was accepted to the university two months prior to the start of classes. Following her acceptance, she and her psychiatrist began to discuss her transition to college. She was encouraged to include parents to assist with finding housing, scholarships, and psychiatric follow-up, but declined as she did not want to further burden them. They were experiencing their own socioeconomic stressors. She agreed to monthly phone sessions with her psychiatrist until she could establish care at the university counseling center. They planned approaches to avoid psychiatric crisis, including reviewing her triggers and signs of relapse. They also planned for ways to address academic struggles: attending the 3-week summer pre-college preparatory program, finding tutoring, and reaching out to her professors once on campus. She planned to get a work-study job to help reduce financial burdens and increase her sense of accomplishment. Noel had her last visit with her psychiatrist the week prior to leaving for college and scheduled an appointment for winter break.

Noel participated in the pre-college preparatory program. However, she felt it was difficult to make friends, finding it hard to connect with the upper and middle class and continuing generation college students. The residence halls were too expensive so she moved to an off-campus apartment to reduce costs. To afford the fees her student loan would not cover, she got an off-campus job which paid more than on-campus work-study jobs. Despite her best efforts to manage school and her 30 h/week job, she began to struggle academically. She did not reach out for help from her professors. When she called home, her mother focused on financial diffi-culties she was having at home, which made Noel feel guilty for leaving. She con-templated going to the student counseling center on campus, but feared that she would be kicked out for her history of fighting that she had not revealed on her application. She eventually called the counseling center but was told there was a 2-month wait and an accompanying fee so she decided not to make an appointment. After the second monthly phone session with her psychiatrist, she felt it was not the same as being seen in person. She determined it would no longer be helpful, so began avoiding her psychiatrist's calls.

By winter break, she felt that she did not belong or deserve to be at the university. Her parents suggested that she take a break from school as they needed financial help and someone to care for the youngest siblings anyway. She missed the previ-ously scheduled in-person psychiatry appointment. She returned to school, but con-tinued to feel hopeless and started to have nightmares and flashbacks to a time when she had been shot, symptoms she had not previously disclosed to her psychiatrist. After failing a midterm exam, she was placed on academic probation. She soon began to cut her arms and legs with a broken piece of glass. She was not sure that she wanted to die, but did not know another way in which to manage her mood. During a routine advising session, her academic advisor noticed the cuts on her arms. Together they called the counseling center from the advisor's office and got an appointment for the following day. After getting established with a psychiatrist there, she was diagnosed with Posttraumatic Stress Disorder (PTSD) and Major Depressive Disorder, recurrent episode, moderate for which she started to attend weekly psychotherapy sessions.

With the help of her psychiatrist, Noel enrolled in the campus' intensive reten-tion program for students at high risk for dropping out. Through this program, she reached out to professors in her academically challenging classes and subsequently her grades began to improve. She was assigned a faculty mentor through the reten-tion program and joined the intramural volleyball team providing her with on-campus peer and faculty supports as well as enhancing her sense of belonging. She processed feelings of guilt she had about leaving home, allowing her to better engage her parents about her adjustment to college life. Noel is now a junior, major-ing in business administration, and attends therapy once per month.

Analysis of Transition

There are several aspects of this case that are predictive of Noel's negative college transition experience. As a first-generation college student (FGCS), it was possible that she would have a difficult transition period regardless of other psychosocial and academic factors. She was academically unprepared; though she participated in the Gifted and Talented program while in middle school, she struggled to pass her classes due to poor effort, particularly when depressed, while in high school. Family stressors, including lack of social or emotional support from her parents and care-giving for younger siblings, contributed as well. She also had limited school-based peer supports given multiple moves and embarrassment over her living conditions. Furthermore, significant economic burdens, including the cost of tuition and famil-ial financial concerns were risk factors. Importantly, Noel initially expressed little personal motivation to attend and excel in college aside from the encouragement from her coach and teachers. Moreover, she had little agency in choosing which college to attend, applying to only one college. Certainly, her history of depression and trauma exposure (which was minimized during the initial treatment) suggested that she might struggle as she began her college career.

Conversely, there are several factors that suggest Noel might have had a positive transition to college. Despite multiple moves and several academic transitions, she was able to participate in a Gifted and Talented program as a child, suggesting she was self-motivated and had independent living skills as noted by teachers. She also demonstrated leadership skills that were noticed by her coach when she was captain of the volleyball team. Furthermore, she was engaged in psychiatric care, doing well, and had insight into how her depression may impact her academic at college. Noel's choice to attend a nearby, mid-size, HBCU suggested that she may have had a more positive outcome. By attending a small university, she was more likely to have faculty and administration as sources of support. Additionally, in choosing to attend an HBCU with other students of color (versus a Predominantly White Institution, PWI) Noel might have had a stronger sense of community. She also chose to attend college where she had established support with her older cousin who was already a student at the university. Finally, in choosing a university that was close to her home, she might have been able to stay connected to social supports, like her guidance counselor, coach, and math teacher, who encouraged her to gradu-ate high school and consider college.

All things considered, Noel had significant difficulties during her first year which are indicative of a suboptimal transition to college. Prior to college, her depression was well managed, but amidst feelings of isolation, acculturation stress, academic challenges, and financial stress, she began to experience worsening of her depressive and PTSD symptoms. These symptoms culminated in recurrent episodes of self-injurious behavior. It is important to note that Noel discontinued care almost imme-diately upon her arrival on campus and did not re-engage in treatment until in crisis at the end of spring semester. During this time period, her significant academic prob-lems resulted in academic probation and the possibility of failing out of school.

Finally, there are a number of aspects of transitioning preparation and planning that could have been approached differently to improve Noel's first year of college. Noel's transition planning was short, occurring only over the course of 2 months despite her being in treatment for nearly 2 years. It would have been prudent for her psychiatrist to address issues of transition earlier in her treatment, even while in the application process. Her psychiatrist could have also approached this by addressing the transition that comes along with graduating high school regardless of her post-graduation plans. In addition to addressing the anticipated financial and academic stressors, Noel would have benefited from discussing her psychological needs during her transition to college. This would include addressing issues of identity, acculturation to the college environment, ways to engender a sense of belonging on campus, and methods to enhance self-efficacy. Despite Noel's trauma history, the possibility of a diagnosis of PTSD was not explored during her pre-college treatment.

Additionally, Noel may have made a more successful transition had issues surrounding her family and social support been addressed. She would have benefited from learning ways to increase social supports, including support from her parents, faculty, and on-campus peers or mentors. If she was able to remain connected to her coach or guidance counselor, she may have sought help from these known supports earlier. Empowering Noel to get her family more involved would have allowed her to have support outside of the college setting, enhanced her parents understanding of the college experience, and helped her cope with feelings of guilt for leaving home.

Another barrier to her success was inherent in services provided by the university. Like other college counseling centers, her university had long wait times for services. Noel's psychiatrist could have assisted in actually connecting her to an on-campus provider prior to her transition. Additionally, the university did not have a way to readily identify students in need of treatment, especially off-campus students. Had her transitioning psychiatrist addressed the availability of resources on *and* off campus, and how to manage her own care (including cost and scheduling an appointment), Noel might have been able to get treatment, even when she could not readily access it and did not feel comfortable using the student counseling center. She might have also been more likely to use on-campus services if she was provided with more psychoeducation on her rights as a student, including issues related to Family Education Rights and Privacy Act (FERPA) and confidentiality.

Clinical Pearls

Clinical Pearls for First-Generation College Students

- FGCSs must quickly adapt to novel social and academic challenges including navigating the application process, finding financial aid, determining a major, and obtaining internships.
- FGCSs are more likely to work full time and often consider themselves an employee first and a student second.
- FGCSs tend to have fewer on-campus supports so college mental health providers and campus advisors should look to enhance academic and social supports through summer bridge, student engagement and retention, and TRIO programs.
- While some FGCSs live at home with family which is a source of support, others might experience feelings of guilt when they are unable to meet familial responsibilities.

Clinical Pearls for All Students

- Conversations about transition should start as early as the college application process.
- Families should be engaged in the process whenever possible.
- Address the academic, financial, and social stressors that a student may face.
- Examine the psychological needs of students including expectations for college, adapting to the college culture, familial expectations, and creating a sense of belonging.
- Have a clearly defined process for transitioning care to another provider, including planning for a psychiatric crisis.
- Institutions of Higher Education (IHE) should have easily accessible mental health services with well-defined directives on how to access and pay for care. Well-supervised trainees can help relieve the burden of wait lists and provide ongoing therapy.
- IHE should have a process to identify students in need of psychiatric services. Faculty and administration should be aware of processes to refer students to these services.

Brief Literature Review

FGCSs are defined as those students whose parents did not attend post-secondary education. Some research expands the definition to include students whose parents did not earn a college degree, but may have attended some college. The most recent national research on FGCSs comes from the National Center for Education Statistics (NCES) and indicates that FGCSs are disproportionately represented by ethnic and racial minorities, in particular African-American and Hispanic students [1, 2]. These students tend to come from low-income families, are female, are more likely to attend a 2-year institution first, and enter college for the first time at a later age than continuing generation students [1, 2]. While each of these characteristics is a risk factor for leaving college before completion, status as a FGCS is also an independent risk factor for attrition [1–3]. Additionally, FGCSs have greater financial constraints, are less likely to be encouraged to attend college by parents and teachers, and have lower aspirations for post-secondary education [2].

Research by Stephens et al. [4] contends that the culture of IHE which are shaped by middle and upper class norms and promote the value of independence. This may contribute to academic difficulties and pose a disadvantage for FGCS from working class backgrounds where interdependence and community is valued instead [4]. For example, FGCS may have interdependent motives for attending college, such as serving as a community role model or the desire to bring honor to the family, which may serve as a source of conflict throughout college [4].

Social, financial, and academic challenges have an impact on the overall mental health and well-being of students. For example, students might feel as though they do not belong or that persons from their background do not deserve to attend college [5]. While FGCSs have nearly equivalent rates of depression, they are more likely to have symptoms of PTSD (possibly because they are more likely to come from a background with trauma) and have lower rates of life satisfaction [6]. FGCSs are less likely to report feelings of stress compared to their counterparts, greatly limiting their access to social supports and other psychological resources [3, 6].

After 5 years, FGCSs are less likely to have attained a degree and more likely to leave college without a degree than their counterparts [2]. However, as indicated by NCES, if FGCSs are able to successfully graduate, they have similar employment rates and average salaries, and are likely to be employed in similar fields of work [2].

Many IHE utilize summer bridge or TRIO programs to provide academic support, financial literacy, career counseling, and social engagement [7]. TRIO programs, such as Upward Bound, Talent Search, or Student Support Services, are federally funded outreach programs and grants that are specifically designed to support disadvantaged students, as early as middle school, as they pursue educational endeavors. Stephens et al. [5] suggests providing a *difference education* intervention in which students are educated about how their backgrounds may impact their college experience, including how their background could be both a strength and a challenge. This intervention improved students' overall well-being, feelings of adjustment to college life, and reduced the amount of reported anxiety [5]. Research suggests that increasing social support is vital to successfully transitioning to college [5]. Social support includes increasing academic support from faculty, enhancing family or peer involvement, and increasing engagement in college campus life. In particular, mentorship provides academic support, access to professional opportunities, and motivation to continue education [3].

FGCSs face unique academic, social, and financial challenges when transitioning to college. However, mental health providers can provide interventions that enhance their overall well-being and increase the likelihood that they will successfully obtain a degree.

Helpful Resources

Resources for Clinicians to Provide to FGCSs

- http://www.1vyg.org/
- http://www.firstgenerationfoundation.org/
- https://firstgraduate.org/
- www.imfirst.org/http://www.firstinthefamily.org/highschool/Introduction.html
- http://www.gocollegenow.org/
- https://sites.ed.gov/whieeaa/files/2016/10/9.15.16-Final-First-Generation-Tool-Kit_WHIEEAAOUS-web-edition.pdf

Sample Mental Health Support Programs for FGCSs

- http://www.clemson.edu/academics/programs/first/
- https://www.brown.edu/campus-life/support/first-generation-students/resources-0

Creating a Difference Education Program

- https://www.insidehighered.com/views/2014/03/18/essay-colleges-can-help-students-talking-about-issues-social-class

Resources for Families

- http://www.firstgenerationfoundation.org/students/parents-of-our-students
- http://www.act.org/content/act/en/education-and-career-planning/resources-for-families.html
- http://ibrinfo.org/what.vp.html
- http://www.affordablecollegesonline.org/college-resource-center/first-generation-college-students/
- http://www.gocollegenow.org/for-students-and-parents/

References

1. Chen X. First generation students in postsecondary education: a look at their college transcripts (NCES 2005-171). Washington, DC: U.S. Department of Education, National Center for Education Statistics, U.S. Government Printing Office; 2005.
2. Choy S. Students whose parents did not go to college: postsecondary access, persistence, and attainment (NCES 2001-126). Washington, DC: U.S. Department of Education, National Center for Education Statistics, U.S. Government Printing Office; 2001.
3. Gibbons M, Woodside M. Addressing the needs of first-generation college students: lessons learned from adults from low-education families. J Coll Couns. 2014;17:21–36.
4. Stephens NM, et al. Unseen disadvantage: how American universities' focus on independence undermines the academic performance of first-generation college students. J Pers Soc Psychol. 2012;102:1178–97.
5. Stephens NM, et al. Closing the social-class achievement gap: a difference-education intervention improves first-generation students' academic performance and all students' college transition. Psychol Sci. 2014;25:943–53.
6. Jenkins SR, et al. First-generation undergraduate students' social support, depression, and life satisfaction. J Coll Couns. 2013;16:129–42.
7. Stebleton MJ, et al. First-generation students' sense of belonging mental health, and use of counseling services at Public Research Universities. J Coll Couns. 2014;17:6–20.

Fostering Transitions to College: Considerations for Youth Aging Out of Foster Care

26

Brian Skehan

Case History

George is a 17-year-old Caucasian male in permanent state custody; parental rights for both parents were terminated when he was age nine. He lived with the same foster parents in a rural town for the 6 years prior to graduating from a therapeutic high school. He had an older adult sister and five known paternal half siblings ranging in age from 11 to 26. His diagnoses included Persistent Depressive Disorder (Dysthymia), Attention-Deficit/Hyperactivity Disorder combined presentation, Post Traumatic Stress Disorder, Generalized Anxiety Disorder, and Intellectual Disability, Mild.

George was born full term with heavy exposure to nicotine during the pregnancy. Speech and gross motor delays were evident and early intervention services were in place before age two. He was identified as a child in need by three separate state social services, beginning at age one, due to frequent moves and concerns for neglect. Breathing difficulties and concern for medical neglect resulted in approximately 20 hospitalizations during the first 5 years of life. He spent the first year of life living with a family friend due to his mother's diagnosis of post-partum depression before returning to live with his mother until the age of five. At that time, he had his first residential placement. There was a history of multiple disrupted attachments that included more than 20 placements, including residential programs, therapeutic foster homes, and attempts at reunification with his biological mother. Parental rights were terminated, and he entered into permanent state custody at age nine. George had a series of different foster home placements until age 13. Each

B. Skehan, M.D., Ph.D.
University of Massachusetts Medical School, Worcester, MA, USA
e-mail: brian.skehan@umassmemorial.org

move resulted in a brief stay in a state-run residential facility until a new home could be identified. This appeared to trigger an increase in reactive attachment symptoms, which typically included destruction of property (plumbing and vehicle damage) and resulted in decreased trust between George and his caregivers. His final foster family also considered relinquishing his care back to the state, but they believed in their ability to help George and ultimately persevered. This led to the first sustained healthy attachment in his life.

Hyperactivity and externalizing behaviors consistent with Attention-Deficit/ Hyperactivity Disorder were first noted at age three and he was treated with a variety of stimulant medications. A diagnosis of Bipolar Disorder was made 4 years later, and he was briefly prescribed valproate for mood stabilization, which was ineffective and was stopped after 6 months. Other historical diagnoses included Reactive Attachment Disorder, Oppositional Defiant Disorder, Pervasive Developmental Disorder, Anxiety Disorder Not Otherwise Specified, and Non-Verbal Learning Disability. Beginning at age seven and throughout high school, he received psychotherapy focused on attachment concerns and medication treatment with a variety of providers at the same community mental health clinic. At the time of his anticipated transition from high school to community college, he was taking methylphenidate ER 54 mg daily, bupropion XL 300 mg daily, and clonidine 0.1 mg twice daily.

School was a relative constant in his life; he attended the same therapeutic day school for 6 years due to behavioral issues in the typical educational setting such as destruction of school property, elopement from the classroom, and verbal outbursts when frustrated. He also had been identified with an intellectual disability and was provided with life skills training in school including management of finances, personal hygiene, and independent living skills—in addition to a modified educational curriculum. Despite this, there were always concerns from his foster mother that the academics were not rigorous enough. She believed that George was capable of achieving more than he was demonstrating at school and that teachers were not challenging him in order to avoid an aggressive or destructive outburst at school which had been common in the past. She also questioned his motivation to do the work as he was often able to complete work with extensive supports in a structured setting but frequently lacked the motivation to do so on his own. His low energy and impaired concentration spanned multiple domains and was evident in his job training during adolescence. He frequently refused to go to his food service job at a local restaurant or ask for additional shifts that he had been allotted per his work agreement. He was typically only motivated to engage in video games or small electronics which were restricted due to his tendency to view developmentally inappropriate content on the internet.

He was on an individualized education program (IEP) throughout his time in school and progressed as planned with his graduation taking place just before his 18th birthday. He required extra time, a personal reader, and multiple attempts to successfully complete the mandatory standardized testing to qualify for graduation. He completed the final exam during the winter of his senior year and obtained his high school diploma. Cognitive testing, school observations, and foster parent reports suggested that he did not possess the necessary skills to live independently without further training. Transition planning, completed as part of his IEP, focused on vocational skills, self-care including hygiene, and developing independence with daily life skills such as cooking, cleaning, and using public transportation. Although he would attend his IEP meetings, George was often resistant to engaging in the skill-building activities, frequently stating that he would continue working with the team until he was 18 and then return to his biological mother so that she could care for him.

From age 13 to 17, his biological mother and extended family were permitted three supervised visits per year. Frequently, these visits would lead to escalation in George's symptoms, and the decision was made to engage his biological mother in therapy. Following extensive attachment work and reconstruction of a "life story," George's mother participated in therapy sessions once per month in addition to the monthly family session with his foster mother starting when George was 15. Due in part to the progress made in these sessions, his biological mother was permitted to have unsupervised visits with George when he was 17 years old. Unfortunately, the state investigated the home that he visited and found it to be unsuitable for a child. Furthermore, his biological mother took him to see his biological father for the first time during one of these visits, without notifying the state, who was the legal custodian. This resulted in termination of all physical contact with his biological parents and his mother was no longer allowed to participate in therapy sessions.

George's future vision was difficult to elicit. He remained ambivalent about pursuing a career or further education following the termination of visits with his mother. He became morbidly obese and neglected his medical care and hygiene. His mother continued to send expensive and desired gifts in the mail and made suggestions through letters and phone calls about a life together once he turned 18. George was eager to reconnect with his mother and, despite encouragement from the clinical treatment team, the state did not allow his mother to be part of supervised sessions nor to participate in meetings to plan for his future.

As contact with his mother decreased, and with graduation 4 months away, George voiced his desire to pursue a trade job in automotives and began to work part time through a job program at a department of public works. He expressed a desire to go to a local community college and remain in supportive housing with his current foster family until age 22. He wanted to have an adult relationship with his biological mother, but, per the wishes of the state, she was not involved in transition planning. He was accepted into an automotive certificate program at the local community college and performed well at two part time automotive mechanic assistant jobs. The college he was accepted to had an excellent reputation for helping those with cognitive, social, and emotional disabilities with the support of a dedicated disability office. Through this office, the school provided access to support groups, extended exam time, assistive technologies, and tutoring. George's team was aware of this and planned to connect him to the disability office when he matriculated. Alternative plans were also considered, including living in the same foster placement and remaining in the therapeutic school until age 22 to continue working on independent life and vocational skills. There was a plan to refer him to the

Department of Developmental Services based on the cognitive testing that was updated just prior to his 18th birthday which would have helped with transition from school-based services to community-based services on his 22nd birthday. He was also given the option of continuing with his care team both at the community mental health center and with his court appointed special advocate, who had been with him since age eight. His depressive symptoms decreased and he had increased motivation. Through diet and support from his foster parents, he lost over 30 pounds and demonstrated good self-care with improved hygiene. His foster mother and school provided support and training focused on managing his finances, maintaining hygiene, and navigating appropriate peer relationships across multiple domains including work, social groups, and romantic relationships.

At midnight on his 18th birthday, his biological mother picked him up at his foster home and he left the state. A few months later, George returned to the clinic to re-establish care and reportedly had been involved with law enforcement several times for operating a motor vehicle without a license. He was no longer employed. Self-care was poor and he had stopped taking all psychiatric medications. He experienced a relatively large number of failed romantic relationships over the preceding months. His biological mother was encouraging him to file for state and federal financial support programs. Although he was working with his former therapist, he was unable or unwilling to attend any appointments with psychiatry despite repeated efforts to engage him in a return to treatment. George made no attempt to attend his certificate program at the community college.

Analysis of Transition

George had a number of strengths predictive of a successful transition to community college. He made significant progress in self-care, maintained good hygiene, and was employed in two different jobs. He was beginning to show increased motivation in attending school and work and was proud of his ability to earn wages and successfully complete the standardized testing required for graduation. He had a secure base of attachment with his foster family and had significantly decreased the frequency and severity of disruptive behaviors in the home. Together, they were able to overcome a number of setbacks, and he remained connected in the same home, school, and community mental health care system for over 5 years. This stable relationship and consistent care provided a foundation that allowed George to achieve his goals of graduating high school and cultivating a consistent relationship with a parental figure.

Unfortunately, George's case also highlights a number of factors that were predictive of a poor outcome. First and foremost, he had significant mental health and learning issues requiring significant support. It is important to recognize that foster youth without these barriers are already less likely to go on to higher education than are their peers. Despite the fact that he was ultimately able to form a stable relationship with his final foster family, he had a history of multiple school transfers and failed foster placements, and was distrustful of authority figures.

George recently demonstrated improvement with life skills, but needed additional supports to assist with autonomy, i.e., obtaining his driver's license and vehicle or practice navigating the bus service to attend college. While he was accepted to the community college, he and his team had done very little in preparation for the transition from his therapeutic school. The disability office at the college was unaware of his intended matriculation and had not been notified by members of George's team, but could have coordinated with his school to make sure accommodations were adequate. George's lack of motivation and poor social skills may have limited his ability to seek out opportunities such as campus tours or meeting with the disability office. It is also possible that his care team and foster mother were anticipating his decision to opt out of services on his birthday and were not willing to force George to participate in some of these activities out of fear that he would reject their suggestions and leave the state with his birth mother. The fantasy of a reunification with his mother was more attractive than developing a more autonomous and self-reliant lifestyle utilizing the foster care system and community college. However, the state's concerns about safety overshadowed this desire, and it was therefore not adequately addressed.

In summary, this case represents a failed transition outcome. George did not follow through on plans for postsecondary education and aborted the transition plan. He experienced a relapse of his depression and stopped medication without medical supervision. Furthermore, he encountered discontinuity of care without health insurance or identified providers.

Close examination of this case highlights the need to begin transition planning early in adolescence especially when there are multiple institutions and stakeholders in place. Improved communication with the school system by the treatment team at an earlier time point may have highlighted adaptive functioning deficits that had persisted and could have been further assessed through updated psychological testing. Additional time in high school with an IEP (up until age 22) could have addressed deficits in social skills, community functioning, and self-care. This option became less attractive to the youth the closer he came to graduation and would likely have negatively impacted his self-worth if presented or even mandated by the legal guardian immediately prior to graduation.

Greater consideration for the youth voice during transition planning could have had major implications in the outcome. Interestingly, George participated in therapy sessions with either his foster mother or biological mother present and rarely had time individually with providers. In fact, his foster mother noted that he was first seen individually by his psychiatrist just after his 17th birthday. George was able to articulate both in his words, and later with his actions, that one of his primary goals was to reconnect with his biological mother. Equal consideration of his priorities and appropriate planning for the eventual outcome may have allowed for establishment of medical and mental health services in his new state and provided much needed supports for the youth and his mother. Transition planning was completed at a late stage with major changes in the plan taking place within the final year. Given the restricted access to his biological mother prior to age 18, an assessment of her ability to support George through this transition and to create an alternative transition plan if he signed out of the state support services was not completed. His transition plan assumed that a child with executive functioning and verbal comprehension deficits would choose to remain in the custody of the state because of the services provided and likely underestimated his intrinsic desire to reconnect with his mother.

Clinical Pearls

- Begin transition planning early in adolescence, especially when there are multiple state agencies and stakeholders involved.
- Close communication between the school system and the clinical team is critical to inform multiple acceptable options for transition planning.
- Foster youth have many barriers to achieving postsecondary education. Alternative plans, including vocational supports, must be considered.
- The youth must have a voice in choosing team members even if other members of the team believe the participation of chosen individuals is not desirable. Keep in mind that 64% of transitional age foster youth report feeling close to their biological mothers and often attempt to reconnect with their families of origin.
- Youth who have been institutionalized have likely had reduced opportunity to practice social skills and peer relationships in an unstructured setting. Anticipating difficulty in navigating social relationships and personal safety in a postsecondary environment is crucial.
- Aging out of foster care results in a dramatic and immediate loss of supports at a critical time in development and transition to adulthood. Youth may be more vulnerable to relapse of mental illness due to loss of supports and increased exposure to additional risk factors like drugs, alcohol, and sexual relationships.
- Updated psychological testing should be completed early in the transition planning if there is reason to believe it may indicate a need for Department of Developmental Services or other supports beyond the transitional period.
- Absence of youth participation in transition planning may indicate that the youth is considering an alternative option that must be considered and hopefully elicited in some capacity by the clinical team.
- The clinical team must assess readiness for transition planning and provide guidance and contacts needed for services should the youth decide against their providers' recommendations.
- Identity formation at this developmental stage favors rejection of authority and the clinical team must be prepared to provide alternative options based on youth preference.

Brief Literature Review

Foster care youth have lower enrollment and graduation rates from college than their peers [1]. Many states offer an expanding list of programming and scholarships to support foster youth and alumni for higher level education [2]. The Higher

Education Opportunity Act expanded upon an earlier law granting youth in foster care access to the TRIO programs—a group of eight federal programs (expanded from the original three) designed to increase access to higher education for financially disadvantaged youth. Although several sources of federal funding are available, one study in California found that less than 4% of foster youth who completed a FAFSA received the three forms of aid that were available to them. Furthermore, state allocation of federal funds designated for youth aging out of foster care who are working towards financial independence varies nationwide. Other youth in foster care may have significant academic struggles upon entering postsecondary education as disadvantaged youth are often clustered in low-performing schools. Foster youth may miss significant parts of the academic year due to suspension, expulsion, or changes in placement—especially if they also suffer from serious mental illness. These students are also less likely to engage in college preparatory courses [3]. Foster youth, especially those that have been institutionalized, may have limited practice and opportunities to advocate for themselves and decreased exposure to adult modeling of educational skills [4]. They will require additional support from their transition team to develop these skills and access necessary resources.

Youth transitioning out of foster care are at risk for a number of other bad outcomes. One study published in 2013 found 36% of 624 respondents had been homeless at least once by age 26. Symptoms of mental health disorders increased the relative risk of becoming homeless over their asymptomatic peers [5]. The Foster Care Independence Act of 1999 (aka the John Chafee Foster Care Independence Program or "Chafee option") gives states the option of providing funding for housing, education, life skills training, and vocational support and mandates that states provide some level of services between the ages of 18 and 21 for youth who have left foster care. The decision on how to utilize these funds remains up to the state and varies greatly nationwide. Adequate insurance to support those with medical and mental health needs can also be problematic. Since 2014, youth that age out of foster care have been eligible for Medicaid services up until age 26 as a result of the Patient Protection and Affordable Care Act. Insurance coverage must be part of the transition plan as the youth will need to enroll for these services and may need to select alternative plans if they plan to change their state of residence or attend college outside of the state where they receive services. There are existing models for collaborative community care for youth with mental health issues once they have reached higher education programs [6]. Establishing care and communication with these stakeholders during the transition process can increase the chances of a smooth transition. A systematic approach for transition that includes anticipatory guidance for health insurance, functional independence, educational supports, vocational programs, medical decision-making, legal matters, and social skills should be completed with the youth and pertinent members of the transition team [7]. Mentoring relationships for foster youth should be considered as they have been shown to have increased chances of positive outcomes and participation in higher education [8]. The transition time period also represents a time when many youth in foster care will reach the legal age of majority and some may choose to reunite with their families of origin, stop psychotropic medications, and terminate treatments [9]. These possibilities should be considered by the treatment team. The youth should have a team discussion regarding these options and be provided with information about potential supports should any of these choices result in an exacerbation of symptoms to avoid adverse outcomes.

Helpful Resources

- https://www.childwelfare.gov/topics/outofhome/independent/.
- http://youth.gov/youth-topics/transition-age-youth.
- https://www2.ed.gov/about/inits/ed/foster-care/youth-transition-toolkit.pdf.
- Casey Life skills: http://lifeskills.casey.org/.

References

1. Salazar AM, Roe SS, Ullrich JS, Haggerty KP. Professional and youth perspectives on higher education-focused interventions for youth transitioning from foster care. Child Youth Serv Rev. 2016;64:23–34.
2. Casey Family Programs. Improving higher education outcomes for students from foster care. Version 2.0. 2010. Available at: http://www.casey.org/supporting-success/. Accessed 6 April 2017.
3. Okpych N. Policy framework supporting youth aging-out of foster care through college: review and recommendations. Child Youth Serv Rev. 2012;34(7):1390–6.
4. Fagan M, Davis M, Denietolis BM, et al. Innovative residential interventions for young adults in transition. Residential interventions for children, adolescents, and families: a best practice guide. East Sussex: Taylor & Francis; 2014. p. 126.
5. Dworsky A, Napolitano L, Courtney M. Homelessness during the transition from foster care to adulthood. Am J Public Health. 2013;103(S2):S318–23.
6. Downs NS, et al. Treat and Teach Our Students Well: College Mental Health and Collaborative Campus Communities. Psychiatr Serv. 2016;67(9):957–63.
7. Unwin BK, Goodie J, Reamy BV, Quinlan J. Care of the college student. Am Fam Physician. 2013;88(9):596–604.
8. Ahrens KR, DuBois DL, Richardson LP, Fan MY, Lozano P. Youth in foster care with adult mentors during adolescence have improved adult outcomes. Pediatrics. 2008;121(2):e246–52.
9. Martel AL, Sood AB. Best practices and resources. In: The Virginia Tech Massacre: strategies and challenges for improving mental health policy on campus and beyond. Oxford: Oxford University Press; 2015. p. 93.

Part IV
Summary

Helping Patients and Families Navigate the Transition to College: Common Themes, Lessons Learned, and Best Practices

27

Adele Martel, Jennifer Derenne, and Patricia K. Leebens

Mental health practitioners (CAP, psychologists, social workers, school counselors, advanced practice nurses, and others) working with adolescents, young adults, and their families have important roles to play in facilitating safe and effective transitions of their patients to college. Clinicians are required to cover many things in the course of routine care, and it is difficult to add yet another set of recommendations to the mix. That being said, there are a number of themes highlighted in the clinical cases included in this book that can be used to guide transition preparation and planning for youth with mental health conditions headed to college.

One overarching theme is that health care transition, in the context of going to college, demands a team effort. Good communication among "transition team" members is essential. The young person, his/her family, high school personnel, treatment providers (or systems) on both sides of the transition, and other designated supporters each have active roles to play in promoting smooth and effective transitions. That said, it is also made apparent through the cases, that the

A. Martel, M.D., Ph.D. (✉)
Division of Child and Adolescent Psychiatry, Department of Psychiatry and Behavioral Sciences, Ann and Robert H. Lurie Children's Hospital of Chicago, Northwestern University Feinberg School of Medicine, Chicago, IL, USA
e-mail: adele.martel@gmail.com

J. Derenne, M.D.
Division of Child and Adolescent Psychiatry, Department of Psychiatry and Behavioral Sciences, Stanford University School of Medicine, Lucile Packard Children's Hospital, Stanford, CA, USA

P.K. Leebens, M.A.T., M.A., M.D.
Child Study Center, Yale School of Medicine, Yale University, New Haven, CT, USA

© Springer International Publishing AG, part of Springer Nature 2018
A. Martel et al. (eds.), *Promoting Safe and Effective Transitions to College for Youth with Mental Health Conditions*, https://doi.org/10.1007/978-3-319-68894-7_27

home-based mental health providers (particularly CAPs given the background of most contributing authors), often find it necessary to take on facilitative roles in the transition process. CAPs serve as consultants to high schools, leaders of the therapeutic team, guides for parents/guardians, and advocates for treatment services on/near campus, all the while treating the patient and hopefully promoting the patient's age-appropriate autonomy.

Another theme is the importance of maintaining a developmental perspective. Some authors acknowledge that turning 18 or acceptance and matriculation to college, though important milestones, does not mean that the young person no longer requires support. We expect our college-bound patients to complete more tasks and mature undertakings (admit to a disability, manage complex mental health needs, navigate a new system of care, etc.) than students without special needs, in the context of an already stressful developmental transition. Offering support and structure before, during, and after transition simply makes developmental sense if it is done with the goal of gradually promoting self-knowledge, self-efficacy, self-reliance, and self-confidence.

Other authors highlight the role of resilience in the transition to college of youth with mental health conditions. They note that before adequate "learning" or "awareness" or "goals adjustment" on the part of the patient and/or family takes place, a failure of sorts has to occur. There may also be changes in treatment and other supports, and alterations in the environment, in response to a suboptimal or "failed" transition. Ultimately, these changes lead to a more successful outcome within a reasonable period of time, either back to the same college, to another college setting, or some other satisfying and more appropriate post high school pathway. Changes that occur over time in the young person, as well as changes in the support system and environment to accommodate the needs of the patient, reflect resilience.

In the process of analyzing their cases, authors discovered that they need to be more active participants in the health care transition process, in parallel with the college application and selection process, as part of their overall ongoing care of their college-bound patients. Their increased participation goes beyond more direct involvement in finding care on or near campus. Clinicians need to be forthcoming and prepared to raise what some might consider unpopular issues such as assessing mental stability, questioning readiness for college, highlighting the reliance or over-reliance on parental and school supports, requiring ongoing care, looking at mental health services when on college tours, considering "non-traditional" post high school education pathways, etc. Furthermore, providers may need to set limits around practicing at a distance including having co-treaters on campus, requiring a certain frequency of appointments, having releases signed, and holding students accountable for decisions and treatment compliance—all in the spirit of patient safety and patient psychoeducation about mental health needs.

Being able to establish measurable outcomes, with the ultimate goal of establishing evidence-informed best practices, has been one obstacle in health care transition research. In this volume, there is also some consensus on how authors "define" or view a suboptimal transition outcome in this specific context. Taking a practical point of view, most authors consider a suboptimal or "failed" transition to college as one in which the student/patient experiences symptom exacerbation, and difficulties functioning in the college environment, which result in one or more of the following outcomes: academic difficulties ranging from underachievement and academic decline to failure with academic probation and/or withdrawal from school; social difficulties including social isolation, inappropriate pastimes, destructive relationships, and turning to substances for coping; need for more intensive level of services (IOP or inpatient hospitalization) and/or medical leave. Given the goal of quality improvement in patient care, it is important for the practitioner to employ strategies to minimize these outcomes.

However, from a more focused health care transition perspective, the lack of continuity of care described in many of the cases would be considered the marker of a suboptimal transition outcome. That is, in the absence of continuous, developmentally attuned health care, symptom exacerbation may go unnoticed, unchecked, and/or not reported, contributing to destabilization and impaired functioning in the new setting. Gaps in continuity of care are more directly related to transition planning and preparation efforts. For example, in some cases, the required services were not available on or near campus. In others, a transition care plan was lacking, inadequate, unrealistic, or not carried out because of poor communication among providers. Some patients chose not to utilize the available resources for reasons of cost, stigma, inadequate understanding of their illness and needs, wishful thinking, desire for autonomy, etc. Other patients had inadequate self-advocacy skills and illness management skills, deterring access to treatment resources and accommodations that were available. Still others had incomplete understanding of their condition particularly as it interfaced with the college environment, underestimating the impact of new stressors and need for a relapse prevention plan. And, in some cases the student, family, and treatment team underestimated the benefits of the structure and accommodations provided at home and high school, so efforts were not made to even look for services in the new setting.

Probably, the most commonly cited explanation for a suboptimal transition is that the treatment team did not devote adequate time and attention to transition planning and preparation. Going to college is viewed as an exciting and happy event; families and treatment teams may not recognize the significant stresses that transition may trigger. Many of the contributing authors expressed that with experience they have come to view the transition to college as a process and not an event, requiring time, effort, intentionality, explicit discussion with patients and families, and a holistic approach.

In cases where the patient presents for initial intake in the weeks and months leading to matriculation, developing a comprehensive care plan may be challenging. Regardless, it is always important to help the patient and family realistically assess the patient's readiness for transition across multiple domains of function. It is not enough to be academically proficient; students must also be able to manage life skills, advocate for themselves, and manage relationships. They must have adequate psychoeducation about their illness, as well as practice managing their own health needs. A carefully thought out diagnostic and biopsychosocial and cultural formulation can serve as a basis for psychoeducation of the patient and parents, assessment of readiness for transition, and individualization of transition preparation and planning.

Anticipatory guidance is a necessary component of transition preparation and planning. It should include discussion of the academic and social milieus of college and how the patient's mental health issues may interface with the college environment. Providers should also anticipate and openly discuss the changes in dynamics that may occur with the transition—the student will be more autonomous, parents will need permission to discuss care with clinicians, and the home clinician may not be the point person moving forward. Raising the issue that the young person, for a variety of reasons, may be tempted to or be planning to stop treatment once away from home, is another valuable anticipatory guidance topic.

In the course of assessing readiness, the patient, family, and treatment team should consider whether the desired institution truly can offer services and resources that are in line with the young person's mental health and academic support needs. Alternative post-secondary options and paths should be explored and discussed honestly, especially if the young person has experienced a more recent mental health complication or setback. Families and schools need to recognize the ways in which the young person will be affected by removing the external support and structure provided by parental support and classroom accommodations. Allowing the student to ask for help and experience natural consequences for decisions can go a long way in helping the student truly understand his/her needs and in encouraging skill development. Teams should also honestly evaluate whether separation from family or moving to a new location might mitigate the student's symptoms, or whether such claims represent magical thinking and desire for a geographic cure.

Finally, lack of a transfer of care plan, or an inadequately developed and communicated plan, is a significant risk factor for suboptimal transition. Students need to know who is in charge of their care when they start college, need to recognize the signs and symptoms of relapse, and need to be securely connected to services proactively, rather than waiting for crisis to strike. Even when patients are stable and seem prepared to meet the challenges of the transition to college, establishing an emergency care plan is a valuable exercise.

Thinking about the campus as a system of care, there are additional interventions that may also help facilitate a positive and effective transition to college. A collaborative team approach characterized by close communication and very clearly defined roles will ensure that all stakeholders are on the same page and can help to create a safety net and set of connections for the patient across campus. Proactively referring students to the ODS ensures that the appropriate documentation is available to approve accommodations and prevents students from delays in accessing appropriate resources. Learning coaches can help students bridge the transition from dependence on school and family to being more independent and self-sufficient. When available, case managers at IHE who are able to navigate the system of care, may be able to facilitate communication and prevent information silos that often impede appropriate treatment.

There are several policies and practices on the "receiving" end that may help smooth transition. Many of the cases illustrate the difficulty setting up appointments for the coming academic year and providing appropriate hand-off when either there is no one available at college counseling centers and disability services during the summer months and/or policies restrict setting up appointments until the academic year. Improving infrastructure and increasing manpower during that time and addressing restrictive policies may be effective strategies to support transition and prevent students from "falling through the cracks." A good hand-off from prior providers is invaluable. Some IHE attempt to normalize mental health issues by asking about them on general health forms, and follow up with those incoming students who disclose mental health concerns; this is a practice that should be more widely adopted. It would also be helpful for college counseling centers to reach out (by text or email) to students who miss appointments in an attempt to engage them in treatment. College mental health professionals should be willing to consult with concerned parents and even involve them in treatment in a developmentally appropriate fashion. University counseling centers should update their websites regularly to make sure that the resources offered are clearly outlined, and they should also be sure to maintain up-to-date referral lists of off-campus providers. Physician extenders like APRNs may be used to triage cases, bridge appointments between the home and campus teams, and support transition. General medical providers at the university's health center (or in the nearby community), if willing, can also be trained to recognize decompensation and consult with the home-based provider. This would be valuable in situations where specialty care is not available, the student has not established appropriate care on or near campus, or when it is deemed important for the patient to remain connected with the home provider but distance is an obstacle. Finally, college counseling centers can continue their excellent work in outreach and efforts to decrease stigma through mental health screenings, orientation events, and advocacy projects on campus.

Despite best efforts on the part of all key stakeholders, some transitions do not proceed in a smooth, safe, or productive fashion. In the face of serious mental illness, all the planning and preparation in the world may not be enough to prevent a negative outcome. At the same time, it is important to recognize that young people with serious mental illness can succeed with knowledge, skills, and the appropriate supports in place. Clinicians should think developmentally, involve family and significant others in appropriate ways, provide good documentation, and resist the urge to become discouraged when there are setbacks along the way. Failures are inevitable and provide opportunities for learning and course-correction when viewed with a resilience mindset.

Overall, it is important for clinicians to recognize that health care transition is a process and not an event. They should understand the rationale for incorporating transition preparation and planning into the ongoing care of all adolescent patients, whether they are headed to post-secondary education or not, and work to develop knowledge and skills to facilitate the transition process. Still, patients, along with their families, make the final decisions. Clinician attitudes which maintain and acknowledge the value of the young person discussing and making decisions about his/her future (self-determination) are more likely to see patients become independent and maximize their potential.

In thinking to the future and as the health care transition research agenda advances, it makes sense for clinicians and IHE to continue their efforts in supporting young people with mental health conditions who are transitioning to college. In turn, practice approaches aimed at quality improvement can be developed into models and programs which can be evaluated and potentially expand the evidence base. Lastly, those clinicians involved with training the next generation of practitioners should advocate for health care transition to be part of training curricula, particularly in those specialties focused on treating children, adolescents, and their families.

Helpful Resources

General Transitioning Resources

- American Academy of Child and Adolescent Psychiatry. Transitioning from high school to college with a psychiatric illness – preparation. http://www.aacap.org/AACAP/Families_and_Youth/Facts_for_Families/FFF-Guide/Transitioning-From-High-School-to-College-With-A-Psychiatric-Illness-Preparation-114.aspx
- American Academy of Child and Adolescent Psychiatry. Starting college with a psychiatric illness. http://www.aacap.org/AACAP/Families_and_Youth/Facts_for_Families/FFF-Guide/Starting-College-with-a-Psychiatric-Illness-115.aspx
- American Academy of Child and Adolescent Psychiatry. Moving into adulthood resource center. http://www.aacap.org/AACAP/Families_and_Youth/Resource_Centers/Moving_Into_Adulthood_Resource_Center/Moving_Into_Adulthood_Resource_Center.aspx
- Connecticut Transition Task Force. 2009. http://www.sde.ct.gov/sde/lib/sde/PDF/DEPS/Special/BuildingABridge.pdf
- National Center for Healthcare transition improvement. http://www.gottransition.org/
- The transition year. http://www.transitionyear.org/
- Transitions Research and Training Center at the University of Massachusetts. http://www.umassmed.edu/transitionsrtc
- Set To Go (A Jed Foundation Program). https://www.settogo.org/
- Starting the conversation: college and your mental health. https://www.nami.org/collegeguide/download
- Your education your future – a guide to college and university for students with psychiatric disabilities (Canadian Mental Health Association). http://www.cmha.ca/youreducation/introduction.html

Tips for Parents and Teens/Young Adults

- How to help new high school grads transition into adulthood. http://www.aap.org/en-us/about-the-aap/aap-press-room/news-features-and-safety-tips/Documents/High_School_Grads_Transition.pdf
- Making the transition to college: a guide for parents. https://med.nyu.edu/child-adolescent-psychiatry/news/csc-news/2015/making-transition-college-guide-parents

- Mental health tips for teens graduating from high school. American Academy of Pediatrics. http://www.aap.org/en-us/about-the-aap/aap-press-room/news-features-and-safety-tips/Pages/Mental-Health-Tips-Teens-Graduating-High-School.aspx
- Transition to college: separation and change for parents and students. https://med.nyu.edu/child-adolescent-psychiatry/news/csc-news/2015/transition-college-separation-and-change-parents-and-students

On-Campus Student Run Advocacy Groups

- ACTIVE MINDS. http://www.activeminds.org/
- ACTIVELY MOVING FORWARD. https://healgrief.org/actively-moving-forward/ (The National Students of AMF Support Network is a nonprofit organization dedicated to supporting college students grieving the illness or death of a loved one)
- NAMI ON CAMPUS. https://www.nami.org/namioncampus

Information for Students with Disabilities

- Boston University Center for Rehabilitation. Higher Education Support Toolkit: assisting students with psychiatric disabilities. http://cpr.bu.edu/wp-content/uploads/2011/09/Higher-Education-Support-Toolkit.pdf
- Bazelon Center for Mental Health Law – CAMPUS MENTAL HEALTH: know your rights (a guide for students who want to seek help for mental illness or emotional distress). http://www.bazelon.org/wp-content/uploads/2017/01/YourMind-YourRights.pdf
- CHOICES – a regional post-secondary planning night/resource for students with disabilities who are college bound (Go to Choices booklets). http://www.post-secondarychoices.org/
- Transitioning from high school to college – help for students with learning disabilities. https://dyslexiaida.org/transitioning-from-high-school-to-college/
- Virginia's College guide for students with disabilities. http://www.doe.virginia.gov/special_ed/transition_svcs/outcomes_project/college_guide.pdf

Websites on Sleep

- http://www.sleepeducation.com/sleep-disorders/insomnia/overview-facts
- http://www.sleepfoundation.org/article/white-papers/how-much-sleep-do-adults-need

Veterans in College

- VA Campus Toolkit. https://www.mentalhealth.va.gov/studentveteran/studentvets.asp

Glossary of Acronyms

AA	Alcoholics Anonymous
ACHA	American College Health Association
ACT	American College Testing
ADA	Americans with Disabilities Act
ADHD	Attention-Deficit/Hyperactivity Disorder
AP	Advanced Placement
ARMS	At-Risk Mental State
ASC	Amphetamine Salt Combination
ASD	Autism Spectrum Disorder
BMI	Body Mass Index
BP I Disorder	Bipolar I Disorder
BPD	Borderline Personality Disorder
CAP(s)	Child and Adolescent Psychiatrist(s)/Psychiatry
CBT	Cognitive Behavioral Therapy
CDC	Centers for Disease Control and Prevention
CME	Continuing Medical Education
CPT	Cognitive Processing Therapy
DBT	Dialectical Behavior Therapy
DSM-5	Diagnostic and Statistical Manual, Edition 5
DSM IV-TR	Diagnostic and Statistical Manual, Edition 4, Text Revision
DUP	Duration of Untreated Psychosis
ED	Emotionally Disturbed or Emotional Disturbance
EF	Executive Functioning/Executive Function(s)
EMDR	Eye Movement Desensitization and Reprocessing
ER	Emergency Room (i.e., Emergency Department)
ExRP	Exposure and Response Prevention
FAFSA	Free Application for Federal Student Aid
FBT	Family Based Therapy
FERPA	Family Educational Rights & Privacy Act
FGCS(s)	First Generation College Student(s)
GAD	Generalized Anxiety Disorder

© Springer International Publishing AG, part of Springer Nature 2018
A. Martel et al. (eds.), *Promoting Safe and Effective Transitions to College for Youth with Mental Health Conditions*, https://doi.org/10.1007/978-3-319-68894-7

GPA	Grade Point Average
HBCU	Historically Black College and University
HCT	Health Care Transition
HFASD	High Functioning Autism Spectrum Disorder
HIPAA	Health Insurance Portability and Accountability Act
IDEA	Individuals with Disabilities Education Act
IEP(s)	Individualized Education Program(s)
IHE	Institution(s) of Higher Education
IOP	Intensive Outpatient Program
LCSW	Licensed Clinical Social Worker
LD	Learning Disability/Disabilities
LGBT(Q)	Lesbian, Gay, Bisexual, Transgender (Queer/Questioning)
LPC	Licensed Professional Counselor
MET	Motivational Enhancement Therapy
MHC	Mental Health Condition(s)
MI	Motivational Interviewing
MLOA	Medical Leave of Absence
MST	Multisystemic Therapy
NCAA	National Collegiate Athletic Association
NCHA	National College Health Assessment
OCD	Obsessive-Compulsive Disorder
ODS	Office of Disability/Disabilities Services
PAD	Psychiatric Advance Directive
PCP	Primary Care Provider
PE	Prolonged Exposure Therapy
PHP	Partial Hospital Program
PTSD	Post Traumatic Stress Disorder
PWI	Predominantly White Institution
SAD	Separation Anxiety Disorder or Social Anxiety Disorder
SAT	Scholastic Aptitude Test
SDM	Shared Decision Making
SMI	Serious Mental Illness
SOC	Student of Concern (Team or Committee)
SRI	Serotonin Reuptake Inhibitor
SSRI(s)	Selective Serotonin Reuptake Inhibitor(s)
TAY	Transitional Age Youth
TF-CBT	Trauma-Focused Cognitive Behavior Therapy
UCC	University Counseling Center
Y-BOCS	Yale-Brown Obsessive Compulsive Scale

Index

© Springer International Publishing AG, part of Springer Nature 2018
A. Martel et al. (eds.), *Promoting Safe and Effective Transitions to College for Youth
with Mental Health Conditions*, https://doi.org/10.1007/978-3-319-68894-7